MCQs for the European Ex
in Core Cardiology

MCQs for the European Exam in Core Cardiology

Second Edition

Edited by

Daniel X Augustine
Consultant Cardiologist, Royal United Hospitals Bath NHS Foundation Trust, UK; Honorary Professor, University of Bath, UK

John Graby
Cardiology Specialist Registrar, Royal United Hospitals Bath NHS Foundation Trust, UK

Ali Khavandi
Consultant Cardiologist, Royal United Hospitals Bath NHS Foundation Trust, UK

Paul Leeson
Professor of Cardiovascular Medicine, Oxford Cardiovascular Clinical Research Facility, University of Oxford & John Radcliffe Hospital, Oxford University Hospitals NHS Foundation Trust, UK

Sri Raveen Kandan
Consultant Cardiologist, Royal United Hospitals Bath NHS Foundation Trust, UK

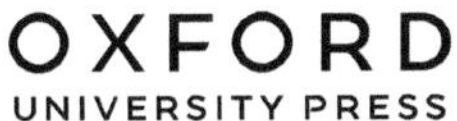

OXFORD
UNIVERSITY PRESS

Great Clarendon Street, Oxford, OX2 6DP,
United Kingdom

Oxford University Press is a department of the University of Oxford.
It furthers the University's objective of excellence in research, scholarship,
and education by publishing worldwide. Oxford is a registered trade mark of
Oxford University Press in the UK and in certain other countries

Published in the United States of America by Oxford University Press
198 Madison Avenue, New York, NY 10016, United States of America

British Library Cataloguing in Publication Data
Data available

Library of Congress Control Number is on file at the Library of Congress

ISBN 978–0–19–879548–3

DOI: 10.1093/med/9780198795483.001.0001

Printed and bound by
CPI Group (UK) Ltd, Croydon, CR0 4YY

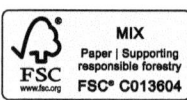

Huge thanks for the support of my wife, Ellie and my junior A team—Zach, Josh, Luke & Yasmin. (DXA)

For Ellen and Huw, and my parents for all the opportunities they provided. (JG)

For my wife Rosalynne, and children, Ilaira and Marisa. (SRK)

PREFACE

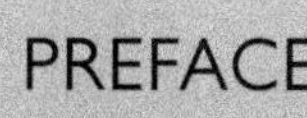

The European Exam in Core Cardiology (EECC) is led by the European Society of Cardiology, in conjunction with the European Union of Medical Specialists and the national cardiac societies. It is designed to assess core cardiology knowledge and is part of an assessment strategy for current specialist trainees in cardiology, our future leaders in cardiology.

MCQs for the European Exam in Core Cardiology contains over 700 multiple choice questions with detailed explanations and links to related ESC guidelines for further reading. Providing a thorough assessment of the reader's knowledge, each chapter has been carefully mapped to the curriculum allowing for focused revision. Written by a team of cardiology registrars and experienced consultants, this resource has been cleverly designed to give you hands-on experience of the level and type of questions you can expect in the exam, as well as high-quality, concise answers possible under time constraints.

Since initiation in 2018, this project has not been without hurdles. The book was restructured in 2020 following the new syllabus launch and since then updated ESC guidelines have been incorporated into the book. There was a hiatus during the COVID-19 pandemic and following ease of restrictions, publishing houses have understandably taken time to reintegrate to allow onward publication. Despite all of this, the contributors to the book have been outstanding and the Editors would like to extend their sincere gratitude to all of our contributors.

We hope this revision aid helps cardiology trainees throughout Europe, our future cardiology leaders.

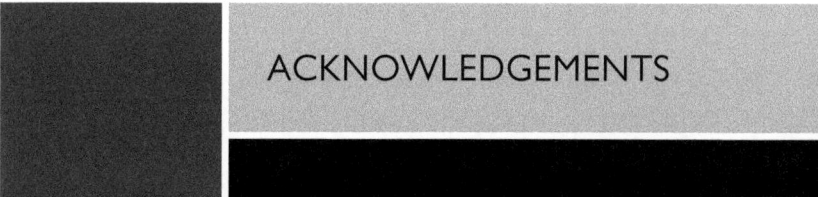

ACKNOWLEDGEMENTS

The editors would like to thank the OUP team for their help during the drafting and processing of the book. A special thanks in particular to James Oates for his support and advice during the whole project.

We would like to thank the following colleagues for contributing images towards the front cover illustration:

Dr Edward Duncan. University Hospitals Bristol and Weston NHS Foundation Trust, UK

Dr Thomas W Johnson. University Hospitals Bristol and Weston NHS Foundation Trust, UK

Dr David Little. Consultant Radiologist, Royal United Hospitals Bath NHS Foundation Trust, UK

CONTENTS

ABBREVIATIONS

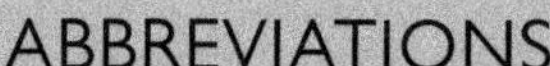

5HIAA	5-hydroxyindoleacetic acid
^{99m}Tc	radioactive technetium-99m
AAA	abdominal aortic aneurysm
AAS	acute aortic syndrome
ABG	arterial blood gas
ABI	ankle-brachial index
ACE	angiotensin converting enzyme
ACE/ACEi	angiotensin converting enzyme inhibitor
ACHD	adult congenital heart disease
ACS	acute coronary syndrome
ACT	activated clotting time
ADA	adenosine deaminase
ADME	absorption, distribution, metabolism, and excretion
AED	automated external defibrillator
AF	atrial fibrillation
AHI	apnoea-hypopnea index
ALCAPA	anomalous origin of the left coronary artery from the pulmonary artery
ALS	advanced life support
ALVC	arrhythmogenic left ventricular cardiomyopathy
ANA	anti-nuclear antibodies
ANCA	anti-neutrophil cytoplasmic antibody
AP	accessory pathway
APS	antiphospholipid syndrome
AR	aortic regurgitation
ARB	angiotensin receptor blocker
ARNI	angiotensin receptor-neprilysin inhibitor
ARVC	arrhythmogenic right ventricular cardiomyopathy
AS	ankylosing spondylitis or aortic stenosis
ASA	American Society of Anesthesiologists
ASD	atrial septal defect
ATP	anti-tachycardia pacing

AV	atrioventricular
AVNRT	atrioventricular-nodal re-entrant tachycardia
AVRT	atrioventricular re-entrant tachycardia
AVSD	atrioventricular septal defect
BAV	bicuspid aortic valve
bd	bis in die (twice daily)
BiPAP	bilevel positive airway pressure
BMD	Becker muscular dystrophies
BMI	body mass index
BMS	bare metal stent
BNP	brain natriuretic peptide
bpm	beats per minute
BrS	Brugada syndrome
BSA	body surface area
CABG	coronary artery bypass graft
CAD	coronary artery disease
CAD-RADS	Coronary Artery Disease Reporting and Data System
CAR	chimeric antigen receptor
CCTGA	congenitally corrected transposition of the great arteries
CCU	coronary care unit
CETP	cholesterylester transfer protein
CFR	coronary flow reserve
CGA	comprehensive geriatric assessment
CGH	comparative genomic hybridization
CIN	contrast-induced nephropathy
CK	creatine kinase
CKD	chronic kidney disease
CL	cycle length
CLI	critical limb ischaemia
CLTI	critical limb threatening ischaemia
CMR	cardiac MRI
CO	cardiac output
COPD	chronic obstructive pulmonary disease
COX	cyclooxygenase
CPAP	continuous positive airway pressure
CPET	cardiopulmonary exercise test
CPR	cardiopulmonary resuscitation
CPVT	catecholaminergic polymorphic ventricular tachycardia
CRP	C-reactive protein

CRT-D	cardiac resynchronization therapy defibrillator
CRT-P	cardiac resynchronization therapy pacemaker
CSA	central sleep apnoea
CSR	Cheyne-Stokes respiration
CT	computed tomography
CTA	computed tomography angiography
CTCA	CT coronary angiogram
CTEPH	chronic thromboembolic pulmonary hypertension
CTO	chronic total occlusion
CTPA	CT pulmonary angiogram
CV	cardiovascular
CVP	central venous pressure
CW	continuous wave
CXR	chest X-ray
CZT	cadmium-zinc-telluride
DAPT	dual antiplatelet therapy
DASH	Dietary Approaches to Stop Hypertension
DBP	diastolic blood pressure
DC	direct current
DCCV	direct current cardioversion
DCM	dilated cardiomyopathy
dcSSc	progressive diffuse cutaneous systemic sclerosis
DES	drug eluting stent
DGH	district general hospital
DLBCL	diffuse large B cell lymphoma
DLCO	diffusing capacity of the lungs for carbon monoxide
DMARDS	disease-modifying anti-rheumatic therapy
DMD	Duchenne muscular dystrophy
DNA	deoxyribonucleic acid
DOAC	direct oral anti-coagulant
DPD	^{99m}Tc-3,3-diphosphono-1,2-propanodicarboxylic acid
DSA	digital subtraction angiography
DSE	dobutamine stress echocardiogram
DVLA	Driver and Vehicle Licensing Agency
DVT	deep vein thrombosis
ECG	Electrocardiogram
ECMO	extra corporeal membrane oxygenation
EDS	Ehlers–Danlos syndrome
EDV	end-diastolic volume

EEG	electroencephalogram
EGE	early gadolinium enhancement
eGFR	estimated glomerular filtration rate
EGM	intracardiac electrogram
ENA	extractable nuclear antigen
EP	electrophysiology
ER	early repolarization
ERI	elective replacement indicator
EROA	effective regurgitant orifice area
ERP	effective refractory period
ESC	European Society of Cardiology
ESKD	end-stage kidney disease
EVAR	endovascular aneurysm repair
FD	Fabry disease
FDG PET	fluorodeoxyglucose-positron emission tomography
FEV1	forced expiratory volume in the first second
FFA	free fatty acids
FFR	fractional flow reserve
FH	familial hypercholesterolaemia
FISH	fluorescent in-situ hybridization
FMD	fibromuscular dysplasia
FMF	familial Mediterranean fever
FOB	faecal occult blood
FOV	field of view
FPO	flash pulmonary oedema
FVC	forced vital capacity
GAD	glutamic acid decarboxylase
GCS	Glasgow Coma Scale
GI	gastrointestinal
GLS	global longitudinal strain
GP	general practitioner
GRACE	Global Registry of Acute Coronary Events
GTN	glyceryl tri-nitrate
HCM	hypertrophic cardiomyopathy
HCN	hyperpolarization-activated cyclic nucleotide-gated
HCQ	hydroxychloroquine
HDL	high density lipoprotein
HFpEF	heart failure with preserved ejection fraction
HFrEF	heart failure with reduced ejection fraction

HITT	heparin-induced thrombocytopenia
HMDP	hydroxymethylene diphosphonate
HMG-CoA reductase	3-hydroxy-3-methyl-glutaryl-coenzyme A reductase
HMOD	hypertension-mediated organ damage
HRCT	high-resolution computed tomography
HRT	hormone replacement therapy
HTA	hereditary thoracic aortopathy
HU	Hounsfield units
IABP	intra-aortic balloon pump
ICD	implantable cardioverter-defibrillator
IDL	low-density lipoprotein cholesterol
IE	infective endocarditis
IHD	ischaemic heart disease
ILR	implantable loop recorder
IMH	intramyocardial haemorrhage
INR	international normalized ratio
IUGR	intrauterine growth restriction
IV	intravenous
IVC	inferior vena cava
IVIG	intravenous immunoglobulin
IVL	shockwave intravascular lithotripsy
IVS	interventricular septum
IVUS	intravascular ultrasound
IwFR	instantaneous wave-free ratio
JVP	jugular venous pressure
K+	potassium
LA	left atrium
LACI	lacunar infarct
LAD	left anterior descending artery
LAO	left anterior oblique
LBBB	left bundle branch block
LCA	left coronary artery
LCSD	left cardiac sympathetic denervation
LCx	left circumflex artery
LDL	low density lipoprotein
LDL-C	low-density lipoprotein cholesterol
LDL-R	low-density lipoprotein receptor
LDS	Loeys–Dietz syndrome

LGE	late gadolinium enhancement
LIMA	left internal mammary artery
LMS	left main stem
LMWH	low-molecular weight heparin
Lp(a)	lipoprotein (a)
LQTS	long QT syndrome
LV	left ventricle
LVAD	left ventricular assist device
LVEDD	left ventricle end diastolic dimension
LVEDP	left ventricular end-diastolic pressure
LVEDVi	LV end-diastolic volume index
LVEF	left ventricular ejection fraction
LVESD	left ventricular end-systolic diameter
LVH	left ventricular hypertrophy
LVOT	left ventricular outflow tract
LVSD	left ventricular systolic dysfunction
MAD	mitral annular disjunction
MALS	median arcuate ligament compression syndrome
MAP	mean aortic pressure
MAT	multifocal atrial tachycardia
MDT	multi-disciplinary team
METS	metabolic equivalents
MI	myocardial infarction
MIBG	iodine-123 metaiodobenzylguandine
MIBI	myocardial perfusion imaging
MPA	main pulmonary artery
MPS	myocardial perfusion scientigraphy
MR	mitral regurgitation
MRA	mineralocorticoid receptor antagonist
MRI	magnetic resonance imaging
MV	mitral valve
MVO	microvascular obstruction
MVR	mitral valve replacement
Na^+	sodium
NASCET	North American Symptomatic Carotid Endarterectomy Trial
NG	nasogastric
NICE	National Institute for Health and Care Excellence
NIHSS	National Institutes of Health Stroke Scale
NMD	neuromuscular dystrophies

NOAC	non-vitamin K oral anticoagulant
NSAIDs	non-steroidal anti-inflammatory drugs
NSTE-ACS	non-ST-segment elevation acute coronary syndrome
NSTEMI	non ST elevation myocardial infarction
NT-proBNP	N-terminal pro-brain natriuretic peptide
NYHA	New York Heart Association
OAC	oral anticoagulants
OCT	optical coherence tomography
od	omne in die (once daily)
OH	orthostatic hypotension
OM	obtuse marginal (coronary artery)
OMT	optimal medical therapy
OP	outpatient
OSA	obstructive sleep apnoea
PA	pulmonary artery
PACI	partial anterior circulation infarct
PAD	peripheral artery disease
PAP	pulmonary artery pressure
PAPVD	partial anomalous pulmonary venous drainage
PAWP	pulmonary artery wedge pressure
PCCD	progressive cardiac conduction disease
PCI	percutaneous coronary intervention
PCIS	post-cardiac injury syndromes
PCSK9 inhibitor	proprotein convertase subtilisin/kexin type 9 inhibitor
PCWP	pulmonary capillary wedge pressure
PDA	posterior descending artery
PE	pulmonary embolism
PEARS	personalized external aortic root support
PEEP	positive end-expiratory pressure
PERC	pulmonary embolism rule-out criteria
PET	positron emission tomography
PFO	patent foramen ovale
PG	pressure gradient
PHT	pulmonary hypertension
PISA	proximal isovelocity surface area
POCI	posterior circulation infarct
PPAR	peroxisome proliferator-activated receptor
PPCI	primary percutaneous coronary intervention

PPCM	postpartum/peripartum cardiomyopathy
PPI	proton pump inhibitor
PPS	psychogenic pseudo syncope
PSA	pacing system analyser
P-SCAD	pregnancy-associated spontaneous coronary artery dissection
PTT	partial thromboplastin time
PVC	premature ventricular contractions
PVD	peripheral vascular disease
PVR	pulmonary vascular resistance
PYP	pyrophosphate
RA	rheumatoid arthritis or right atrium
RAAS	renin angiotensin aldosterone system
ras	renal artery stenosis
RBBB	right bundle branch block
RCA	right coronary artery
RCT	randomized controlled trial
RER	respiratory exchange ratio
RIHD	radiation-induced heart disease
RNV	radionuclide ventriculography
RRR	relative risk reduction
RRT	renal replacement therapy
RV	right ventricle
RVEDP	right ventricular end-diastolic pressure
RVEF	right ventricular ejection fraction
RVOT	right ventricular outflow tract
RVSP	right ventricular systolic pressure
SADS	sudden arrhythmic death syndrome
SAM	systolic anterior motion
SAVR	surgical aortic valve replacement
SBP	systolic blood pressure
SCD	sudden cardiac death
SGLT	sodium-dependent glucose cotransporters
S-ICD	subcutaneous implantable cardioverter-defibrillator
SLE	systemic lupus erythematosus
SPAP	systolic pulmonary artery pressure
SPECT	single-photon emission computed tomography
SpO2	oxygen saturations
SSFP	steady-state free precession
STEMI	ST elevation myocardial infarction

SV	stroke volume
SVG	saphenous vein grafts
SVR	systemic vascular resistance
SVT	supra ventricular tachycardia
TAAD	thoracic aortic aneurysm and dissection
TACI	total anterior circulation infarct
TAPSE	tricuspid annular plane systolic excursion
TAVI	transcatheter aortic valve implantation
TBI	toe brachial index
tds	three times per day
TIA	transient ischaemic attack
TIMI	thrombolysis in myocardial infarction
TOE	transoesophageal echocardiogram
TPG	transpulmonary gradient
TPVI	transcatheter pulmonary valve implants
TPW	temporary pacing wire
TR	tricuspid regurgitation
TRAPS	tumour necrosis factor receptor-associated periodic fever
TS	tuberous sclerosis
TTE	transthoracic echocardiogram
TTR	transthyretin
TURP	transurethral resection of the prostate
TV	tricuspid valve
uIFN-γ	unstimulated interferon-gamma
UKOSS	UK Obstetric Surveillance System
ULN	upper limit of normal
V	velocity
VA	ventricular arrhythmia or ventriculoarterial
VE/VCO2 slope	minute ventilation/carbon dioxide production
vEDS	vascular Ehlers–Danlos syndrome
VF	ventricular fibrillation
VHD	valvular heart disease
VSD	ventricular septal defect
VT	ventricular tachycardia
VTE	venous thromboembolism
WCC	white cell count
WPW	Wolf–Parkinson–White
WU	Wood units

CONTRIBUTORS

Joanna Abramik, Cardiology Specialist Registrar, Bristol Heart Institute, University Hospitals Bristol NHS Foundation Trust & Severn Deanery, UK

Patrizia Aruta, Policlinico University Hospitals "G. Rodolico-San Marco," Division of Cardiology San Marco Hospital, Catania, Italy

Daniel X Augustine, Consultant Cardiologist Royal United Hospitals Bath NHS Foundation Trust, Honorary Professor, University of Bath, UK

Luigi P. Badano, Professor of Cardiovascular Medicine, University of Milano-Bicocca, Italy

Richard Baker, Consultant Cardiologist, Musgrove Park Hospital, Somerset NHS Foundation Trust, UK

Joyee Basu, Cardiology Specialist Registrar, John Radcliffe Hospital, Oxford, UK

Lesley-Anne Bissell, Consultant Rheumatologist & Honorary Senior Lecturer, Leeds Teaching Hospitals NHS Trust and University of Leeds, Leeds, UK

Richard Bond, Consultant Cardiologist and Cardiac Electrophysiologist, Gloucestershire Royal Hospital NHS Foundation Trust, UK

Paul Brady, Cardiology Specialist Registrar, Bristol Heart Institute, University Hospitals Bristol NHS Foundation Trust & Severn Deanery, UK

Marcus Brooks, Consultant Vascular Surgeon, North Bristol NHS Trust, UK

Stewart Brown, Cardiology Specialist Registrar & Research Fellow, Musgrove Park Hospital, Somerset NHS Foundation Trust & Severn Deanery, UK

Alexander Carpenter, Cardiology Specialist Registrar and MRC Clinical Research Training Fellow, Bristol Heart Institute, University Hospitals Bristol NHS Foundation Trust & Severn Deanery, UK

Mimi Z. Chen, Consultant Endocrinologist & Honorary Senior Lecturer, St. George's University Hospitals NHS Foundation Trust & St. George's, University of London, UK

James Choulerton, Consultant Stroke Physician, Royal United Hospital Bath NHS Foundation Trust, UK

Andrew Clark, Professor of Cardiology, Hull York Medical School, UK

Gerry Coghlan, Consultant Cardiologist, Royal Free Hospital, London, UK

Stephanie Curtis, Consultant Cardiologist, University Hospitals Bristol and Weston NHS Foundation Trust, UK

Gemina Doolub, Cardiology Specialist Registrar, Severn Deanery, UK

Mark Elliott, Cardiology Specialist Registrar, North East Thames Deanery, UK

Tim Fairbairn, Consultant Cardiologist, Liverpool Heart and Chest Hospital, UK

Mazaya Fawzy, Ameenathul Mazaya Fawzy, Cardiology Specialist Registrar, West Midlands Deanery, UK

Hossam Fayed, Structural Heart Fellow, Kings College Hospital, London and Hon. Clinical Lecturer, Institute of Cardiovascular Science, University College London, London, UK

Christopher Nicholas Floyd, Visiting Senior Lecturer in Clinical Pharmacology & Therapeutics, King's College London, UK

Phillip Freeman, Interventional cardiologist and Cardiac MRI, Aalborg University Hospital, Denmark

Arjun K Ghosh, Consultant Cardiologist, Cardio-Oncology Services at Barts Heart Centre, St Bartholomew's Hospital and Hatter Cardiovascular Institute, University College London Hospital, London, UK

Ben Gibbison, Associate Professor in Cardiac Anaesthesia & Intensive Care, University of Bristol, UK

Konstantinos Gkastaris, Consultant in Diabetes and Endocrinology, St. Luke's Hospital, Panorama, Thessaloniki, Greece

Adam Graham, Consultant Cardiologist, Nottingham University Hospitals NHS Trust, UK

Abdul Hameed, Consultant Cardiologist & Honorary Senior Lecturer, Sheffield Teaching Hospitals Trust & Hull University Teaching Hospitals NHS Trust, UK

James Harper, Consultant Respiratory Physician, Royal United Hospitals Bath NHS Foundation Trust, Bath, UK

Benjamin J Hudson, Consultant Cardiothoracic Radiologist, Royal United Hospitals Bath NHS Foundation Trust, UK

Sarah Hudson, Consultant Cardiologist, Wye Valley NHS Trust, UK

Georgios Kaltsakas, Consultant Respiratory Physician and Honorary Senior Lecturer Guy's and St Thomas' NHS Foundation Trust & King's College London, UK

Sri Raveen Kandan, Consultant Cardiologist, Royal United Hospitals Bath NHS Foundation Trust, UK

Boon Lim, Consultant Cardiologist, Imperial College Healthcare NHS Trust, UK

Mark Mariathas, Consultant Cardiologist, Bristol Heart Institute, University Hospitals Bristol NHS Foundation Trust, UK

Nav Masani, Consultant Cardiologist, Cardiff & Vale University Health Board, UK

Ursula McHugh, Consultant Anaesthetist, St James's Hospital, Dublin, Ireland

Victoria McKay, Consultant in Cardiovascular Clinical Genetics, Liverpool Centre for Genomic Medicine & Liverpool Heart and Chest NHS FT, UK

Dan McKenzie, Consultant Cardiologist, Royal United Hospitals Bath NHS Foundation Trust

Vishal S Mehta, Cardiology Specialist Registrar, North East Thames Deanery, UK

Florence Mouy, Internal Medicine Trainee, Royal United Hospitals Bath NHS Foundation Trust & Severn Deanery, UK

Denisa Muraru, Cardiologist, University of Milano-Bicocca, Istituto Auxologico Italiano, IRCCS, San Luca Hospital, Milan, Italy

David Murphy, Cardiology Specialist Registrar & Research Fellow, Royal United Hospitals Bath NHS Foundation Trust & Severn Deanery, UK

Patrick B Murphy, Consultant in Sleep, Ventilation and Respiratory Medicine, Reader in Respiratory Medicine, King's College London, London, UK

Angus Nightingale, Consultant Cardiologist, Bristol Heart Institute, University Hospitals Bristol NHS Foundation Trust, UK

Dimitra Nikoletou, Associate Professor in Exercise Rehabilitation, St George's University of London, London, UK

Victoria North, Consultant Cardiologist (Congenital Heart Disease), Bristol Heart Institute, University Hospitals Bristol NHS Foundation Trust, UK

Chiara Palermo, Cardiac Sonographer, University of Padua, Azienda Ospedale-Università Padova, Padua, Italy

Dimitrios Panagopoulos, Clinical Electrophysiology Research Fellow, Imperial College Healthcare NHS Trust, London, UK

Hiten Patel, Consultant Cardiologist, Eastbourne District General Hospital, UK

John D Pauling, Consultant Rheumatologist & Honorary Senior Lecturer, Department of Rheumatology & Translational Health Sciences, North Bristol NHS Trust & University of Bristol, Bristol, UK

Dimitrios Poulikakos, Consultant Renal Physician Salford Royal NHS Foundation Trust & Honorary Senior Lecturer, Salford Royal NHS Foundation Trust & University of Manchester, UK

Bernard Prendergast, Consultant Cardiologist, St Thomas' Hospital and Cleveland Clinic London, London, UK

Majd Protty, WCAT Clinical Lecturer in Interventional Cardiology, Cardiff University, Cardiff, UK

Mahim Qureshi, NIHR Academic Clinical Lecturer, University of Bristol, UK

Dan Raine, Consultant Cardiologist and Electrophysiologist, Norfolk and Norwich University Hospital, UK

Kim Rajappan, Consultant Cardiologist and Cardiac Electrophysiologist, John Radcliffe Hospital, Oxford University Hospitals NHS Foundation Trust, UK

James Redfern, Consultant Cardiologist, Countess of Chester Hospital, UK

Rhian Richardson, Specialty Doctor in Cardiology, Royal United Hospital Bath NHS Foundation Trust, Bath, UK

Jonathan Rodrigues, Consultant Cardiothoracic Radiologist, Royal United Hospitals NHS Foundation Trust, Honorary Senior Lecturer, Department of Health, University of Bath, Chief Medical Officer and Co-Founder, Heart & Lung Imaging LTD

James Rosengarten, Consultant Cardiologist, East Kent Hospitals University NHS Foundation Trust, UK

Nikant Sabharwal, Consultant Cardiologist, John Radcliffe Hospital, Oxford University Hospitals NHS Foundation Trust, Oxford, UK

Eva Sammut, Consultant Cardiologist, Bristol Heart Institute, University Hospitals Bristol NHS Foundation Trust, UK

Helen Sims, Geriatric and Stroke Specialist Registrar, North Bristol NHS Trust & Severn Deanery, UK

S M Afzal Sohaib, Consultant Cardiologist, St Bartholomew's Hospital, London, & King George Hospital, Essex, UK

Graham Stuart, Consultant Cardiologist (Congenital heart Disease) & Honorary Associate Professor in Sports and Exercise Cardiology, Bristol Heart Institute & Bristol Royal Hospital for Children, University Hospitals Bristol NHS Foundation Trust & University of Bristol, UK

Jay Suntharalingam, Consultant Respiratory Physician, Royal United Hospitals Bath NHS Foundation Trust

Elena Surkova, Senior Clinical Fellow in Cardiovascular Imaging, Guy's and St Thomas' NHS Foundation Trust, London, UK

Patricia Taraborrelli, Syncope Nurse Specialist, Imperial College Healthcare NHS Trust, London, UK

Katharine Thomas, Clinical Research Fellow, University of Oxford, Oxford, UK

James Tomlinson, Cardiology Specialist Registrar, Royal United Hospitals Bath NHS Foundation Trust, Bath, UK

Diana Vassallo, Resident Specialist Nephrology, Department of Medicine, Mater Dei Hospital, Malta

Ruta Virsinskaite, Clinical Research Fellow in Pulmonary Hypertension, National Pulmonary Hypertension Service, Royal Free London NHS Foundation Trust, London, UK

Oliver Watkinson, Consultant Cardiologist, Royal United Hospitals Bath NHS Foundation Trust, UK

Thomas White, Cardiology Specialist Registrar, Royal United Hospital Bath NHS Foundation Trust & Severn Deanery, UK

Howell Williams, Cardiology Specialist Registrar, Bristol Heart Institute, University Hospitals Bristol NHS Foundation Trust & Severn Deanery, UK

David Wilson, Consultant Cardiologist, Worcestershire Acute Hospitals NHS Trust, UK

Abbas Zaidi, Consultant Cardiologist, Cardiff & Vale University Health Board, UK

chapter 1

IMAGING

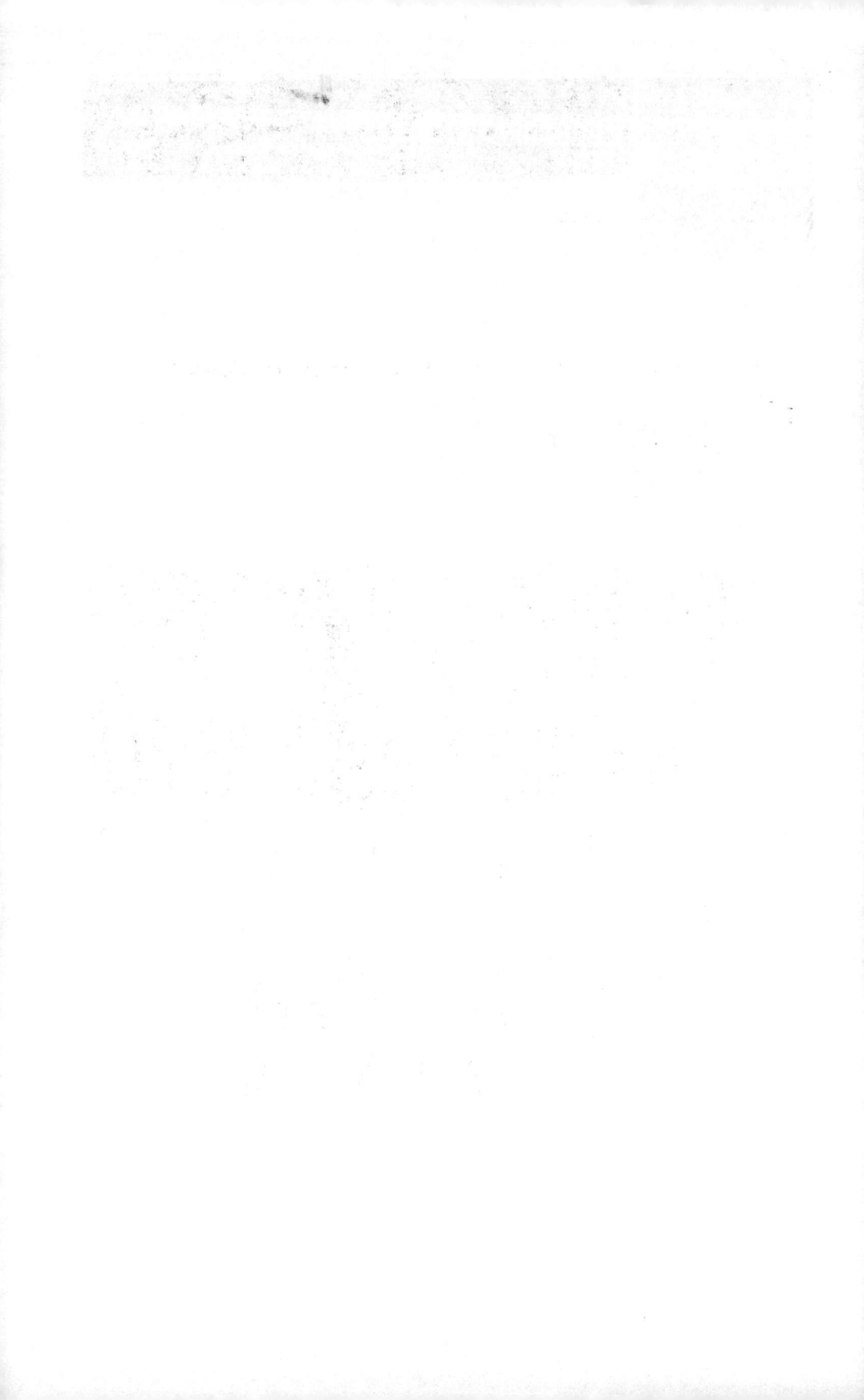

chapter 1.1

ECHOCARDIOGRAPHY

QUESTIONS

1. Tricuspid valve can be seen in all of the following views (Figure 1.1.1) except:

A. Parasternal long-axis view
B. Parasternal RV inflow view
C. Parasternal short axis view at great vessels level
D. Apical RV-focused four-chamber view
E. Subcostal four-chamber view

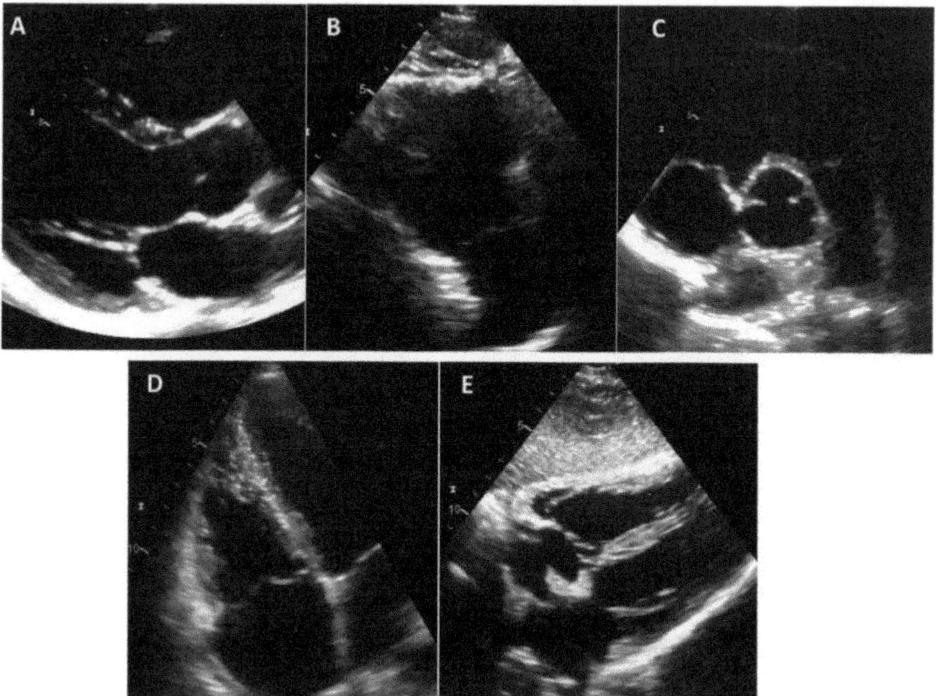

Figure 1.1.1

2. **Which of the following structures is not considered to be a normal finding?**

   A. Eustachian valve
   B. Crista terminalis
   C. Moderator band
   D. Subaortic membrane
   E. Chiari network

3. **A 66-year-old patient with a history of myocardial infraction due to LAD occlusion and regional wall motion abnormalities on previous transthoacic echocardiograpy was referred for echocardiography follow up.**

   Based on the 2D echo images provided (Figure 1.1.2), what is your conclusion regarding the LV thrombus?

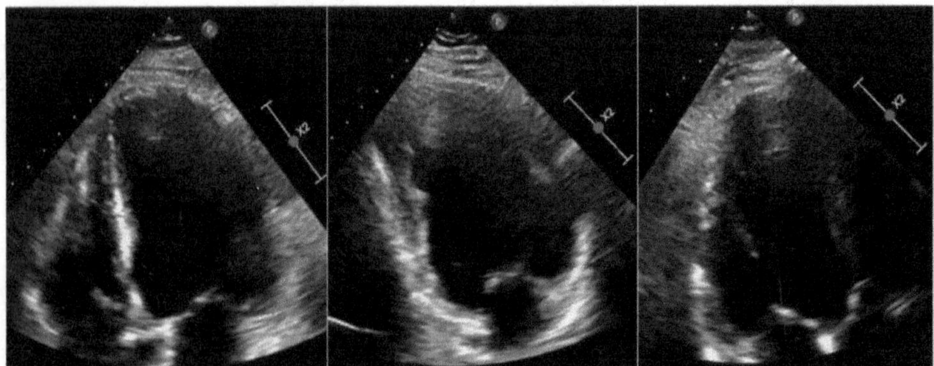

Figure 1.1.2

   A. There is a thrombus in LV apex
   B. The LV thrombus can be ruled out
   C. LV thrombus cannot be excluded; transoesophageal echocardiography is needed to confirm the diagnosis
   D. LV thrombus cannot be excluded; microbubble agitated saline test is needed to confirm the diagnosis
   E. LV thrombus cannot be excluded; contrast echocardiography is needed to confirm the diagnosis

4. A 60-year-old female patient underwent a surgical ASD closure and tricuspid annuloplasty 6 months previously. She has longstanding atrial fibrillation. She was referred for a follow-up echo. On TTE examination, there was a residual atrial septal defect with continuous left-to-right shunt (peak pressure gradient 17 mmHg and mean pressure gradient 12 mmHg). The IVC was dilated but collapsing >50% with inspiration (Figure 1.1.3).

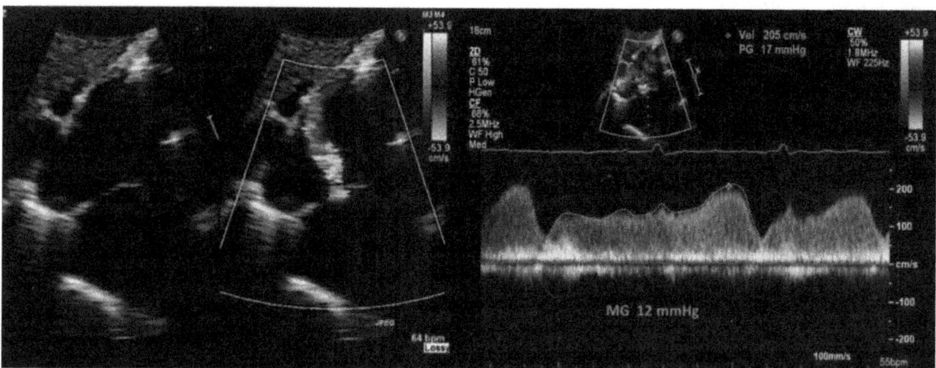

Figure 1.1.3

These findings reflect:

A. LV systolic dysfunction
B. LV diastolic dysfunction
C. RV systolic dysfunction
D. RV diastolic dysfunction
E. Increased risk of paradoxical embolism

5. A 64-year-old female with a history of pulmonary hypertension due to systemic sclerosis undergoes surveillance echocardiography (Figure 1.1.4). The echocardiographic parameters of RV function are shown below:

- TAPSE 1.9 cm
- S' 11 cm/s
- FAC 28%
- RV GLS −18%
- 3DE EF 37%

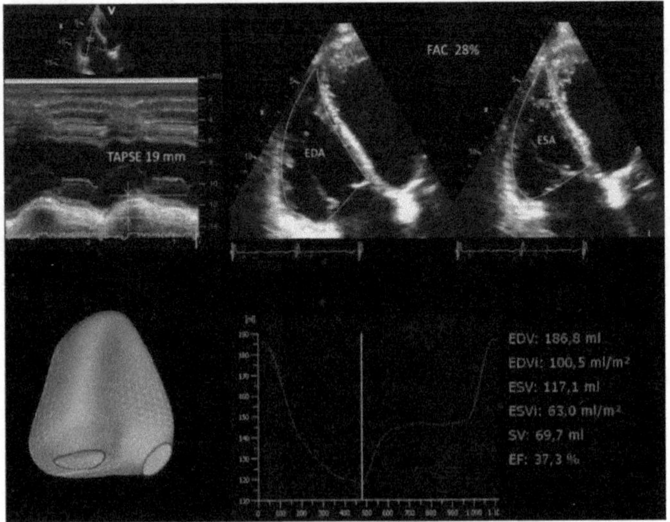

Figure 1.1.4

How would you describe the RV global systolic function?

A. Hyperdynamic
B. Preserved
C. Reduced
D. Unable to comment on RV global systolic function based on the data provided
E. None of the above

6. An 81-year-old male patient with a history of degenerative aortic stenosis has developed symptoms of heart failure. He attends for a TTE examination. Valve parameters and Doppler trace is shown in Figure 1.1.5.

LVOT diameter 2.4 cm

LVOT VTI 22 cm

Aortic valve VTI 123 cm

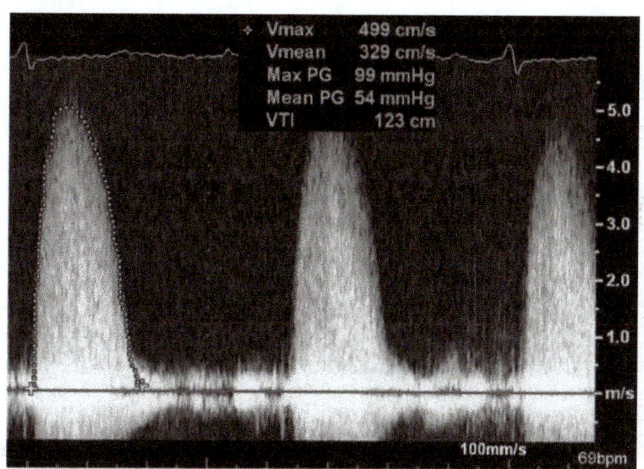

Figure 1.1.5

What is the calculated aortic valve area (AVA)?

A. 1.0 cm²
B. 0.9 cm²
C. 0.8 cm²
D. 0.7 cm²
E. 0.65 cm²

7. A 68-year-old gentleman with breathlessness was referred for echocardiography by a cardiologist who noticed a new systolic murmur at the apex. Rupture of the posterior mitral valve chordae with flail of posterior mitral valve leaflet is seen on the echocardiogram (Figure 1.1.6).

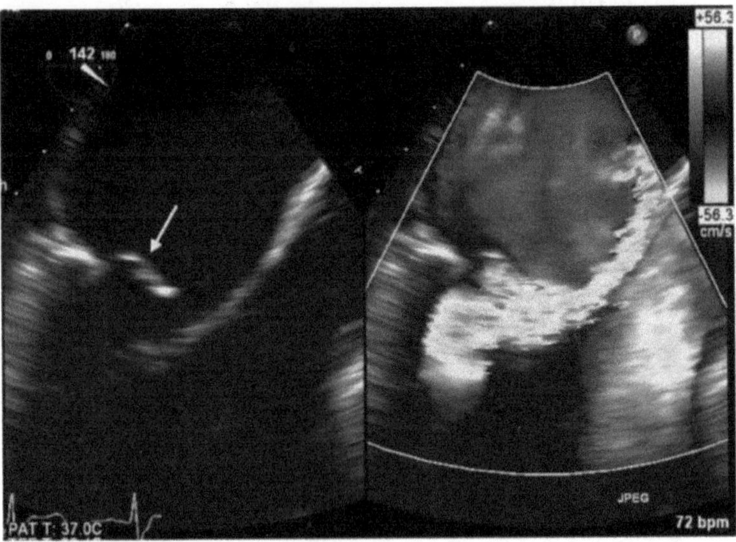

Figure 1.1.6

Which of the following echocardiographic parameters is not consistent with severe mitral regurgitation?

A. Vena contracta diameter = 6 mm
B. PISA radius = 1.2 cm
C. Effective regurgitant orifice = 48 mm²
D. Regurgitant volume = 74 ml
E. Systolic flow reversal in pulmonary veins.

8. A 67-year-old patient post of following CABG developed hypotension and tachycardia. An urgent echocardiogram demonstrated a pericardial effusion. The diagnosis of cardiac tamponade was made during echocardiographic exam (Figure 1.1.7):

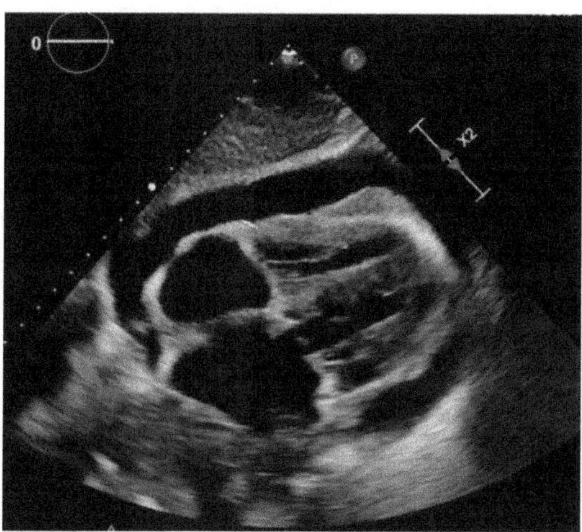

Figure 1.1.7

Which one of the following echocardiographic is most suggestive of cardiac tamponade?

A. RV systolic collapse
B. LA early collapse in ventricular diastole
C. LV systolic collapse
D. RA early collapse in ventricular systole
E. Normal RA size and inspiratory collapse

9. The regurgitant volume in mitral regurgitation (Figure 1.1.8) is not altered by which of the following:

A. Type of mitral regurgitation
B. VTI of mitral regurgitant jet
C. Heart rate
D. Systolic ejection period
E. Effective regurgitant orifice area

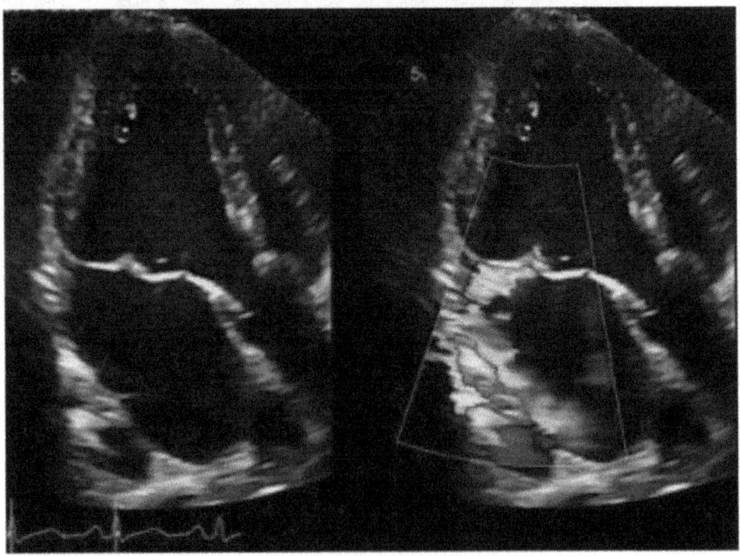

Figure 1.1.8

10. A 46-year-old woman with a history of rheumatic fever in childhood was referred for echocardiography due to clinical suspicion of severe mitral stenosis. TTE revealed mitral stenosis, and trivial mitral and trivial aortic regurgitation (Figure 1.1.9).

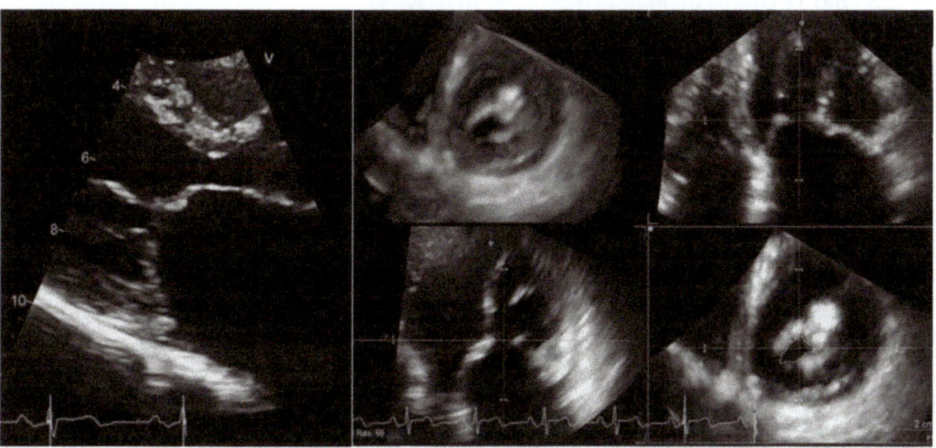

Figure 1.1.9

LVOT diameter = 2.2 cm; LVOT VTI = 23 cm; MV VTI = 80 cm.

What was the calculated MV area?

A. 1.2 cm^2
B. 1.1 cm^2
C. 1.0 cm^2
D. 0.9 cm^2
E. MV area cannot be calculated using these parameters

11. A 73-year-old gentleman with known chronic heart failure has moderate tricuspid regurgitation with regurgitant jet max velocity of 4.2 m/sec, and IVC diameter of 2.5 cm during expiration and 1.8 cm during inspiratory sniff (Figure 1.1.10).

What is the estimated mean RA pressure?

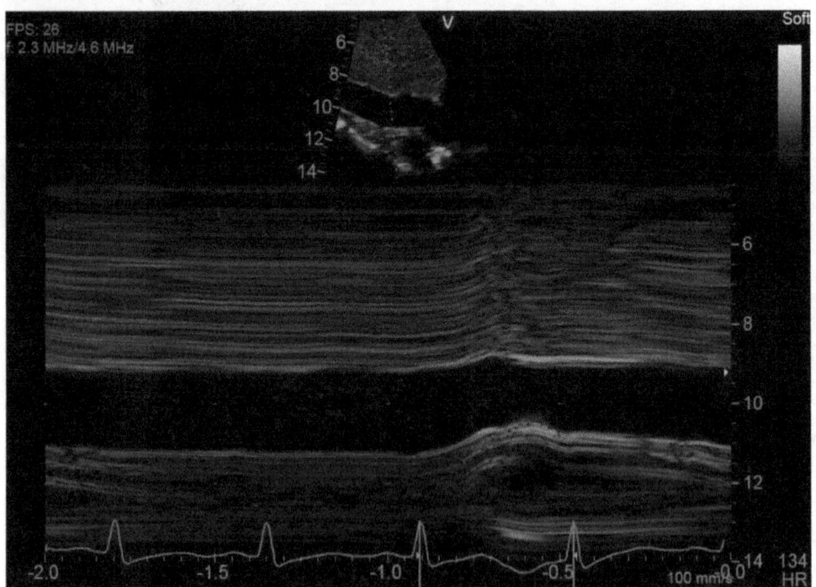

Figure 1.1.10

A. 3 mmHg (range, 0–5 mmHg)
B. 8 mmHg (range, 5–10 mmHg)
C. 15 mmHg (range, 10–20 mmHg);
D. Cannot be estimated;
E. None of the above

12. All of the following statements regarding the echocardiographic assessment of aortic stenosis are true except:

A. Patients with severe aortic stenosis and preserved LVEF usually have a mean gradient across the aortic valve ≥ 40 mmHg
B. Patients with severe aortic stenosis and low LVEF may have mean aortic valve gradient < 40 mmHg
C. Patients with 'paradoxical' low flow, low gradient aortic stenosis usually have stroke volume index > 35 ml/m²
D. AVA index < 0.6 cm²/m² represents severe AS
E. Peak aortic valve gradient assessed by CW Doppler echocardiography is usually higher than peak-to-peak gradient measured in catheterization laboratory

13. In which of the following circumstances you would expect to see normal motion of IVS on M-mode most frequently (Figure 1.1.11)?

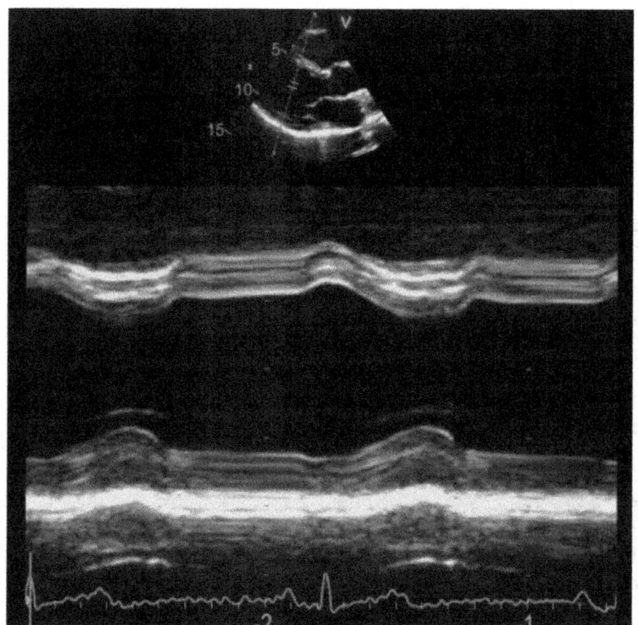

Figure 1.1.11

A. LBBB
B. RV pacing
C. Severe tricuspid regurgitation with right ventricular volume overload
D. Aortic valve replacement
E. Moderate aortic regurgitation

14. Which of the following parameters is recommended for routine echocardiographic assessment of LA size in clinical practice (Figure 1.1.12)?

A. LA antero-posterior diameter
B. LA length in four-chamber view
C. LA area
D. LA volume single-plane
E. LA volume biplane

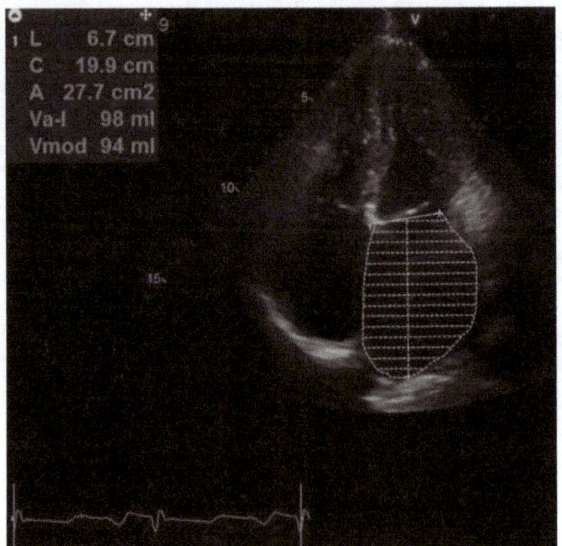

Figure 1.1.12

15. Which of the following conditions would usually be associated with the lowest indexed LV mass?

A. Severe aortic stenosis
B. Severe aortic regurgitation
C. Severe mitral stenosis
D. Severe mitral regurgitation
E. VSD with significant left-to-right shunt

16. All of the following echocardiographic findings (Figure 1.1.13) are typical in patients with dilated cardiomyopathy except:

A. LV EDV index > 112 ml/m^2
B. Thinning of the LV walls
C. Reduced LV EF
D. Spherical shape of the LV
E. 'Apical sparing'

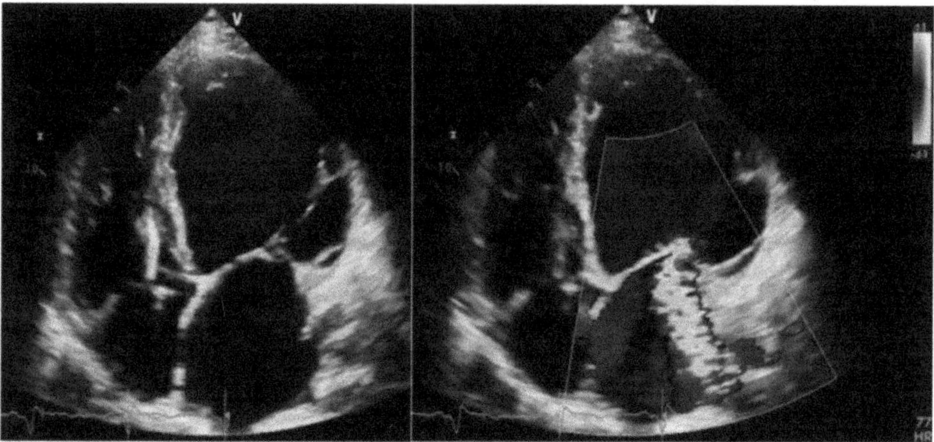

Figure 1.1.13

17. Major 2D echocardiographic criteria of arrhythmogenic RV cardiomyopathy (Figure 1.1.14) include regional RV akinesia, dyskinesia, or aneurysm and which one of the following:

A. RVOT diameter in parasternal long-axis view ≥32 mm (≥19 mm/m^2)
B. RVOT diameter in parasternal short-axis view ≥32 mm (≥19 mm/m^2)
C. TAPSE <18 mm
D. FAC ≤35%
E. McConnell's sign

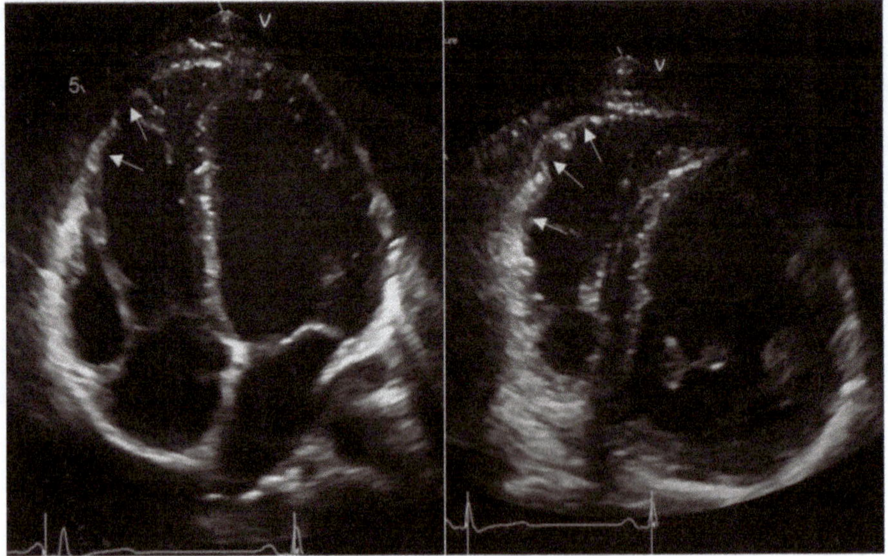

Figure 1.1.14

18. An 18-year-old patient with a perimembranous ventricular septal defect (VSD) has a blood pressure of 140/80 mmHg and a VSD jet peak velocity of 5 m/sec (Figure 1.1.15):

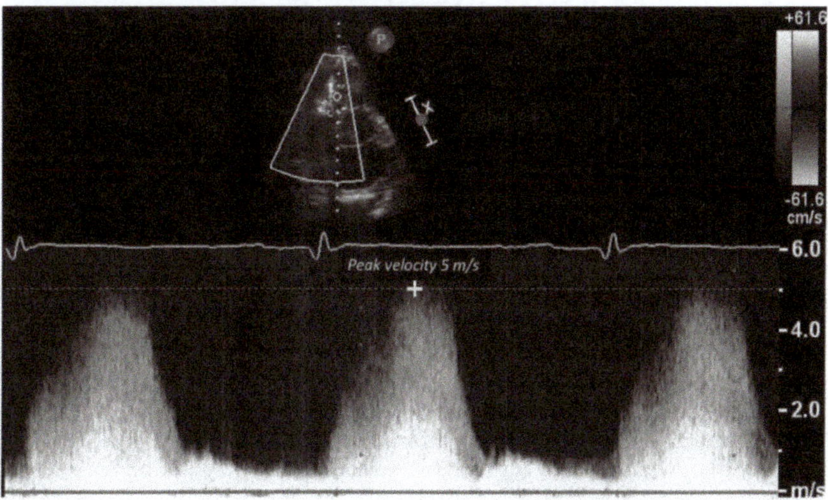

Figure 1.1.15

What is the RV systolic pressure?

A. 40 mmHg
B. 80 mmHg
C. 120 mmHg
D. 135 mmHg
E. 150 mmHg

chapter

1.1

ECHOCARDIOGRAPHY

ANSWERS

1. A. In a standard parasternal long-axis view tricuspid valve cannot be visualized. All other views are suitable for visualization of tricuspid valve.

2. D. Subaortic membrane is a pathological structure and may lead to subaortic stenosis, while all others are normal structures which may mimic masses in right heart chambers.

3. E. From the 2D echo images there is a suspicion of apical thrombus; however, the image quality is suboptimal, and it may be a near field clutter artefact mimicking an LV thrombus in the apex. Contrast echocardiography using left heart contrast agents is the echocardiographic method of choice for the assessment of left ventricular apical thrombus. It's clear from the contrast images provided (Figure 1.1.A1), that the LV is free from thrombus on this particular patient.

A micro bubble agitated saline test would not be useful in this case as agitated saline provides opacification of right cardiac chambers only. Transoesophageal echocardiography is not the modality of choice to assess left ventricular apical thrombus.

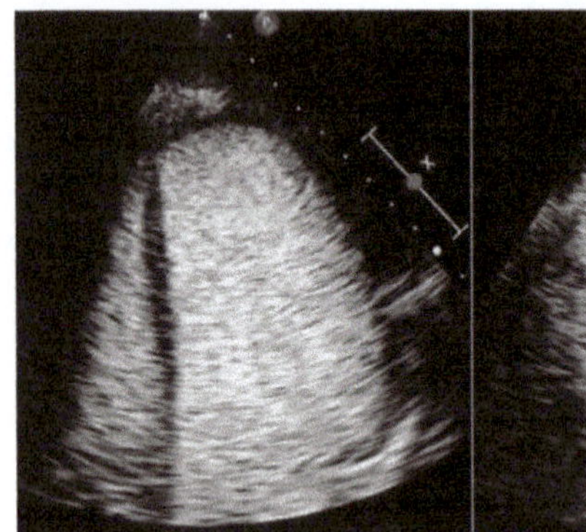
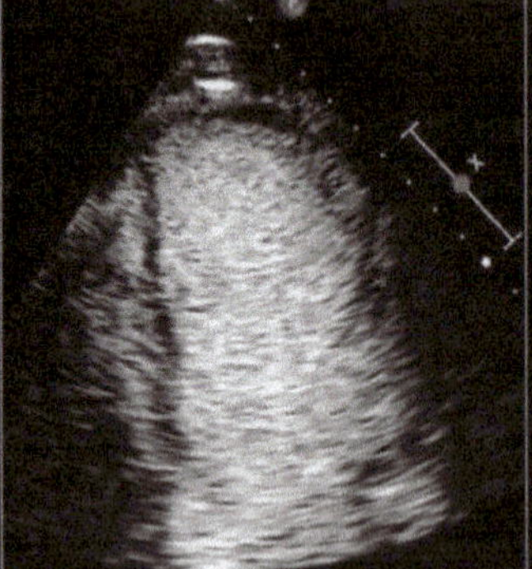
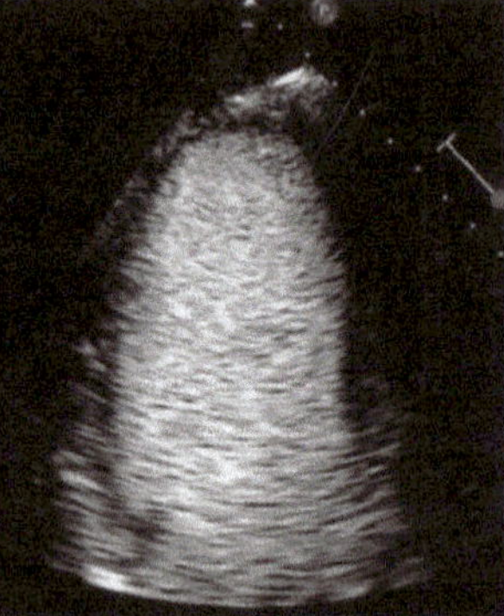

Figure 1.1.A1

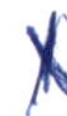

4. B. The mean left atrial (LA) pressure can be calculated as the sum of mean pressure across the ASD plus right atrial pressure. If the IVC is dilated but collapsing >50% with inspiration, we assume that the right atrial pressure is 8mmHg. Therefore, LA pressure = 12 + 8 = 20 mmHg. This is elevated LA pressure which is a sign of LV diastolic dysfunction. Other findings confirming LV diastolic dysfunction in this patient are presented on the images below: short MV deceleration time; presence of L-wave on mitral inflow Doppler signal and TR peak velocity >2.8 m/s (Figure 1.1.A2).

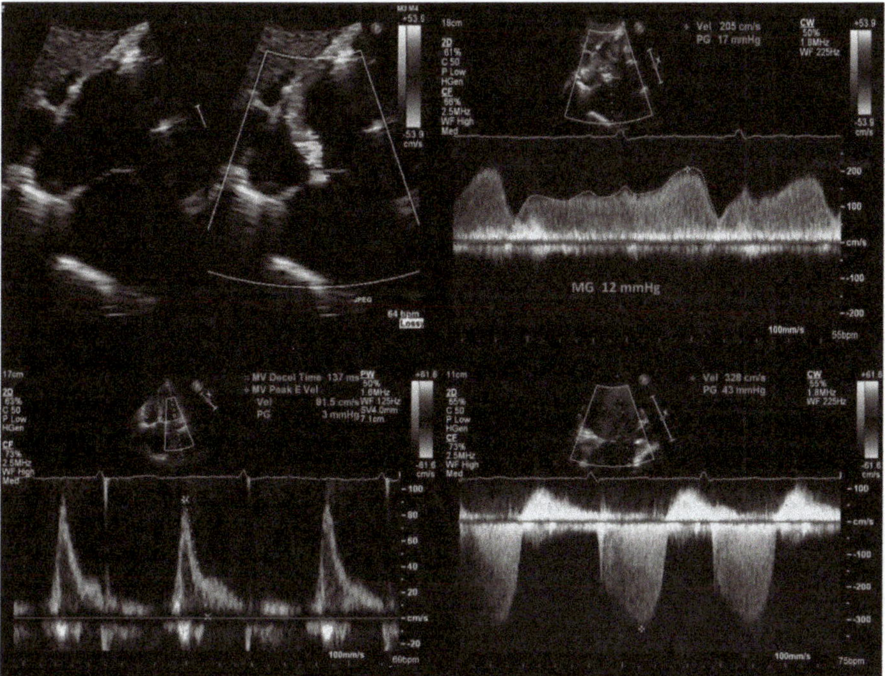

Figure 1.1.A2

From the information and images provided, it's not possible to make any conclusions about LV systolic function, or RV systolic and RV diastolic function.

Paradoxical thromboembolism is unlikely in this case because the shunt is left to right.

5. C. 3DE EF is the only echocardiographic parameter which reflects true global systolic RV function. The lower limit for 3DE RV EF is >45% which means. Therefore, this patient has impaired RV systolic function. TAPSE, S', and GLS are markers of longitudinal function only and should not be used in isolation to assess the global systolic function. FAC reflects both longitudinal and radial contraction (reference value >35%). However, it's important to remember that FAC neglects the contribution of RVOT and is limited to the part of RV seen in the RV-focused four-chamber view.

6. C. AVA can be calculated by continuity equation using the following formula:

AVA = (LVOT VTI × LVOT area) / Aortic valve VTI

LVOT area = $\pi \times$ (LVOT diameter/2)^2

In this case AVA =0.8 cm^2 and is indicative of severe aortic stenosis.

7. A. 2DE vena contracta ≥ 7mm (or >8 mm for biplane measurement) is suggestive of severe mitral regurgitation.

All other parameters satisfy the current echocardiographic criteria of severe organic mitral regurgitation.

8. D. Early systolic collapse of the RA and diastolic collapse of the RV free wall are important signs of cardiac tamponade.

9. A. Regurgitant volume can be calculated using the following formula: R Vol = EROA × VTI_{MR}

It is directly proportional to the effective regurgitant orifice area (EROA), velocity time integral of regurgitant jet (VTI_{MR}), while VTI_{MR} itself is directly proportional to systolic ejection period, and reversely proportional to heart rate.

Regurgitant volume does not depend on the type of mitral regurgitation.

10. B. Since there is only trivial mitral and aortic regurgitation, the flow through LVOT will be equal to the flow through the mitral valve. Consequently, a continuity equation can be used to calculate MV area by the following formula:

MV area = LVOT area × LVOT VTI / MV VTI,

where LVOT VTI and MV VTI – velocity time integrals of flow through LVOT and MV, respectively. LVOT area = π × (LVOT diameter/2)2

MV area = π × 1.12 × 23 / 80 = 1.1 cm^2

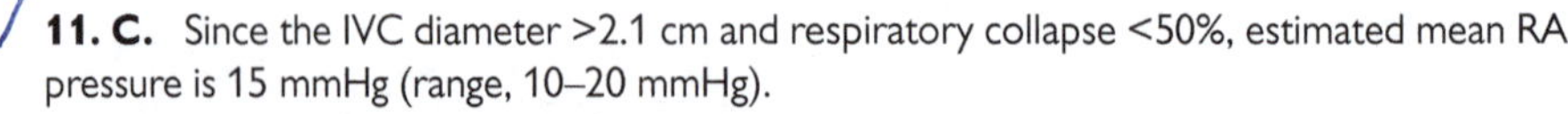

11. C. Since the IVC diameter >2.1 cm and respiratory collapse <50%, estimated mean RA pressure is 15 mmHg (range, 10–20 mmHg).

Mean RA pressure is estimated at 3mmHg (1–5 mmHg) if IVC dimension is <2.1 cm and respiratory collapse >50%.

In any other possible combinations, the RA pressure is estimated at 8 mmHg (5–10 mmHg).

12. C. 'Paradoxical' low flow, low gradient aortic stenosis occurs in patients with small hypertrophied LV resulting in SV index <35 ml/m^2 despite normal LV EF.

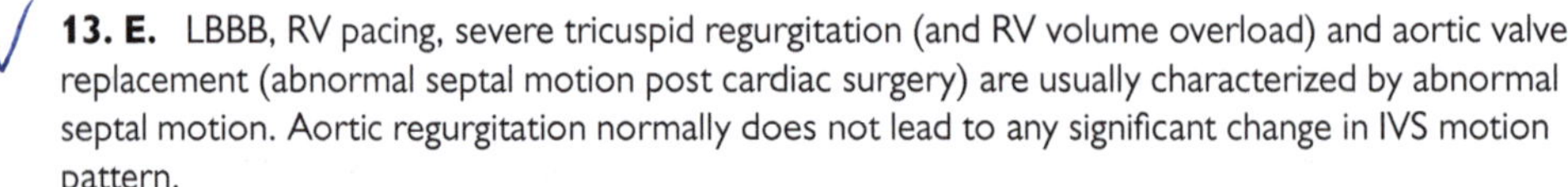

13. E. LBBB, RV pacing, severe tricuspid regurgitation (and RV volume overload) and aortic valve replacement (abnormal septal motion post cardiac surgery) are usually characterized by abnormal septal motion. Aortic regurgitation normally does not lead to any significant change in IVS motion pattern.

14. E. According to current guidelines, 2D echocardiographic assessment of LA volume by biplane method of discs or area-length method is the preferred approach for quantification of LA size.

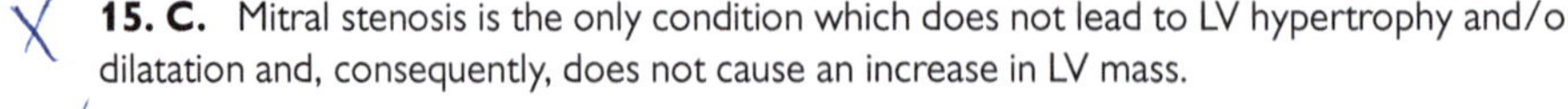

15. C. Mitral stenosis is the only condition which does not lead to LV hypertrophy and/or dilatation and, consequently, does not cause an increase in LV mass.

16. E. 'Apical sparing' is a regional pattern in 2D speckle-tracking echocardiography longitudinal strain frequently observed in patients with cardiac amyloidosis, but not with dilated cardiomyopathy (Figure 1.1.A3):

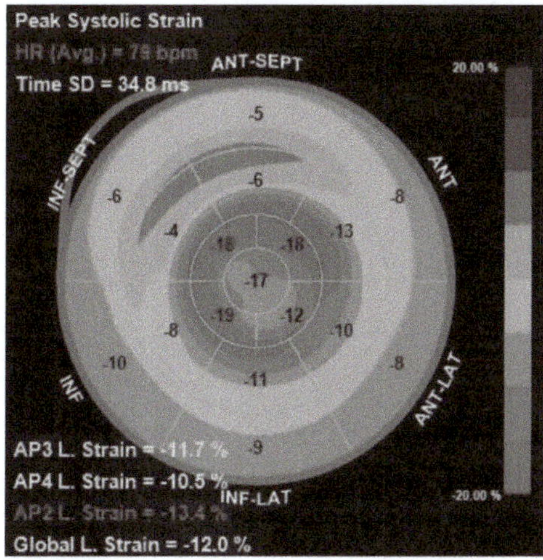

Figure 1.1.A3 All other options are correct.

17. A. Major 2D echocardiographic criteria of arrhythmogenic RV cardiomyopathy include regional RV akinesia, dyskinesia or aneurysm and one of the following:

- RVOT diameter in parasternal long-axis view ≥32 mm (≥19 mm/m^2), or
- RVOT diameter in parasternal short-axis view ≥36 mm (≥21 mm/m^2), or
- FAC ≤33%.

TAPSE is a parameter of RV longitudinal systolic function; however, it is not a criterion for arrhythmogenic RV cardiomyopathy. McConnell's sign is a distinct regional pattern of RV dysfunction, with akinesia of the mid free wall but normal motion at the apex described in patients with acute pulmonary embolism.

18. A. Pressure gradient (PG) between the left and right ventricle can be calculated from VSD jet peak velocity (V) using the following formula:

PG = 4V2

PG = 4 × 25 = 100 mmHg

If LV systolic pressure is 140 mmHg, then RV systolic pressure is 140 – 100 = 40 mmHg.

chapter 1.2

CARDIAC MAGNETIC RESONANCE IMAGING

QUESTIONS

1. **A 54-year-old man with troponin-positive chest pain and unobstructed coronaries is undergoing CMR imaging for assessment of possible cause for the elevated troponin. The MR technologists show you the following image (Figure 1.2.1):**

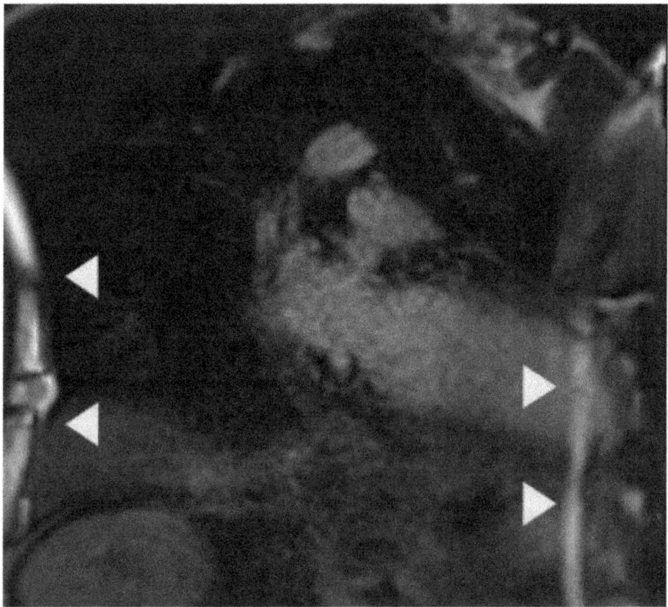

Figure 1.2.1

Which single response will not reduce this particular artefact?

A. Decrease field of view (FOV)
B. Perform phase-oversampling
C. Swap phase and frequency directions
D. Use selective tissue saturation bands
E. Use a surface coil

2. **A medical student on their cardiology rotation asks you if there are any circumstances when it is not safe to perform a CMR.**

   Regarding CMR safety, which single response is an absolute contraindication to CMR performed at 1.5 tesla?

   A. Bio-prosthetic aortic valve replacement < 6 weeks ago
   B. Drug-eluting stent in the left anterior descending artery (LAD) < 24 hours ago
   C. Implantable loop recorder in situ
   D. Intra-ocular metallic foreign body
   E. Legacy dual chamber cardiac pacemaker (VVI)

3. **A 66-year-old man with prior history of ischaemic heart disease and coronary artery bypass (LIMA to LAD, SVG to RCA and SVG to OM1) 5 years ago for stable angina presents with re-emergent angina. An adenosine stress perfusion CMR is requested to assess for inducible ischaemia.**

   Which single response is not an absolute or relative contraindication to IV adenosine?

   A. Consumption of caffeine within 6 hours
   B. Use of long-acting nitrate
   C. Use of dipyridamole
   D. Third degree AV block
   E. Severe asthma

4. **A 58-year-old man with a past medical history of type 2 diabetes mellitus, obesity, and hyperlipidaemia, presents with new onset shortness of breath on exertion and orthopnoea. Serum NT-proBNP is elevated. Echocardiography is limited by poor acoustic windows but demonstrates moderate LV systolic impairment. A CMR is performed to assess for the underlying aetiology of the heart failure.**

   Which one of the following late gadolinium enhancement (LGE) patterns suggests an ischaemic cardiomyopathy?

   A. Anteroseptal subepicardial LGE
   B. Global subendocardial LGE
   C. Mid to apical inferior subendocardial LGE
   D. Septal midwall LGE
   E. Inferolateral midwall LGE

5. A 67-year-old woman with past medical history of arterial hypertension and type 2 diabetes mellitus complains of central chest pain on exertion, relieved with rest. She undergoes CT coronary angiography that demonstrates a mid LAD artery moderate stenosis (50–69% stenosis). The patient undergoes an adenosine stress perfusion CMR for further assessment.

Which one of the following findings in the mid LAD territory on CMR would not be associated with gain in regional function following revascularization?

A. Hypokinesia that resolves on low-dose dobutamine
B. Hypokinesia with inducible perfusion defect with no LGE
C. Hypokinesia with < 25% transmural subendocardial LGE
D. Inducible perfusion defect with no regional wall motion abnormality or LGE
E. Myocardial thinning < 5 mm with no LGE

6. An 18 year old woman collapses whilst running during a football match. She makes an immediate and spontaneous recovery without intervention but is admitted to hospital for further investigation. Her 12-lead ECG and telemetry are normal. High sensitivity troponin T is normal (<14 ng/L). On dedicated questioning, she admits to occasionally feeling lightheaded during strenuous exercise. A CT coronary angiogram is performed and demonstrates the right coronary artery arises from the left-facing coronary cusp and passes between the main pulmonary artery and ascending aorta to reach the right atrioventricular groove with normal left main stem origin and other proximal coronary anatomy.

Regarding CMR stress testing, which of the following types should be considered?

A. Adenosine stress perfusion CMR
B. Dipyridamole stress perfusion CMR
C. Dobutamine stress CMR
D. Regadenoson stress perfusion CMR
E. CMR stress testing not indicated

7. A 62-year-old woman with arterial hypertension, hyperlipidaemia, and obesity undergoes adenosine stress perfusion CMR for typical angina symptoms.

Which one of the following perfusion findings represents clinically significant myocardial ischaemia?

A. Transient subendocardial hypoperfusion on stress as the LV first opacifies
B. Subendocardial hypoperfusion on stress with matching subendocardial LGE
C. Subendocardial hypoperfusion on stress without LGE in < 1 segment.
D. Global subendocardial hypoperfusion on stress
E. >75% transmural subendocardial LGE in proximal LAD territory

8. A 82-year-old man presented with chest pain radiating to his left arm for 2 hours. A 12-lead ECG demonstrates 2 mm ST depression in V1-4 with T-wave inversion. High sensitivity troponin T is 120 ng/L. He is treated for a NSTEMI and undergoes in-patient angiography, which reveals severe triple vessel CAD. Echocardiography demonstrates LV dilatation with global systolic impairment and LVEF 35%. CMR is performed to determine the extent of viable myocardium to guide revascularization strategy.

Which one of the following findings suggests the myocardial segment is non-viable?

A. Indian ink artefact on SSFP cine imaging
B. Severe hypokinesia
C. Subendocardial LGE with >75% transmural extent
D. Transmural inducible perfusion defect without matching LGE
E. Wall thickness <5 mm

9. You read the research protocol for an interventional study in acute ST elevation MI using CMR-defined area at risk, myocardial salvage, and infarct size as end-points.

Which of the following statements is incorrect?

A. Area at risk and infarct size can be determined by T1 mapping
B. Area at risk correlates with the extent of culprit territory oedema
C. Infarct size correlates with the extent of culprit territory LGE
D. Pre and post intervention CMR are needed to estimate myocardial salvage
E. Reperfusion injury can contribute to oedema following revascularization

10. A 54-year-old man presents with shortness of breath following a severe episode of anterior chest pain that started 12 hours previously and lasted for several hours. He is diagnosed with a late presentation acute anterior ST elevation MI. He undergoes primary percutaneous angioplasty to the LAD. A CMR is performed the following day for prognostication.

Which one of the following is diagnostic of intramyocardial haemorrhage (IMH)?

A. High signal in the midwall on LGE
B. High signal in the myocardium on SSFP cine imaging
C. Low signal in the LV cavity on early gadolinium enhancement
D. Low signal in the myocardium on T2*-weighted imaging
E. Low signal in the subendocardium on LGE

11. A 54-year-old man presents with shortness of breath since a severe episode of anterior chest pain that started 12 hours previously and lasted for several hours. He is diagnosed with a late presentation acute anterior ST elevation MI. He undergoes primary percutaneous angioplasty to the LAD. CMR is performed the following day for prognostication.

Which one of the following is incorrect?

A. IMH is a predictor of adverse clinical outcomes
B. IMH occurs more frequently than MVO
C. IMH prevalence peaks around 2 day post reperfusion
D. MVO decreases with time post-revascularization
E. MVO is a predictor of adverse LV remodelling

12. A 48-year-old woman with paroxysmal atrial fibrillation presents with chest pain with ST depression in V1–V3 with T-wave inversion, following a long-haul flight. High sensitivity troponin T was 72 ng/L and repeat 3 hours later was 79 ng/L. She is treated as a non-ST elevation MI and undergoes in-patient catheter angiography. This reveals unobstructed coronary arteries. A CMR is preformed which reveals focal mid anteroseptal subendocardial LGE.

Which one of the following is not a differential diagnosis in the LGE pattern?

A. Coronary artery side branch occlusion
B. Deep myocardial bridge
C. Deep vein thrombus and patent foramen ovale
D. Left atrial appendage thrombus embolism
E. Plaque event with spontaneous recanalization

13. A 76-year-old woman experiences central chest pain associated with ST elevation. The pain developed shortly after she received bad news. Catheter angiography demonstrates unobstructed coronary arteries but characteristic regional wall motion abnormality on LV-gram of Takotsubo cardiomyopathy. High sensitivity troponin T on admission was 110 ng/L and repeat 3 hours later was 114 ng/L. Takotsubo cardiomyopathy is suspected and a CMR was performed.

Which one of the following is not compatible with the diagnosis of Takotsubo cardiomyopathy?

A. Apical to basal LGE gradient
B. High myocardial signal on SSFP cines
C. Left ventricular outlet obstruction
D. Mid to apical systolic ballooning
E. Pericardial effusion

14. A previously fit and well 44-year-old man presents with central chest following a prodromal viral illness. His ECG reveals anterolateral T-wave inversion. High sensitivity troponin T is 44 ng/L and repeat 3 hours later is 47 ng/L. Catheter angiography reveals normal coronary arteries. A clinical diagnosis of peri-myocarditis is suspected and a CMR is performed.

Which one of the following patterns of LGE is compatible with myocarditis?

A. Anteroseptal subepicardial LGE
B. Inferolateral transmural LGE
C. Global subendocardial LGE
D. RV insertion point LGE
E. Septal subendocardial LGE

15. A 72-year-old woman with previous history of tuberculosis presents with gradual onset shortness of breath, leg and ankle swelling, and fatigue. Prior CT of the thorax has demonstrated some pericardial calcification. Echocardiographic windows were poor. A CMR is performed.

Which one of the following is not a CMR feature of constrictive pericarditis?

A. Biatrial dilatation
B. Inferior vena cava engorgement
C. Pericardial thickening
D. Interventricular septal flattening during systole
E. Transient leftward septal deviation on deep inspiration

16. A 46-year-old woman with history of palpitations undergoes an echocardiogram that demonstrates right ventricular enlargement. A CMR is performed to assess further. This demonstrates the left upper lobe pulmonary vein drains into the left brachiocephalic vein but there is normal drainage of the other pulmonary veins.

Which one of the following in not associated with partial anomalous pulmonary venous drainage?

A. Pulmonary hypertension
B. Right-to-left shunt
C. Scimitar syndrome
D. Superior sinus venosus atrial septal defect
E. Turner's syndrome

17. A 24-year-old woman with history of palpitation and frequent extra-systoles of right ventricular outflow tract morphology on 12-lead ECG undergoes CMR as part of the diagnostic work-up for arrhythmogenic right ventricular cardiomyopathy/dysplasia.

Which one of the following is not a major or minor criterion for arrhythmogenic right ventricular cardiomyopathy/dysplasia according to the 2010 Modified Task Force criteria?

A. Right ventricular indexed end diastolic volume >110 ml/m^2
B. Right ventricular dyssynchrony
C. Right ventricular ejection fraction <40%
D. Right ventricular LGE
E. Right ventricular systolic regional wall motion abnormality

18. A 49-year-old man experiences exertional syncope. An echocardiogram demonstrates asymmetric septal thickness 20 mm. Hypertrophic cardiomyopathy is suspected and a CMR is performed for diagnostic and prognostic purposes.

Which one of the following is not a predictor of adverse cardiovascular morbidity or mortality?

A. Apical aneurysm
B. Presence of LGE
C. Resting LVOT gradient >30 mmHg
D. Systolic anterior motion of the anterior mitral valve
E. Wall thickness ≥ 30 mm

19. A 44-year-old woman presents with chest pain, with lateral T-wave inversion. High sensitivity troponin T was 42 ng/L and repeat 3 hours later was 49 ng/L. Catheter angiography reveals unobstructed coronary arteries. A CMR is negative for acute myopericarditis.

Which one of the following is not a potential extracardiac cause of acute chest pain that would be discernible on CMR?

A. Cholecystitis
B. Oesophageal reflux
C. Pleural effusion
D. Pulmonary embolism
E. Right lower lobe consolidation

chapter 1.2

CARDIAC MAGNETIC RESONANCE IMAGING

ANSWERS

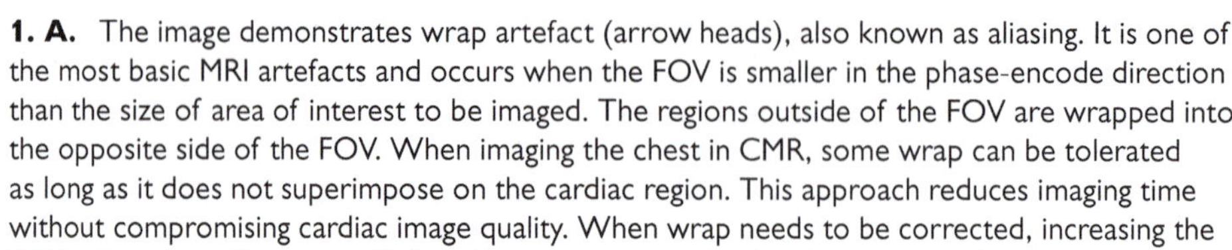

1. A. The image demonstrates wrap artefact (arrow heads), also known as aliasing. It is one of the most basic MRI artefacts and occurs when the FOV is smaller in the phase-encode direction than the size of area of interest to be imaged. The regions outside of the FOV are wrapped into the opposite side of the FOV. When imaging the chest in CMR, some wrap can be tolerated as long as it does not superimpose on the cardiac region. This approach reduces imaging time without compromising cardiac image quality. When wrap needs to be corrected, increasing the FOV will reduce aliasing as will the other options described in the question above.

2. D. Most medical prostheses used nowadays will be made from MRI compatible materials but confirmation should always be sought directly from the manufacturer. Generally, MRI is deferred for 6 weeks after surgery, but this should be reassessed on a case-by-case basis for the risk-to-benefit ratio. Large registry datasets demonstrate that it is generally safe to perform MRI with legacy pacemakers but strict safety protocols need to be adhered to. It should also be appreciated that whilst it may be safe to perform CMR in the context of an MRI compatible pacemaker, they may be resultant artefacts from the device and/or leads that impairs diagnostic image quality. Finally, it should be appreciated that prostheses that are considered MR safe at 1.5 tesla field strength may not be at higher 3 tesla field strength.

3. B. Adenosine can result in AV nodal conduction block and should be avoided in the context of sick sinus syndrome, high grade second-degree AV block, and third-degree AV. Dipyridamole potentiates the action of adenosine. Methylxanthine (e.g. caffeine in coffee, theophylline in tea, and theobromine in chocolate) are competitive inhibitors with adenosine. An increased dose of adenosine may be required but there is also the risk of a false-negative study if adenosine stress perfusion CMR is performed within 6 hours of consumption of any of these substances. Owing to its bronchoconstriction side effects, adenosine is contraindicated in moderate–severe asthma. Whilst adenosine results in vasodilatation, concomitant use of other vasodilator anti-anginal medications is not a contraindication.

4. C. The ischaemic-necrotic ischaemic wavefront starts at the subendocardium, progressing to the epicardium. Consequently, a subendocaridal pattern of LGE is compatible with prior MI. The transmural extent correlates with the severity of the MI. However, a global subendocardial LGE pattern, not confined to an anticipated epicardial coronary artery territory, suggests a non-ischaemic aetiology, such as amyloidosis, systemic sclerosis, and post cardiac transplantation in the appropriate correct clinical context. The presence of subepicardial LGE raises the possibility of prior myocarditis. Midwall LGE is a feature of non-ischaemic cardiomyopathy with a septal location well recognized in idiopathic dilated cardiomyopathy and basal inferolateral midwall location is a classic reported finding in Anderson-Fabry's disease.

Mahrholdt H, Wagner A, Judd RM, et al. Delayed enhancement cardiovascular magnetic resonance assessment of non-ischaemic cardiomyopathies. Eur Heart J, **26**, 1461–74 (2005). doi: 10.1093/eurheartj/ehi258.

5. D. Demonstrating an inducible perfusion defect confirms the diagnosis of angina. However, in the absence of regional wall motion abnormality there will be no regional regain in function with revascularization, but potentially improvement in anginal symptoms. Transmurality of subendocardial LGE is a useful determinant of regional regain in function following resvascularization in ischaemic cardiomyopathy. Generally, transmural infarcts <25% will regain function. Demonstrating viability with a low-dose dobutamine protocol can help identify those who will respond to revascularization. Revascularization is associated with regional regain of function in myocardial segments that are hibernating, which is a state of metabolic downregulation in the context of chronic ischaemia. Hibernating myocardium can be seen in cases of regional wall motion abnormality that demonstrate inducible perfusion defect but no significant ischaemic-pattern LGE. Hibernating myocardium may be thinned but can regain function and wall thickness if there is no associated infarction. However, more recently, work has raise the question of the role of revascularisation with PCI over optimal medical therapy in ischaemic cardiomyopathy.

Perera D, Clayton T, O'Kane PD, et al. Percutaneous revascularization for ischemic left ventricular dysfunction. N Engl J Med, **387**(15), 1351–60 (2022). doi: 10.1056/NEJMoa2206606. Epub 2022 Aug 27.

6. E. The value of stress testing in anomalous coronary arteries with inter-arterial course is limited by both false-positive and false-negative results. Importantly, vasodilator mechanisms for stress, such as adenosine, dipyridamole, and regadenoson, are unlikely to mimic the pathophysiological state that causes symptoms in such coronary anomalies. The absence of inducible ischaemia in the coronary territory of concern cannot be viewed as reassuring.

7. D. Global subendocardial hypoperfusion on adenosine stress perfusion can be seen in the context of balanced three-vessel ischaemia. Dark rim artefact is common and describes the findings of a transient low endocardial border signal during the early phase of myocardial perfusion. It disappears quickly and may be discernible on the second pass of contrast too. The extent of myocardium affected by inducible ischaemia needs to be >1 segment to be significant in terms deriving symptomatic benefit of revascularization. A perfusion defect can occur in the area of ischaemic-pattern LGE but if the extent of hypoperfusion matches the infarct, there is no evidence of peri-infarct ischaemia. Likewise, there may be a large territory of prior MI but this does not necessarily equate to clinically significant inducible myocardial ischaemia.

8. C. Transmural extent of subendocardial LGE is the best CMR predictor of viability, with >75% transmural involvement the segment is very unlikely to remain viable. Indian ink artefact on SSFP cine images can be seen in cases of lipomatous metaplasia of prior infarct but does not infer lack of viability. Severe regional wall motion abnormality and myocardial thinning can occur in segments that may remain viable, as long as there is no significant transmural subendocardial LGE. Such segments are likely to be hibernating. The transmurality of inducible ischaemia does not necessarily predict whether a segment is viable, in the absence of matching transmural LGE.

9. D. The area at risk is the volume of myocardium that is endangered during an acute coronary artery occlusion. CMR performed within a couple of days after acute ST elevation MI is able to document the area at risk with oedema-weighted sequences such as T2-STIR and T2 mapping. The infarct core size can be estimated by LGE and the difference in the volumes between the area at risk and infarct size represents the amount of myocardium that has been salvaged by revascularization. Reperfusion injury can result in culprit coronary artery territory oedema, particularly in the cases of delayed revascularization. Native T1 mapping has been shown to be able to detect area at risk and the infarct size can be determined from post-contrast T1 mapping

10. D. IMH is diagnosed as low myocardial signal on T2 and/or T2* weighted imaging, owing to the paramagnetic effects of iron within the bleed. Microvascular obstruction is the imaging correlate of no-reflow on angiography and is diagnosed as myocardial signal void on post gadolinium sequences, both EGE and LGE. A signal void in the LV cavity on EGE and LGE is consistent with LV thrombus. Occasionally, laminar LV thrombus can be challenging to distinguish from MVO and underlying infarct is a risk factor for both.

11. B. Following ST elevation MI, CMR may demonstrate no MVO or IMH, MVO only or MVO and IMH. The prevalence of MVO is higher than the prevalence of IMH. MVO is a predictor of adverse LV remodelling post-MI but IMH, not MVO, has been demonstrated to be a predictor of a composite end-point of death and/or heart failure admission. IMH prevalence peaks around 2 days post-revascularization and MVO gradually decreased in prevalence with time from revascularization.

12. B. The subendocardial LGE pattern implies an ischaemic pattern insult. In the context of unobstructed coronary arteries, this could be due to a small side branch occlusion or a plaque event with subsequent recanalization by the time of angiography. An embolic MI is a consideration. The source may be a left atrial or left ventricular thrombus. In the context of a patent foramen ovale, a paradoxical systemic arterial embolism can occur from a venous thrombosis. Myocardial bridging is a not infrequent normal variant finding. The coronary compression can sometimes be striking in systole but more coronary perfusion occurs in diastole. Myocardial bridging itself is unlikely to result in MI.

13. A. Takotsubo may be associated with an apical to basal myocardial oedema gradient but is typically not associated with any LGE. High signal on SSFP cine images in the areas of classical regional wall motion abnormality may be seen as a reflection of myocardial oedema. The hyperdynamic basal contractility can result in left ventricular outflow tract obstruction, but if this occurs it is usually transient.

14. A. Patterns of LGE compatible with myocarditis include midwall and subepicardial LGE. LGE may be patchy and does not necessarily respect major epicardial coronary artery territories. The ischaemic-necrotic wave front progresses from subendocardium to epicaridium. Hence subendocardial to transmural LGE are compatible with MI of differing extent. Global subendocardial LGE could in theory represent triple-vessel ischaemic pattern LGE, but should prompt other diagnostic considerations, such as amyloidosis. It can also be seen post-heart transplant. RV insertion point LGE has been reported in the context of hypertrophic cardiomyopathy and pulmonary hypertension but may also be seen in otherwise normal ventricles.

15. D. Interventricular septal flattening during systole is a feature of right ventricular pressure loading, e.g. in the context of pulmonary hypertension. Abnormal septal motion may be present in the context of constrictive pericarditis but this is best assessed with dynamic breathing and real-time cines, with high temporal, but lower spatial, resolution than SSFP cines. Upon deep inspiration, a transient leftward septal deviation is noted as a result of decreased intrathoracic pressure and increased venous return predominantly from the lower body resulting in a transient higher RV pressure within the confines of the constricted pericardium resulting in the abnormal septal motion.

16. B. Partial anomalous pulmonary venous drainage has a predilection for the right lung. It results in a left-to-right shunt of oxygenated blood returning from the lungs. There is a recognized association with Turner's syndrome and scimitar syndrome. Partial anomalous pulmonary venous drainage from the right upper lobe to the inferior aspect of the superior vena cava is associated with a superior sinus venosus atrial septal defect. Pulmonary hypertension is a recognized complication.

17. D. CMR criteria are one component of the 2010 modified task force criteria for ARVC/D. They are as follows:

Major

- Regional RV akinesia or dyskinesia or dyssynchronous RV contraction

AND one of the following

- RV indexed end diastolic volume $\geq$110 ml/m^2 (men) or $\geq$100 ml/m^2 (women)
- RV ejection fraction $\leq$40%

Minor

- Regional RV akinesia or dyskinesia or dyssynchronous RV contraction

AND one of the following

- RV indexed end diastolic volume $\geq$100 to $<$110 ml/m^2 (men) or $\geq$90 to $<$100 ml/m^2 (women)
- RV ejection fraction $>$40 to $\leq$45%

Tissue characterization of the RV wall is on the basis of histology only. Presence of LGE does not feature in the 2010 modified task force criteria.

18. D. Both the presence and extent of LGE are predictors of adverse cardiovascular events, with $>$15% LV mass subtended by LGE a predictor of sudden cardiac death. Apical aneurysm predisposes the patient to apical thrombus formation and risk of thromboembolic stroke. Systolic anterior motion itself if not a reported independent predictor of adverse cardiovascular events in HCM.

19. B. Extracardiac findings at CMR are common and may be clinically important. Sometimes they can help make the cardiac diagnosis, e.g. in the case of sarcoidosis. In other cases, the extracardiac pathology may be the cause of the symptoms. Oesophageal reflux itself will not be detectable on CMR. However, a hiatus hernia, which could predispose to this might be evident. It should be realized that the risk factors for atherosclerosis are also risk factors for malignancy, which may be evident on CMR.

Rodrigues JCL, Lyen SM, Loughborough W, et al. Extra-cardiac findings in cardiovascular magnetic resonance: what the imaging cardiologist needs to know. J Cardiovasc Magn Reson, **18**(26), 1–21 (2016).

chapter 1.3

CARDIAC COMPUTED TOMOGRAPHY

QUESTIONS

1. A 79-year-old female is being investigated for severe aortic regurgitation. An echocardiogram suggests a dilated aortic root. An ECG-gated CT is performed as the gold standard non-invasive investigation to assess aortic calibre.

Which measurement technique is recommended to attain accurate and reproducible measurements from the CT dataset?

A. End systolic; inner to inner
B. End systolic; outer to outer
C. End diastolic; inner to inner
D. End diastolic; outer to outer
E. Mid systolic; outer to outer

2. A 26-year-old female is due to under cardiac CT but is keen to minimize her radiation exposure. With regards to cardiac CT and radiation dose reduction techniques, which of the following could be deployed to decrease the radiation dose the most?

A. Retrospective ECG gating without tube current modulation
B. Retrospective ECG gating with 25% tube current modulation
C. Retrospective ECG gating with 4% tube current modulation
D. Prospective ECG gating with low kVp technique with reference tube current
E. Prospective ECG gating with high kVp technique with reference tube current

3. A 73-year-old male is being investigated for aortic stenosis. Echo demonstrates an indexed stroke volume of 30 ml/m^2, LVEF 45%, an aortic valve gradient of 35 mmHg, and an aortic valve area of 0.9 cm^2. Low dose dobutamine echo shows no contractile reserve. A CT calcium score of the aortic valve is performed.

Which specific threshold Agatston AV calcium score does severe aortic stenosis become very likely?

A. 500
B. 1000
C. 2000
D. 3000
E. 4000

4. A 48-year-old female has been referred for investigation of her chest pain with a CT coronary angiogram. She will require administration of glyceryl trinitrate spray to aid analysis.

Which of the following are NOT contraindications to administration of GTN?

A. Concomitant sildenafil administration
B. Severe aortic stenosis
C. Hypertrophic cardiomyopathy with LV outflow tract obstruction
D. Concomitant use of isosorbide mononitrate
E. Pericardial tamponade

5. A 52-year-old male has been referred for investigation of his chest pain with a CT coronary angiogram. The patient is in sinus rhythm with a heart rate of 85 bpm. He will require administration of intravenous beta blockade to optimize his heart rate prior to scanning.

Which of the following are NOT contraindications to administration of beta blockade?

A. Third-degree heart block
B. Concomitant use of verapamil
C. Concomitant use of ivabradine
D. Acute uncontrolled heart failure
E. Poorly controlled asthma

6. A 69-year-old male who has previously undergone a mechanical aortic valve replacement has an echocardiogram for recurrent breathlessness. This demonstrates restricted leaflet motion. A cardiac CT is requested as a complementary test to investigate further.

Which of the following parameters makes pannus more likely than thrombus?

A. Leaflet thickening with attenuation of >145 HU
B. Occurrence within 3 months after surgery
C. Periprosthetic mass/thickening above the prosthesis
D. Irregularly shaped mass attached to the leaflet or hingepoint
E. No contrast enhancement

7. A 62-year-old obese man with a previous mitral valve replacement, atrial fibrillation, and chronic obstructive pulmonary disease (COPD) is referred for a CT coronary angiogram.

Which of the following patient factors are NOT associated with challenging coronary angiogram scan acquisition?

A. High body mass index
B. Cardiac arrhythmia
C. Symptomatic respiratory disease
D. Metallic implants
E. Low R-R variability

8. You are reporting a CT coronary angiogram in a 54-year-old man and want to classify the degree of stenosis in accordance with CAD-RADS 2.0 international guidance.

Which of the following statements regarding the specific categorization of luminal stenosis is correct?

A. Minimal stenosis = 0–30% luminal narrowing
B. No stenosis = 0–5% luminal narrowing
C. Severe stenosis = >60% luminal narrowing
D. Moderate stenosis = 40–80% luminal narrowing
E. Mild stenosis = 25–49% luminal narrowing

9. A 56-year-old man has presented with an acute coronary syndrome three months after having had a CT coronary angiogram. What have recent studies suggested might be evident on coronary CT angiograms to indicate a high risk of future ACS events, independent of the severity of stenosis of a particular coronary plaque—so-called high-risk plaque?

A. Negative remodelling
B. Napkin ring sign
C. High attenuation plaque
D. Coarse calcification
E. Proximal left circumflex plaque

10. A 42-year-old male is undergoing a CT coronary angiogram. He is in sinus rhythm, but refractory to rate-lowering medication, and maintains a heart rate of 86 bpm.

Which of the following strategies would be the most appropriate to obtain diagnostic images?

A. Increase tube current
B. Increase gantry rotation time
C. Increase tube voltage
D. Prospective ECG-triggered multiphase systolic acquisition
E. Increase intravenous contrast dose

11. You are interpreting a CT coronary angiogram in a 72-year-old man with suspected CAD. There are numerous densely calcified coronary plaques producing partial volume effect/blooming artefact.

Which of the following methods will best aid accurate interpretation in this scenario?

A. Increasing window width
B. Increase slice thickness
C. Soft reconstruction kernel
D. Widening reconstruction field of view
E. Decrease tube potential

12. A morbidly obese 63-year-old male attends for a CT coronary angiogram.

Which factor could you adjust to increase the quality and chances of a diagnostic CT coronary angiogram?

A. Lower tube voltage
B. Decrease iodinated contrast strength
C. Decrease tube current
D. Increase contrast flow rate
E. Decrease slice thickness

13. A 41-year-old female is referred for a CT coronary angiogram following an inability to fully visualize the coronary anatomy on invasive catheter angiography. You report a coronary artery anomaly. In classifying this anomaly, which of the following are not usually associated with haemodynamic compromise, i.e. shunting, ischaemia or sudden cardiac death?

A. ALCAPA (anomalous origin of the left coronary artery from the pulmonary artery)
B. Anomalous RCA arising from the left coronary sinus with interarterial course
C. Left main stem coronary artery atresia
D. Anomalous LCx arising from RCA with retro-aortic course
E. Anomalous LAD arising from the right coronary sinus with interarterial course

14. A 69-year-old female undergoes an echocardiogram which demonstrated a pericardial effusion.

Which of the following characteristics does CT *not* provide superior assessment to echocardiographic assessment?

A. Adhesions
B. Effusion content
C. Calcification
D. Pericardial thickness
E. Effusion detection

15. A 67-year-old man has been referred for a coronary artery calcium score.

With regards to coronary artery calcium scoring, which one of the following statements is true?

A. Only calcified plaques ≥1 mm^2 are included in the Agatston score
B. An Agatston score of 0 excludes a flow-limiting stenosis
C. Coronary artery calcification only occurs in intimal atherosclerosis
D. Only iso-osmolar intravenous iodinated contrast should be used
E. Pixels of >50 HU are included in the Agatston score

16. A 58-year-old man presenting to the emergency department with severe chest pain radiating to the back undergoes a gated CT aortogram. The scanning protocol includes a non-contrast study of the thorax, followed by an arterial phase CT of the thoracic and abdominal aorta.

Which of the following pathologies is the non-contrast study most useful in detecting?

A. Penetrating atherosclerotic ulcer
B. Intramural haematoma
C. Location of dissection flap
D. Involvement of arch branches
E. Compression of true lumen

17. You are asked your opinion on a non-coronary cardiac CT for a 54-year-old man who has been identified with an abnormal lesion adjacent to the heart. A region of interest measurement displays a mean attenuation of minus (-) 70 HU.

Which tissue type is the lesion likely to be comprised of?

A. Bone
B. Calcification
C. Fat
D. Muscle
E. Water

18. An 81-year-old female with atrial fibrillation undergoes a cardiac CT for recent onset of atypical chest pain. This demonstrates hypoenhancement in the tip of the left atrial appendage which could represent thrombus. You consider repeating the study.

An alteration in which parameter would best help confirm or refute the presence of thrombus?

A. Decrease contrast volume
B. Increase scan delay after contrast
C. Increase tube voltage
D. Increase pre-scan beta blockade
E. Scan in expiration

19. A patient is referred for a transcatheter aortic valve implantation (TAVI) CT planning study.

Which features on the CT study favour surgical aortic valve replacement over a TAVI?

A. Short distance between coronary artery ostia and aortic valve annulus
B. Porcelain aorta
C. Patent coronary artery bypass grafts
D. Chest deformity and/or thoracic scoliosis
E. Good iliac and subclavian artery access

20. A 45-year-old male with stable chest pain of recent onset undergoes a CT coronary angiogram. This demonstrates a moderate (50–69%) severity stenosis in the proximal LAD. An FFR CT analysis is performed.

Which of the following statements regarding FFR CT are FALSE?

A. FFR CT analysis requires high quality CT imaging to be performed accurately
B. Well validated against invasive FFR, performing better than any other non-invasive imaging test
C. FFR CT values of <0.80 can be considered safe to defer from PCI
D. FFR CT analysis requires hyperaemia for analysis
E. FFR CT analysis performs well in patients with high Agatston scores

21. You are reviewing the CT coronary angiogram of 62-year-old woman, but there is evidence of significant motion artefact.

What are the most likely reasons for motion artefact in cardiac CT?

A. Elevated heart rate
B. Prolonged scanning time
C. Variable heart rate
D. Poor compliance with breathing instructions
E. Low gantry rotation time

22. A 52-year-old man is undergoing a coronary CT angiogram and contrast opacification is poor.

Which of the following parameters do NOT aid good contrast opacification of the coronary arteries in cardiac CT?

A. Iterative reconstruction
B. Low tube voltage study
C. Spectral computed tomography
D. Low iodine concentration intravenous contrast
E. Test bolus technique

23. A 48-year-old female undergoes a CT coronary angiogram for atypical chest pain. No coronary artery atherosclerosis is identified, but the pulmonary venous anatomy is abnormal.

Which of the following statements regarding partial anomalous pulmonary venous drainage is correct?

A. Anomalous pulmonary venous drainage of the left superior pulmonary vein is commonly associated with a superior sinus venosus atrial septal defect
B. Are more commonly left sided
C. Result in a right-to-left shunt
D. The anomalous pulmonary vein can drain into the azygos vein
E. The most common associated congenital heart defect is a patent ductus arteriosus

24. A 51-year-old patient undergoes a CT examination for investigation of non-acute chest pain and dyspnoea. A recent echocardiogram raised the possibility of pulmonary hypertension.

Which of the following CT features are NOT associated with pulmonary hypertension?

A. Mosaic lung attenuation
B. Right ventricular hypertrophy
C. Right ventricular dilation
D. Reflux of contrast into the hepatic veins
E. Aorta: main pulmonary artery ratio of 1.3:1

25. A 39-year-old male undergoing a CT coronary angiogram, on review is found to have a congenitally bicuspid aortic valve (BAV).

Which of the following statements regarding bicuspid aortic valve are FALSE?

A. The most common complication is aortic stenosis
B. A Sievers type 0 BAV has one raphe
C. When one raphe is present, the most commonly involved cusps are the left and right
D. Coarctation of the aorta needs to be excluded
E. CT is more accurate than transoesophageal echocardiography in providing anatomical classification

chapter 1.3

CARDIAC COMPUTED TOMOGRAPHY

ANSWERS

1. C. The 2023 Multimodality imaging in thoracic aortic diseases: a clinical consensus statement from the European Association of Cardiovascular Imaging and the European Society of Cardiology working group on aorta and peripheral vascular diseases recommend the inner-to-inner-edge technique in end diastole, using double oblique reconstructions perpendicular to the axis of blood flow at the aortic segment being measured.

2023 Multimodality imaging in thoracic aortic diseases: a clinical consensus statement from the European Association of Cardiovascular Imaging and the European Society of Cardiology working group on aorta and peripheral vascular diseases. Eur Heart J Cardiovasc Imaging, **24**(5), e65–e85 (2023). doi: 10.1093/ehjci/jead024.

2. D. Whilst dose modulation in retrospective ECG-gated studies can reduce doses, retrospectively acquired helical/spiral CT studies have higher radiation doses than prospectively acquired studies, and they should be reserved only for special circumstances. Lowering the tube potential/kVp can also significantly reduce radiation dose, with more modern scanners able to compensate for potential increased image noise by dynamically changing tube current (mA).

Strategies for radiation dose reduction in nuclear cardiology and cardiac computed tomography imaging: a report from the European Association of Cardiovascular Imaging (EACVI), the Cardiovascular Committee of European Association of Nuclear Medicine (EANM), and the European Society of Cardiovascular Radiology (ESCR). Eur Heart J, **39**, 286–96 (2018).

3. D. Aortic Valve Calcium score thresholds:

Severe aortic stenosis very likely: men ≥3,000; women ≥1,600

Severe aortic stenosis likely: men ≥2,000; women ≥1,200

Severe aortic stenosis unlikely: men <1,600; women <800

Vahanian A, Beyersdorf F, Praz F, et al.; ESC/EACTS Scientific Document Group. 2021 ESC/EACTS Guidelines for the management of valvular heart disease. Eur Heart J, **43**(7), 561–632 (2022). doi: 10.1093/eurheartj/ehab395

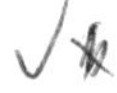

4. D. GTN combined with phosphodiesterase inhibitors can lead to profound systemic hypotension. GTN can exacerbate outflow obstruction in hypertrophic cardiomyopathy. The vasodilator effect of GTN can reduce preload and cardiac output, and theoretically cause severe hypotension in patients with severe aortic stenosis or pericardial tamponade.

5. C. Even cardio-selective beta blockers can precipitate bronchospasm in patients with severe/poorly controlled asthma. Beta blocker in third-degree heart block can potentiate a fatal arrhythmia. The negative inotropic effects of beta blockade can exacerbate cardiac failure in the acutely unwell patient. The combination of verapamil and beta blocker can have a synergistic negative inotropic, chronotropic, and dromotropic effect which can lead to conduction disorders, heart failure, and hypotension.

6. A. CT now has a major role in the management of patients with suspected mechanical valve prosthetic obstruction. Whilst urgent surgery is a management option for both pannus and thrombus, thrombolysis is an alternative option for valve thrombosis. Features on CT that favour pannus are CT attenuation of >145 HU; usually 12 months after surgery; circular mass extending from the sewing ring, located beneath the prosthesis, can enhance and can contain calcification.

Thrombus meanwhile tends to have an attenuation of <145 HU; can occur above or below the prosthesis; tends to attach to the leaflet or hingepoint and does not tend to enhance.

Moss AJ, Dweck MR, Dreisbach JG, et al. Complementary role of cardiac CT in the assessment of aortic valve replacement dysfunction. Open Heart, **3,** e000494 (2016).

7. E. Several patient factors can lead to intrinsic challenges in CT coronary angiogram acquisition. Judicious protocoling, evolving scanner technology, patient coaching, and clinician education can alleviate many of these factors:

High BMI: can lead to poor signal to noise ratio and poor contrast resolution, with markedly increased radiation doses which still may lead to suboptimal studies.

Cardiac arrhythmia: may require scanning protocols intrinsically associated with higher radiation doses (retrospective scanning, padded prospective scanning). Irregular rhythms can lead to misregistration artefact due to changes in position of the heart (and coronaries) on successive cardiac cycles/scan blocks.

Poor breath-holding: most common cause of motion artefact leading to step and blurring (which can simulate coronary stenoses).

Metal artefact: the lower energy X-rays are filtered out by the dense material, leading to artefactually lower attenuation values which may simulate disease.

8. E.

0% no	plaque or stenosis
1–24%	minimal stenosis or plaque with no stenosis
25–49%	mild stenosis
50–69% stenosis	moderate stenosis
70–99% stenosis	severe stenosis
100% stenosis total	coronary occlusion

CAD-RADS™ 2.0 - 2022 Coronary Artery Disease-Reporting and Data System: An Expert Consensus Document of the Society of Cardiovascular Computed Tomography (SCCT), the American College of Cardiology (ACC), the American College of Radiology (ACR), and the North America Society of Cardiovascular Imaging (NASCI). J Cardiovasc Comput Tomogr, **16**(6), 536–57 (2022). doi: 10.1016/j.jcct.2022.07.002.

9. B. High risk plaque is associated with increased risk of future ACS events. Two or more high-risk features are required to designate a particular plaque as high risk in the CAD-RADS 2.0 classification.

i) Spotty calcium: punctate calcium within a plaque

ii) Napkin ring sign: central low attenuation plaque with a peripheral rim of higher CT attenuation.

iii) Positive remodelling: ratio of outer vessel diameter at the site of plaque divided by the average outer diameter of the proximal and distal vessel greater than 1.1.

iv) Low attenuation plaque: non-calcified plaque with internal attenuation less than 30 HU.

CAD-RADS™ 2.0 - 2022 Coronary Artery Disease-Reporting and Data System: An Expert Consensus Document of the Society of Cardiovascular Computed Tomography (SCCT), the American College of Cardiology (ACC), the American College of Radiology (ACR), and the North America Society of Cardiovascular Imaging (NASCI). J Cardiovasc Comput Tomogr, **16**(6), 536–57 (2022). doi: 10.1016/j.jcct.2022.07.002.

10. D. For most scanning protocols a heart rate of ≤60 bpm is optimal for imaging the coronary arteries. The higher the heart rate is, the shorter the duration of ventricular diastole (where cardiac motion is usually at its lowest at low heart rates).

At heart rates above 65 bpm, a padded acquisition may be required, which allows reconstruction of multiple phases of the cardiac cycle. The different coronary arteries (and different segments) can be reviewed at different time points and a full assessment of coronary disease made, even if this is not at the same point in the cardiac cycle.

One option is to obtain data in a late systolic phase of the cardiac cycle (between 110 and 380 milliseconds from the R wave. which optimizes the study for higher and irregular heart rates.

Increasing gantry rotation time increases the time it takes to acquire data, and therefore decreases the temporal resolution of the study.

White, SK, Castellano E, Gartland N, et al. Quality assurance in cardiovascular CT: a practical guide. Clin Radiol, **71**, 729–38 (2016).

11. A. Partial volume effect can occur when individual voxels contain tissue of ≥ 2 different attenuations. If one of the tissues has a very high attenuation (e.g. calcium) the average (high) of the attenuation value of that voxel will be assigned to the entire voxel, therefore the size of a small, but very dense focus can be overestimated. This is termed blooming and can be problematic when interpreting coronary arteries with densely calcified plaques, and may lead to indeterminism or overestimation of luminal stenosis.

Increasing window width will aid reduction in blooming.

Decreasing slice thickness and decreasing field of view will improve spatial resolution and decrease blooming. Sharp reconstruction kernels will also aid interpretation.

Nicol E, Stirrup J, Kelion AD, & Padley SP. (eds.) Cardiovascular computed tomography. (2011). OUP Oxford.

12. D. High BMI can lead to poor signal to noise ratio and poor contrast resolution.

Increasing contrast strength provides better contrast opacification and thus better contrast resolution. Increasing contrast flow rate will result in a higher peak contrast enhancement and better contrast resolution.

Increasing tube voltage increases X-ray energy and thus penetration. Increasing tube current increases the X-ray beam intensity.

Decreasing slice thickness will make the image appear 'noisier'.

13. D. ALCAPA usually presents in the neonatal period, results in left-to-right shunt and steal of blood flow from the myocardium.

Interarterial anomalous coronary arteries course between the aorta and pulmonary trunk—associated with sudden cardiac death, thought due to either compression of the coronary artery between the two great vessels and/or due to increased risk of slit-like orifice which can occlude.

LMS atresia is a rare finding, but clearly of clinical significance.

LCx arising from the RCA/RCS with a retro-aortic course is not felt haemodynamically significant. It is of importance when considering aortic valve surgery/implantation.

Shriki JE, Shinbane JS, Rashid MA, et al. Identifying, characterizing, and classifying congenital anomalies of the coronary arteries. Radiographics, **32**, 453–68 (2012).

14. A. Given the volume coverage, detection of a pericardial effusion is superior with CT. Calcification, characterizing the contents (density) of the effusion and measuring the thickness of the pericardium are all superior with CT owing to the better contrast and spatial resolution.

Bogaert J, Francone M. Pericardial disease: value of CT and MR imaging. Radiology, **267**, 340–56 (2013).

15. A. For a calcified plaque to be included in the Agatston calcium score, the minimum area needs to be ≥1 mm^2. The standardized threshold attenuation value for the inclusion of a plaque in the Agatston score is ≥130 HU. A coronary calcium score is an unenhanced study. Coronary artery calcification can also occur in chronic renal disease, where the coronary artery media can become calcified. Whilst a calcium score of 0 confers a low cardiovascular event rate (<1%/year), significant, flow limiting non-calcified plaques can be present in this patient group.

16. B. Acute intramural haematoma can be considered to be part of the spectrum of disease processes in acute aortic syndrome (along with aortic dissection and penetrating atherosclerotic ulcer). It is due to localized haematoma within the medial layer of the aorta. It is likely due to rupture of one of the vasa vasorum vessels supplying the aortic wall. It usually appears on unenhanced CT as a crescentic, high attenuation focus within the wall of the aorta. Following the administration of IV contrast, these can be challenging to appreciate when opposed by high attenuation iodinated contrast material.

17. C. The range covered by CT coronary angiography will include the lower portions of the mediastinum, lungs, and chest wall, as well as the uppermost abdomen. A sound knowledge of the anatomy of these structures and good appreciation of normal and abnormal appearances is required when reporting cardiac CT. The attenuation characteristics of abnormal structures encountered can be very useful in helping determine the likely tissue composition.

By definition pure water has a value of 0 HU. Fat is less dense than water, appearing of lower attenuation (-50 to -100 HU). Lungs, when healthy, are largely aerated. They therefore do not attenuate X-rays significantly in comparison with an attenuation of approximately -750 to -900 HU. Soft tissue without IV contrast generally has an attenuation value of +20 to +60 HU. Calcification tends to exceed +100 HU, with bone (dependent on location and underlying mineral density) usually in the range of +300 to +1000 HU.

18.B. Poor contrast enhancement due to stasis of blood in the left atrial appendage can occur quite commonly in patients with AF undergoing cardiac CT. Whilst these patients are clearly at risk of developing thrombus, consideration should be given to artefactual filling defects—so-called pseudothrombus. If suspected, either prior to commencement of the cardiac CT, or upon live review, a repeat delayed study through the left atrial appendage can be performed. In the case of pseudothrombus, the extra delay can allow extra time for contrast to mix with unopacified blood in the left atrial appendage, allowing opacification of the cavity and exclusion of genuine thrombus.

19. A. Pre-TAVI CT evaluation is essential to assess the aortic root dimensions and anatomy, relationship to the coronary ostia, valve anatomy, and calcification, as well as the anatomy and any disease of the access routes (femoral/iliac/subclavian/LV apex). A short distance between the annulus and coronary ostia risks occlusion of the ostia when the implant is deployed.

2021 ESC/EACTS Guidelines for the management of valvular heart disease. Eur Heart J, **43**(7), 561–632 (2022). doi: 10.1093/eurheartj/ehab395.

Blanke P, Weir-McCall JR, Achenbach S, et al. Computed tomography imaging in the context of transcatheter aortic valve implantation (TAVI)/transcatheter aortic valve replacement (TAVR): An expert consensus document of the Society of Cardiovascular Computed Tomography. J Cardiovasc Comput Tomogr, **13**(1), 1–20 (2019). doi: 10.1016/j.jcct.2018.11.008.

20. C. Several studies have demonstrated good correlation between invasive and CT-derived FFR measurements. As with anatomical CT coronary angiography this relies heavily on high quality diagnostic images to provide accurate analyses. One of the major benefits of the technology is its ability to derive accurate and determinate results even in the presence of heavily calcified plaques. FFRct requires GTN administration for validated results. FFRct values of >0.80 are associated with very low event rates when managed medically and deferred from PCI.

Fairbairn TA, Nieman K, Akasaka T, et al. Real-world clinical utility and impact on clinical decision-making of coronary computed tomography angiography-derived fractional flow reserve: lessons from the ADVANCE Registry. Eur Heart J, **39**(41), 3701–11 (2018). doi: 10.1093/eurheartj/ehy530

21. E. Low gantry rotation time is intrinsically linked to good temporal resolution. Elevated heart rates increase cardiac motion and decrease ventricular diastole duration. Poor compliance with scan instructions and prolonged scan time increase the risk of breathing artefact.

22. D. Several factors can affect good contrast opacification of the coronary arteries. Low iodine concentration IV contrast will reduce contrast enhancement and higher concentration preparations are preferred. Low tube voltages close to the k-edge of iodine (70–80 kVp) either individually or as part of spectral imaging can increase the attenuation of IV contrast media. Iterative reconstruction processes reduce image noise and increase contrast enhancement without specific radiation dose penalty. Test bolus and bolus tracking techniques both provide bespoke timing of cardiac CT acquisition to aid peak enhancement of the coronary arteries.

Scholtz JE, Ghoshhajra B. Advances in cardiac CT contrast injection and acquisition protocols. Cardiovasc Diagn Ther, **7**, 439–51 (2017).

23. D. Partial anomalous pulmonary venous drainage (PAPVD) results in a left-to-right shunt. They are more commonly right sided. Right-sided PAPVD are commonly associated with superior sinus venosus atrial esptal defects. Atrial septal defects are the most commonly associated congenital heart defect.

Lyen S, Wijesuriya S, Ngan-Soo E, et al. Anomalous pulmonary venous drainage: a pictorial essay with a CT focus. J Congenital Cardiol, **1**(1), 7 (2017).

24. E. There are several features of pulmonary hypertension that can be identified on CT. RV dilation, RV hypertrophy, and reflux of contrast into the IVC are all associated with elevated right-sided pressures. A dilated MPA and MPA greater in diameter then the ascending aorta are positive predictors of pulmonary hypertension.

25. B. Sievers type 0 BAV has two cusps with zero raphes. Type 1 BAV has one raphe joining together two under-developed cusps and type 2 BAV has two raphes joining together the two under-developed cusps with the one fully-developed cusp.

Ko SM, Song MG., Hwang HK. Bicuspid aortic valve: spectrum of imaging findings at cardiac MDCT and cardiovascular MRI. Amer J Roentgenology, **198**, 89–97 (2012).

chapter 1.4

NUCLEAR TECHNIQUES

QUESTIONS

1. **Ultra-low dose stress only myocardial perfusion scientigraphy (MPS) with a cadmium-zinc-telluride (CZT) camera can regularly expose a patient to what level of dose (mean)?**

   A. 10–15 mSv
   B. 0.5–1.5 mSv
   C. 2.0–5.0 mSv
   D. 5.0–10 mSv
   E. 0.1–0.5 mSV

2. **An 82-year-old man has noted increasing shortness of breath over the past year in addition to peripheral oedema. An echocardiogram is performed, which shows hypertrophy of both ventricles and a small pericardial effusion. Amyloidosis is suspected.**

   Which PET tracer can be used in amyloidosis?

   A. ^{18}F-FDG
   B. ^{18}F-florbetapir
   C. ^{18}F-NaF
   D. ^{18}F-FMISO
   E. ^{18}F-choline

3. **A 21-year-old man with a background of pulmonary stenosis was treated with a transcatheter pulmonary valve replacement (Melody valve). Several months later he felt generally unwell, with fatigue, chills, and fevers. On admission to hospital, he was noted to have raised inflammatory markers.**

   Which of the following investigations is particularly useful in the detection of prosthetic valve endocarditis?

   A. FDG PET
   B. CMR
   C. TTE
   D. ECG
   E. CT

4. Which pharmacological stress agent is given as a bolus rather than a continuous infusion during myocardial perfusion scintigraphy?

A. Regadenoson
B. Dobutamine
C. Adenosine
D. Dipyridamole
E. Adrenaline

5. Which isotope does not require a cyclotron for production?

A. ^{201}Thallium
B. ^{82}Rubidium
C. ^{15}Oxygen-water
D. ^{13}Nitrogen-ammonia
E. ^{11}Carbon-acetate

6. What is the dose limit of radiation for UK employees per year in mSv?

A. 10
B. 15
C. 20
D. 25
E. 30

7. When handling radioactive isotopes for diagnostic imaging, which of the following is not mandatory?

A. Badge monitoring
B. Lead shielding of isotopes
C. Valid certification of operators
D. Radiation warning signs
E. Protective clothing

8. A 52-year-old woman with breast cancer is due to start trastuzumab (Herceptin). She is otherwise fit and well. Her oncologist is concerned regarding the cardiotoxic nature of this chemotherapy and requests an accurate and reproducible method of assessing LV function.

Which method of imaging does not use endocardial edge detection to calculate ventricular function?

A. Echocardiography
B. CT
C. CMR
D. Radionuclide ventriculography
E. MPS

9. A 68-year-old man was referred for coronary angiography due to chest pain on exertion. He had an inferior STEMI six years ago with PCI to RCA and two further NSTEMIs in the intervening years. He also had a history of type 2 diabetes and hypercholesterolaemia. Coronary angiography revealed a blocked RCA stent (likely CTO), with collaterals from the LAD. It also revealed moderate to severe stenosis of the proximal circumflex. Prior to revascularization, further imaging is requested to assess myocardial viability.

Which test is the gold standard for assessment of myocardial viability?

A. FDG-PET
B. Thallium MPS
C. CMR with late gadolinium enhancement
D. Dobutamine echocardiography
E. Radionuclide ventriculography

10. Which test carries the highest radiation dose?

A. RNV
B. PET-CT
C. Cardiac perfusion SPECT
D. CT coronary angiogram
E. Cardiac MIBG

11. An 84-year-old woman reports increasing shortness of breath and fatigue over the past six months. She has a past medical history of hypertension but is otherwise well. An echocardiogram is performed, which revealed dilated cardiomyopathy, diastolic dysfunction, and a pericardial effusion, which was suggestive of cardiac sarcoidosis.

Which is the best method of imaging for the detection of disease activity in cardiac sarcoidosis?

A. MPS
B. CMR
C. Echocardiogram
D. CT
E. FDG-PET

12. A 62-year-old man with a background of hypertension and hypercholesterolaemia is referred to clinic with atypical angina. You arrange a myocardial perfusion scan, which is normal even at high workload. You review him in clinic to discuss the results.

What can you tell him regarding his annual cardiovascular adverse event rate?

A. Less than 0.1%
B. Less than 1%
C. Less than 3%
D. Less than 4.8%
E. Less than 6.7%

13. A 55-year-old woman is referred to clinic with typical angina. She has a background of hypertension, type 2 diabetes, and is a current smoker. You decide to refer her for a myocardial perfusion scan and explain this to her; however, she is concerned about the radiation dose required.

By approximately how much does the lifetime risk of cancer increase following a typical myocardial perfusion scan?

A. 1:25,000
B. 1:2,500
C. 1:250
D. 1:25
E. 1:2.5

14. A 72-year-old man with a background of ischaemic heart disease with previous MI, ischaemic cardiomyopathy (LVEF 25%), and hypertension is due a cholecystectomy due to gallstones. He reports atypical chest pain and a worsening of his usual shortness of breath and is referred for cardiac assessment prior to surgery. Myocardial perfusion scintigraphy is requested. On the day of the scan, he arrives in the department, and reports dull chest pain that started at rest that morning. He is also diaphoretic, nauseated, and short of breath.

For which of the following would investigation with myocardial perfusion scintigraphy be less helpful?

A. Assessment of atypical chest pain
B. Assessment of residual ischaemic burden post MI
C. Risk assessment before non-cardiac surgery
D. Risk stratification in heart failure
E. Acute coronary syndrome with ongoing ischaemic symptoms

15. A 68-year-old man with chest pain and shortness of breath on exertion was referred for myocardial perfusion scintigraphy. He had a background of hypertension, type 2 diabetes, and obesity.

MPS can provide information on regional wall motion abnormalities and left ventricular function through which method?

A. ECG gating
B. Increasing the dose of the isotope given
C. Extending duration of infusion of stressor
D. Using a CZT camera rather than a NaI camera
E. MPS cannot be used to provide information on these properties

16. A 72-year-old man with a past medical history of ischaemic heart disease with previous STEMI develops shortness of breath and peripheral oedema, along with a raised BMI. Echocardiography reveals a left ventricular ejection fraction of 30%. For further prognostic information regarding his heart failure, he is referred for further imaging. Prognostic information can be provided through cardiac uptake of a particular isotope via sympathetic innervation.

Which isotope is this?

A. ^{99m}Technetium pertechnetate
B. ^{201}Thallium
C. ^{82}Rubidium
D. ^{123}Iodine metaiodobenzylguandine
E. ^{18}Fluorine-fluorodeoxyglucose

17. A 62-year-old woman with stage 4 ovarian cancer experiences sudden shortness of breath with pleuritic chest pain and attends A&E for further investigation.

Which of the following is not recognized as a method of investigating her a pulmonary embolism?

A. Planar V/Q
B. CTPA
C. Magnetic resonance angiography
D. V/Q SPECT
E. RNV

18. A 65-year-old man with a background of asthma is referred to your clinic by the respiratory team due to central chest pain which occurs on exertion and resolves at rest. He also has a background of hypertension, obesity, and epilepsy.

Which stress agent for myocardial perfusion scintigraphy is not contraindicated in moderate airways disease?

A. Dipyridamole
B. Adenosine
C. Regadenoson
D. All of these
E. None of these

19. A 67-year-old man was referred to clinic prior to a planned Whipple's procedure for pancreatic cancer. He reports typical angina and has a past medical history of type 2 diabetes, hypertension, hypercholesterolaemia, and a raised BMI. MPS was performed, which suggested that this patient is high risk.

Which of these results on MPS is not an indicator of high-risk patients?

A. Lung uptake of thallium
B. Transient ischaemic dilatation
C. End-systolic volume of more than 70 ml
D. Bronchospasm
E. 10% myocardial ischaemia

20. A 58-year-old man reports chest pain on exertion on a background of hypertension, hypercholesterolaemia, COPD, and a lifelong history of smoking.

What feature seen during MPS is an independent predictor of cardiac mortality?

A. Blunted heart rate in response to vasodilator stress
B. Hypertension in response to vasodilator stress
C. An exercise capacity of 10 metabolic equivalents
D. A normal stress study
E. Non-response to dipyridamole

21. A 60-year-old woman reports chest pain and breathlessness on exertion. She has a background of obesity, chronic kidney disease, and has had a previous gastrectomy and right knee replacement. She also reports claustrophobia.

Which of these conditions is a relative contraindication to technetium-99m myocardial perfusion scintigraphy?

A. Obesity
B. Claustrophobia
C. Metal implants
D. Renal dysfunction
E. Gastrectomy

22. An 87-year-old woman reports a history of progressive shortness of breath and peripheral oedema. Echocardiography reveals biventricular hypertrophy with a preserved ejection fraction suggestive of amyloidosis.

Which is the best non-invasive test for the diagnosis of ATTR amyloidosis?

A. Transoesophageal echocardiography (TOE)
B. Cardiac MRI (CMR)
C. Myocardial perfusion scintigraphy
D. DPD scintigraphy
E. FDG-PET

23. A 79-year-old man is awaiting a total right knee replacement. He has a background of hypertension, is an ex-smoker, and reports that his brother died of a myocardial infarction at 45 years old. He also reports intermittent chest pain not related to exertion. He is referred for MPS to assess his cardiac risk pre-operatively.

What is the preferred method of stressor in myocardial perfusion scintigraphy?

A. Mental
B. Physiological
C. Adenosine
D. Dobutamine
E. Dipyridamole

24. A 66-year-old woman is referred for MPS due to chest pain on exertion. She has a background of peripheral vascular disease, hypertension, and asthma. She takes aspirin, dipyridamole, ramipril, bisoprolol, inhalers, and theophylline. She also reports that she drinks several cups of coffee a day.

Which of the following substrates do not need to be avoided prior to myocardial perfusion scintigraphy?

A. Coffee
B. Oral dipyridamole
C. Bisoprolol
D. Ramipril
E. Theophylline

25. A 59-year-old man with a background of brittle asthma, hyperlipidaemia, hypertension, and severe aortic stenosis was referred for myocardial perfusion scintigraphy due to exertional chest pain. An ECG showed left bundle branch block. He is known to have second-degree heart block. The patient attends the scan with a mostly empty cup of coffee in his hand.

For which of the following is administration of adenosine not contraindicated?

A. Known reversible severe airways disease
B. Severe aortic stenosis
C. Consuming their usual morning cup of coffee
D. Known second degree heart block
E. Known left bundle branch block

26. A 58-year-old man with a background of obesity, smoking, and hypercholesterolaemia reports typical angina associated with dyspnoea and is referred for MPS. These polar plots demonstrate a stress and rest myocardial perfusion scintigram using a ^{99m}Tc tracer.

Which statement best represents the MPS scan?

A. Fixed apical perfusion defect
B. Hypertrophic cardiomyopathy
C. Transient ischaemic dilatation
D. No perfusion defect (normal scan)
E. Partly reversible apical perfusion defect

27. An 81-year-old woman with a recent diagnosis of breast cancer is referred to your clinic prior to surgery. She has been referred due to T-wave inversion on her ECG and shortness of breath on exertion. She has a background of hypertension and a strong family history of ischaemic heart disease. MPS is performed. These polar plots demonstrate a stress and rest myocardial perfusion scintigram using a ^{99m}Tc tracer.

Which statement best represents the MPS scan?

A. This patient is low risk for non-cardiac surgery
B. Optimal medical therapy is the best option
C. Transient ischaemic dilatation
D. Multi-vessel coronary disease is present
E. Severe circumflex artery stenosis

28. A 53-year-old man awaiting bariatric surgery was referred due to a strong family history of ischaemic heart disease, hypercholesterolaemia, type 2 diabetes, and a raised BMI in addition to shortness of breath on exertion. MPS was performed. These polar plots demonstrate a stress and rest myocardial perfusion scintigram using a ^{99m}Tc tracer.

Which statement best represents the MPS scan?

A. This patient is low risk for non-cardiac surgery
B. The anterior wall is ischaemic
C. The lateral wall is a non-viable infarct
D. Multi-vessel coronary disease is present
E. Severe circumflex artery stenosis is present

chapter

1.4

NUCLEAR TECHNIQUES

ANSWERS

1. B. MPS uses images generated through the emission of photons from either technetium-99m (^{99m}Tc) or thallium-201 (^{201}Tl) isotopes. These are detected by a gamma camera. Traditionally NaI crystals were used inside the gamma camera. However, CZT cameras are a newer form of gamma camera with much shorter acquisition times and improved image quality. Subsequently the amount of radiation patients are exposed to has fallen to around 0.5–1mSv.

2. B. 18F-florbetapir was initially developed for use in imaging Alzheimer's disease, as it binds tightly to beta-amyloid. However, it has subsequently been found to be of use in imaging for cardiac amyloidosis. The other tracers are also PET tracers but with different uses. Fluorodeoxyglucose (FDG) is radiolabelled glucose, which is preferentially taken up by active metabolic areas due to increased glucose metabolism. It is therefore able to detect intra- and extra-cardiac inflammation. Sodium fluoride (NaF) is taken up primarily by bone. 18F-choline is useful in imaging patients with prostate cancer. 18F-fluoromisonidazole (FMISO) is used as a tracer for tumour hypoxia.

3. A. Though TOE is often used for the diagnosis of endocarditis, it can be challenging to identify vegetations in the presence of prosthetic valves. FDG-PET uses radiolabelled glucose to detect areas of inflammation through increased glucose metabolism. It can be very useful in the detection of prosthetic valve endocarditis, and has emerged in the latest diagnostic algorithms for prosthetic valve endocarditis. It can be less useful in patients who have recently undergone cardiac surgery or in patients with septic emboli in the brain. ECG, though useful in monitoring patients with endocarditis, has no role in the diagnosis of endocarditis. CT and CMR are unable to provide sufficient temporal resolution to consistently and accurately identify vegetations, though CT can often be useful in the detection of abscesses and pseudoaneurysms.

4. A. Regadenoson is a newer cardiac specific A2a receptor antagonist which is given as a non-weight adjusted bolus. Due to adenosine's much shorter half-life of 10 seconds, it is instead given as a continuous infusion. Dipyridamole and dobutamine are also given as continuous infusions, with half-lives of 20 minutes and 2 minutes respectively. Adrenaline is not used as a stress agent during myocardial perfusion scintigraphy.

5. B. ^{82}Rubidium is obtained from its parent radionuclide ^{82}strontium, which has a half-life of 4 weeks. An on-site cyclotron is therefore not required. ^{82}Rubidium, which has a half-life of 75 seconds, is taken from the generator and administered to the patient directly. ^{15}Oxygen has a half-life of two minutes, ^{13}nitrogen has a half-life of ten minutes, and ^{11}carbon has a half-life of 20 minutes. ^{201}Thallium has a half-life of seventy-three hours but is generatedin acyclotron.

6. C. The annual dose limit is 20 mSv per year for UK employees. This limit is defined in UK legislation. Employers must restrict employee exposure to well below these limits where this is reasonably practicable. Badge monitoring is mandatory but rarely reveals excessive exposure during routine clinical practice.

7. E. Badge monitoring, lead shielding of isotopes, valid certification of operators, and radiation warning signs are all required when handling radioactive isotopes for diagnostic imaging. Doctors and technologists performing the tests do not need to wear any protective clothing apart from everyday clinical gloves when handling isotopes. Badge monitoring is mandatory but rarely reveals excessive exposure during routine practice.

8. D. Radionuclide ventriculography uses planar (fixed head) imaging to reproducibly measure the LVEF. It relies on accurately quantifying radiolabelled red blood cells in their passage through the LV and RV cavity. The blood pool is pre-treated with stannous pyrophosphate, which diffuses into red blood cells. The blood pool is then labelled using technetium-99m, which binds to the stannous ions inside cells. Multiple gated cardiac cycles are acquired and merged to give an accurate and reproducible assessment of overall LV function. Echocardiography, CT, CMR, and MPS all use endocardial edge detection to calculate ventricular function.

9. A. FDG-PET is considered the gold standard for assessment of myocardial viability. PET (positron emission tomography) uses 18F-fluoroeoxyglucose (FDG) to detect changes in glucose metabolism. These changes are an indicator of myocardial viability. This test is usually combined with an assessment of myocardial perfusion. Perfusion-metabolic mismatches indicate hibernating viable myocardium that could benefit from revascularization. Thallium MPS, CMR with late gadolinium enhancement, and dobutamine stress echocardiography can all be used for assessment of myocardial viability, but are less sensitive. Radionuclide ventriculography uses radiolabelled red blood cells in the in their passage through the left ventricle to reproducibly measure LVEF and has no significant role in the assessment of myocardial viability.

10. B. PET-CT is a form of hybrid imaging. SPECT and PET offer information regarding function and perfusion of the heart, and CT and MRI provide detailed information of the anatomy of heart. Combining these data sets improves diagnostic yield; however, this leads to higher doses of radiation exposure to the patient, varying between 2 and 20 mSv. This increased radiation dose does require justification. CT/MRI or SPECT/PET alone carries a lower radiation dose than hybrid imaging, as does RNV and cardiac MIBG.

11. E. FDG-PET can identify intracardiac and extracardiac inflammation and can be used to monitor disease activity and response to therapy, especially in the absence of a biochemical marker. While echocardiogram and CMR are useful diagnostic tools in the assessment of cardiac sarcoidosis, these imaging modalities cannot demonstrate whether disease activity is present. Myocardial perfusion scintigraphy has no role in the diagnosis or management of sarcoidosis, but can reveal myocardial perfusion defects caused by sarcoidosis. Though CT can be very useful for detecting pulmonary sarcoidosis, it is of limited use in cardiac sarcoidosis.

12. B. There have been a number of detailed studies assessing the prognosis of a patient with a normal myocardial perfusion scan. A normal myocardial perfusion scan result confers an annual cardiovascular adverse event rate of less than 1% per annum per medium-to-high pre-test probabilities. In low-to-medium risk patients this prognostic benefit is conferred for at least 5 years. Patients with a normal MPS and an exercise capacity of more than ten metabolic equivalents (METS) have a cardiac death rate of <1% a year.

13. B. A typical myocardial perfusion scan exposes the patient to 6–14 mSv of ionizing radiation (dependent on the type of isotope used). The annual UK background radiation exposure is 2.6 mSv. The lifetime risk of cancer is approximately 30%. Given a dose equivalent of 8 mSv, the lifetime risk of cancer would increase by 1:2667 (0.0004%) on a background lifetime cancer risk of 30%.

14. E. Myocardial perfusion scintigraphy is indicated in the assessment of atypical chest pain, residual ischaemic burden post MI, and for risk stratification in both non-cardiac surgery and heart failure. However, myocardial perfusion scintigraphy should not be performed in patients with acute coronary syndrome with ongoing ischaemic symptoms, as pharmacological stress to the heart is contraindicated during acute myocardial infarction.

15. A. MPS can provide information on regional wall motion abnormalities and left ventricular function through ECG gating. Using a CZT camera rather than a NaI camera reduces acquisition times and radiation dose and improves image quality. However, it does not provide additional information compared to a NaI camera. Increasing the dose of the isotope given and extending the duration of the infusion of the stressor does not provide additional information on regional wall motion abnormalities and left ventricular function in the absence of ECG gating.

16. D. Iodine-123 metaiodobenzylguandine (MIBG) works through cardiac uptake via sympathetic innervation. Sympathetic nerve terminals are more sensitive than myocardium to ischaemia. MIBG is labelled with an isotope and works as a false neurotransmitter to the sympathetic nervous system. It identifies areas of myocardium that have been denervated through myocardial injury or ischaemia, which remain denervated even after revascularization. Lack of cardiac uptake is a marker of adverse prognosis for sudden cardiac death and progression of heart failure in patients with LV systolic dysfunction. The other isotopes mentioned do not act as a false neurotransmitter and so do not provide information on sympathetic innervation.

17. E. All methods aside from RNV can be used to investigate pulmonary embolism (PE), though with varying levels of availability across hospitals. Computed tomography pulmonary angiography (CTPA) is the investigation of choice in those patients suspected to have a PE. Isotope lung scanning such as planar V/Q and V/Q SPECT can also be performed, and may be favoured in certain circumstances. MRA can also be used for investigating PE and does not require either contrast or ionizing radiation. However, use of this modality may be limited by availability. Radionuclide ventriculography provides accurate and reproducible information regarding left and right ventricular ejection fraction but is unable to provide information regarding PE.

18. C. Stressors for myocardial perfusion scintigraphy are usually either physiological or pharmacological. The vasodilator stress agents are adenosine, dipyridamole, or regadenoson. Dipyridamole reduces the uptake and inhibits breakdown of endogenous adenosine. Adenosine acts on A1 receptors to cause coronary vasodilatation. Both of these tracers can cause bronchospasm and are contraindicated in moderate airways disease. Regadenoson is a newer cardiac specific A2a receptor antagonist which can be used in patients with mild or moderate airways disease due to much lower rates of bronchospasm. Dobutamine can also be used as an alternative pharmacological stress agent.

19. D. Bronchospasm is a side effect of adenosine, dipyridamole, and, to a lesser extent, regadenoson, and is not a high risk feature. Lung uptake of thallium is an indirect indictor of high risk. An end-systolic volume of more than 70 ml confers a worse prognosis, especially if the ejection fraction is <45% (cardiac death rate 7.9% a year). Ischaemic defects greater than 10% of the myocardium are associated with a 4.8% annual cardiac death rate. LV dilatation post stress (transient ischaemic dilatation) is an adverse sign and provides incremental prognostic value over quantitative SPECT.

20. A. A blunted heart rate in response to vasodilator stress is an independent risk factor of cardiac mortality. Hypertension in response to vasodilator stress is a normal response and will reach its peak at maximal exercise capacity. A normal stress study would indicate that this patient was at low risk of cardiac mortality. Demonstrating an exercise capacity of 10 metabolic equivalents (or 10 METS) would also indicate that this patient was very low risk for cardiac mortality. Non-response to dipyridamole is not associated with cardiac mortality.

21. E. Gastrectomy reduces the take up and bio-distribution of technetium-99m. This therefore affects the myocardial uptake of technetium-99m, reducing the sensitivity of the test. Renal dysfunction, metal implants, claustrophobia, and obesity are not contraindications to myocardial perfusion scintigraphy.

22. D. ^{99m}Tc-3,3-diphosphono-1,2-propanodicarboxylic acid (DPD) is taken up by myocytes in the presence of transthyretin (TTR) amyloidosis and has an almost 100% positive predictive value in the absence of a monoclonal protein in the serum and urine. 18F-fluorodeoxyglucose (FDG) is taken up by areas of increased glucose metabolism. Uptake is not affected by the presence of TTR amyloidosis, and so FDG can provide no diagnostic information regarding ATTR amyloidosis. TOE and CMR, though able to provide important structural information, are unable to provide diagnostic clarity regarding the subtype of amyloidosis. Myocardial perfusion scintigraphy cannot be used in the diagnosis of amyloidosis.

23. B. Physiological stressors are the preferred method as this most closely replicates real world conditions. It provides information on symptoms, heart rate, blood pressure, and ECG data which cannot be as easily assessed with pharmacological stressors. The pharmacological stressors are either vasodilator stressors (adenosine, dipyridamole, or dobutamine) or beta agonists (dobutamine). Mental stressors are not recommended as a form of stressor for MPS.

24. D. Caffeine and theophyllines antagonize dipyridamole, adenosine, and regadenoson and should therefore be avoided prior to administration. Bisoprolol may reduce the severity of myocardial ischaemia as it limits heart rate. Taking oral dipyridamole prior to MPS reduces the efficacy of vasodilator stress and should be discontinued. Ramipril does not antagonize stressors or reduce sensitivity or specificity and therefore does not need to be avoided prior to MPS.

25. E. Patients with known left bundle branch block can safely receive adenosine. Patients with second- or third-degree heart block should not be given adenosine due to the inhibitory effect of adenosine on the atrioventricular (AV) node causing transient block. Patients with severe airways disease cannot receive adenosine due to the risk of bronchospasm. Caffeine (in coffee) antagonizes adenosine and so should be avoided 24 hours prior to administration. Patients should not receive pharmacological stress with very severe or critical aortic stenosis.

26. E. This scan (Figure 1.4.A1) shows reduced perfusion in the apex at rest. The area of reduced perfusion at the apex is increased during stress. This indicates a partially reversible apical perfusion defect. A fixed apical perfusion defect would demonstrate equal areas of reduced perfusion during both rest and stress. Patients with hypertrophic cardiomyopathy may show perfusion defects on MPS, but these would usually be seen primarily in the septum. Transient ischaemic dilatation would show an apparent increase in left ventricular volume during stress compared to rest. This is not a normal study, as a normal study would show no perfusion defect during either rest or stress.

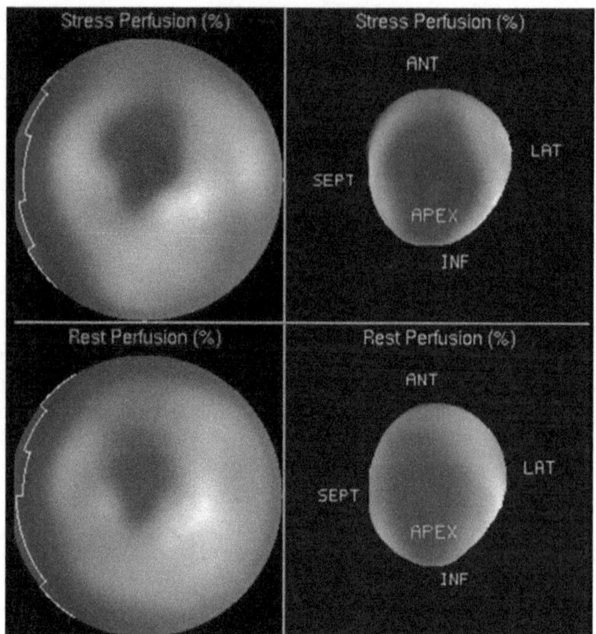

Figure 1.4.A1

27. D. This shows multi-vessel coronary disease (Figure 1.4.A2). At rest, there is reduced perfusion seen at the apex of the inferior wall. At stress, there is also reduced perfusion anterolaterally, demonstrating a large burden of ischaemia. Given this, the patient is likely to benefit from intervention rather than optimal medical therapy as a first line treatment. Severe circumflex artery stenosis would show lateral wall ischaemia only which is not seen on this scan. Transient ischaemic dilatation is not seen on this scan and would appear as an apparent increase in left ventricular volume during stress compared to rest. This patient would not be low risk for non-cardiac surgery given the large burden of ischaemia seen.

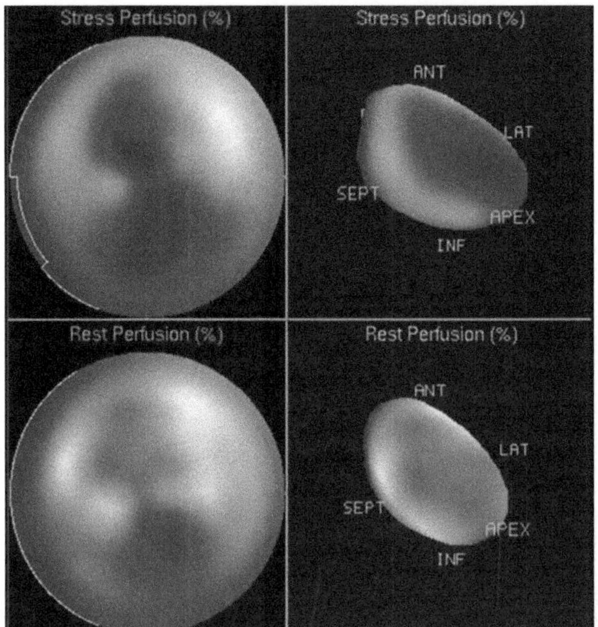

Figure 1.4.A2

28. E. This MPS shows reduced perfusion in the inferolateral territory at stress, but with a marked improvement in perfusion at rest (Figure 1.4.A3). This territory corresponds to the area supplied by the circumflex artery, and suggests severe circumflex artery stenosis. If the lateral wall were a non-viable infarct, there would be reduced perfusion both during stress and at rest. There is good perfusion to the anterior wall during both stress and rest, suggesting that the anterior wall is not ischaemic. No other territory other than the lateral territory shows reduced perfusion, so this scan does not suggest multi-vessel coronary disease. Due to a suggestion of severe circumflex artery stenosis, with visually a large burden of ischaemia, this patient would not be considered low risk for non-cardiac surgery.

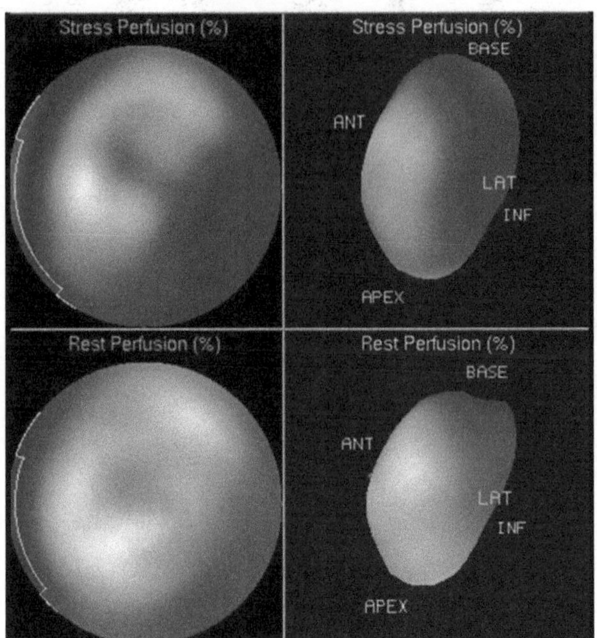
Stress Perfusion (%)
Stress Perfusion (%)
BASE
ANT
LAT
INF
APEX
Rest Perfusion (%)
Rest Perfusion (%)
BASE
ANT
LAT
INF
APEX

Figure 1.4.A3

chapter 2

CORONARY ARTERY DISEASE

chapter 2.1

ACUTE CORONARY SYNDROME

QUESTIONS

1. A 56-year-old gentleman has been admitted with a NSTE-ACS, he had subsequent PCI to his LAD artery. Forty-eight hours following the procedure he develops severe chest pain and anterior ST elevation on his ECG. He has urgent coronary angiography which shows thrombotic occlusion of his LAD stent.

What type of myocardial infarction has he suffered?

A. Type 1
B. Type 2
C. Type 3
D. Type 4a
E. None of the above

2. A 65-year-old male presents with central chest pain lasting 2 hours. ECG reveals T-wave inversion in leads V1–V4. His baseline hs-cTn level is 549 ng/L (normal reference range <40 ng/L).

How should he now be managed?

A. Invasive coronary angiography
B. Rule out other differential diagnoses
C. CT coronary angiogram
D. Repeat hs-cTn level in 3 hours
E. None of the above

3. A 45-year-old lady has presented with central crushing chest pain. Her 12-lead ECG reveals ST depression in V5+V6, her hs-cTn level on admission is 2240 ng/L (normal reference range <40ng/L) and on risk assessment her GRACE score is 180. She is currently in a non-PCI centre.

What is the appropriate management plan for this lady?

A. Conservative medical management
B. Non-invasive ischaemia testing
C. Immediate transfer to a centre that offers PCI
D. Transfer to a centre that offers PCI with a view to invasive treatment within 24 hours
E. None of the above

4. An 85-year-old gentleman has been admitted with a NSTE-ACS. He has a background of CVA, AF (non-valvular), and hypertension. Prior to admission he was on bisoprolol, ramipril, and apixaban. A decision is made to manage this gentleman conservatively with medical management.

What is the most appropriate antithrombotic treatment strategy on discharge?

A. Stop apixaban and commence aspirin and clopidogrel for 12 months.
B. Apixaban as monotherapy.
C. Triple therapy for 6 months followed by apixaban and clopidogrel for 6 months.
D. HAS-BLED score should first be calculated.
E. Apixaban plus clopidogrel for 12 months.

5. The same gentleman prior to his discharge has three further episodes of chest pain with dynamic anterior ST-depression on his 12-lead ECG. A decision is made to assess his coronaries and he subsequently has PCI (DES) to his proximal LAD. In addition, he has significant bystander disease in his RCA. As part of your risk assessment a HAS-BLED score is done, his score is 4.

What is the most appropriate regime of antiplatelet therapy?

A. Triple therapy (apixaban, aspirin and clopidogrel) for 4 weeks followed by apixaban plus clopidogrel for 11 months.
B. Aspirin and clopidogrel for 4 weeks followed by apixaban plus clopidogrel for 11 months
C. Aspirin plus ticagrelor for 12 months.
D. Triple therapy for 6 months followed by apixaban and clopidogrel for 6 months.
E. None of the above.

6. A 75-year-old gentleman has been admitted with an anterior STEMI. He has a drug eluting stent implanted into his proximal LAD artery. Unfortunately, it later transpires that he requires urgent abdominal surgery that cannot be delayed.

What advice would you give to the surgeons?

A. Under no circumstances can this gentleman have his abdominal surgery.
B. He will be discharged on aspirin so that he can have his abdominal surgery.
C. A minimum of 3 months of dual antiplatelet therapy is recommended.
D. A minimum of 1 month of dual antiplatelet therapy is recommended.
E. Surgery must be performed on dual antiplatelet therapy.

7. A 69-year-old lady has been admitted with a NSTE-ACS. Coronary angiography has revealed severe three-vessel disease that is not amenable to PCI. A decision is made to refer her for inpatient CABG. She develops further severe chest pain when on the CCU with evidence of infero-lateral ST depression, she is currently still on aspirin and clopidogrel.

How should this lady be managed?

A. Further coronary angiography and attempt PCI.
B. Stop clopidogrel and undergo CABG in 5 days.
C. Stop clopidogrel and undergo CABG in 7 days.
D. Urgent CABG irrespective of antiplatelets
E. Stop clopidogrel and undergo CABG within 24 hours.

8. A 70-year-old gentleman has presented with NSTE-ACS. Coronary angiography has revealed three-vessel disease. He is haemodynamically stable and pain free. Following a MDT discussion he is referred for CABG. He is currently on aspirin and ticagrelor.

How should he now be managed?

A. Stop aspirin and ticagrelor and undergo CABG within 24 hours.
B. Stop ticagrelor and undergo CABG in 5 days.
C. Undergo CABG within 24 hours
D. Urgent CABG irrespective of antiplatelets
E. Stop ticagrelor and undergo CABG in 7 days.

9. A 55-year-old smoker comes direct to the cath lab with severe chest pain and ST segment depression in the precordial leads. The optimal access route is:

A. Right femoral artery without ultrasound guidance to gain quick arterial access in an unstable patient
B. Distal radial access (snuff box)
C. Brachial access
D. Ulnar arterial access
E. Radial artery access

10. A patient is being treated for STEMI with primary PCI.

Which of the following is the recommended anticoagulation therapy in the cath lab?

A. Bivalirudin
B. Fondaparinux
C. ACT guided heparin
D. Cangrelor
E. Subcutaneous enoxaparin

11. The majority of acute coronary syndromes have plaque rupture as the underlying cause.

Which statement is most correct?

A. Plaque rupture is an inflammatory condition that can be helped with clarithromycin treatment
B. Plaque rupture susceptibility can be easily predicted by OCT and treated effectively with percutaneous coronary intervention
C. Plaque rupture may occur in more than one site and this is one of the reasons why longer-term antiplatelet drugs are effective after an MI
D. Increased nitric oxide levels is one of the fundamental underlying causes of cardiovascular disease
E. Is characterised by the fracture of fibro-calcific plaques as seen on OCT imaging

12. A 34-year-old active woman presents to the emergency room with intermittent chest pain that started whilst she was taking part in a 5-km semi-competitive run about 10 days earlier with a nursing colleague. She has no particular cardiovascular risk factors beyond her father having an MI at the age of 64. She is 167-cm tall with a BMI of around 24. No previous history and a negative troponin. Her ECG is normal and the last episode of chest pain was around 3 days ago. Her symptoms sound ischaemic. Your investigations should consider / be directed towards:

A. Typical stable angina
B. Investigation is not necessary, the symptoms are probably psychosomatic
C. Antidepressant treatment
D. Potential spontaneous coronary artery dissection
E. This is likely a thoracic aortic dissection with involvement of the aortic valve and coronary arteries.

13. An 85-year-old man presents with acute chest pain with dynamic anterior ST depression on his ECG. He is known to have moderate renal failure and paroxysmal atrial fibrillation. He has also had a previous TIA. Echocardiography shows normal left ventricular function and no significant valvular abnormality.

How quickly should he receive a coronary angiogram?

A. He shouldn't receive an angiogram he is elderly and is unlikely to gain benefit
B. Within 24 hours
C. Within one week
D. He should be treated like a primary PCI with no further investigations needed
E. It is probably better to do a CT coronary angiogram and consider medical treatment

14. The same 85-year-old man is now on the cath lab table and has been found to have a severe mid LAD stenosis. We are now discussing his treatment options in terms of antiplatelet therapy.

Which answer is most correct?

A. Continuous GP IIB.IIIa inhibitor infusion and a referral for CABG
B. Ticagrelor for one year and lifelong aspirin and proceed to a PCI with a drug eluting stent (type is not of critical importance)
C. Clopidogrel and aspirin together with a bare metal stent to his LAD
D. Clopidogrel and aspirin together with a specific drug eluting stent
E. Antiplatelet therapy alone, no stent

15. A 57-year-old man presents with an anterior STEMI and comes direct to the cath lab for a primary PCI within 6 hours of pain onset. He is found to have an acutely occluded proximal LAD artery together with a stable (non-culprit) severe proximal lesion in a large circumflex artery. The optimal strategy is:

A. Because he is young, acute referral to CABG for a LIMA to LAD and a graft to his circumflex artery
B. Primary PCI to LAD and a trial of anti-anginal therapy for his circumflex lesion
C. Primary PCI to LAD and pressure wire assessment of his circumflex artery
D. Primary PCI to LAD and PCI to circumflex under the same admission
E. PCI to his circumflex, no indication to treat the LAD as it is a completed infarct

16. A 70-year-old man comes acutely to the cath lab with anterior ST elevation a BP of 85 mmHg systolic, pH 7.2 and a lactate of 9 mmol/L. He is found to have an occluded LAD and a chronic total occlusion of his right coronary artery. His left ventricular function is severely impaired. The most correct strategy is.

A. Acute CABG
B. Treat the LAD and RCA CTO immediately, this will improve the clinical situation
C. Open the LAD and consider left ventricular support.
D. Perform an echo to rule out aortic dissection
E. If the patient survives there is good evidence to perform a CTO PCI procedure to open up the RCA

17. Figure 2.1.1 is from a coronary angiogram of a 50-year-old woman with acute onset chest pain and intermittent ST elevation.

What is the most likely diagnosis?

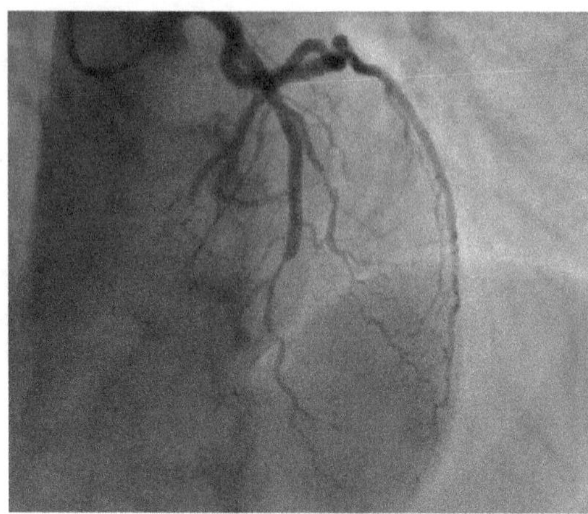

Figure 2.1.1

A. Normal
B. Severe atherosclerotic disease
C. Coronary embolus
D. Spontaneous coronary artery dissection
E. STEMI

18. A 45-year-old smoker presents with chest pain. There is no obvious ischaemia on his resting 12-lead ECG. His troponin level on admission is 60 ng/L.

Which of the following statements are true?

A. Medical therapy alone never has a role
B. In patients with high-risk features angiography should be undertaken within 24 hours
C. Always try to stabilize a patient with unstable clinical symptoms with medical treatment prior to invasive angiography
D. Younger patients with low GRACE scores never need early angiography
E. The rate of stroke during angiography is considerable (>5%)

19. In the context of a patient with a new diagnosis of NSTE-ACS and no other co-morbidities, which answer is correct?

A. Start the patient on an infusion of heparin
B. In patients with ongoing pain a glycoprotein inhibitor is indicated whilst waiting for a diagnostic angiogram
C. The GRACE score is irrelevant in guiding the timing and type of investigation
D. Fondaparinux is indicated on the day of the invasive angiogram
E. Offer a loading dose of aspirin 300 mg as soon as possible

20. A 79-year-old man with stable angina is found to have significant left main stem disease. Following MDT discussion, he is offered PCI. In left main stem coronary intervention, the following is true:

A. Intravascular imaging with IVUS is rarely indicated to guide optimal treatment as long as big stents are used

B. A provisional approach (one stent) when possible is superior to two stent bifurcation treatments

C. When comparing CABG to PCI, CABG is always superior to PCI in LMS treatment

D. Coronary pressure measurements are never indicated due to there being two large vessels after the bifurcation

E. Lifelong dual antiplatelet therapy is always indicated

chapter

2.1

ACUTE CORONARY SYNDROME

ANSWERS

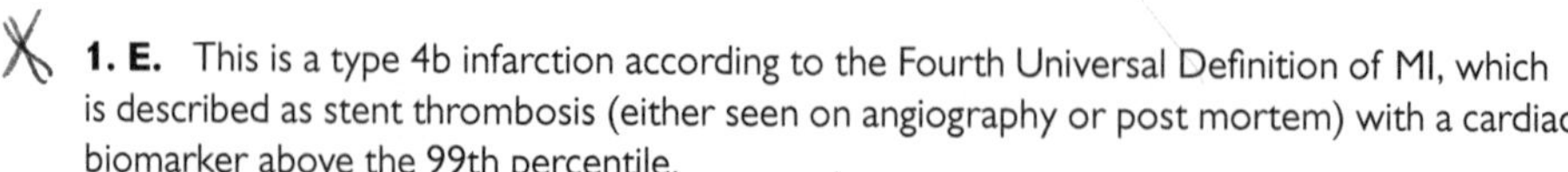

1. E. This is a type 4b infarction according to the Fourth Universal Definition of MI, which is described as stent thrombosis (either seen on angiography or post mortem) with a cardiac biomarker above the 99th percentile.

2. A. The most likely diagnosis here is a NSTE-ACS. This gentleman has a hs-cTn level more than five times above the ULN. Therefore, according to the ESC guidelines he should receive invasive coronary angiography as a first-line investigation barring any contraindications.

3. D. Based on the information available this lady falls in the high risk group. She has hs-cTn compatible with an MI, ST depression on her ECG, and her GRACE score is above 140. As she is in a high risk group she should receive invasive treatment within 24 hours.

4. E. For patients with NSTE-ACS who require long term anticoagulation, the ESC guidelines recommend treatment with a DOAC, e.g. apixaban (long term) plus an antiplatelet (either aspirin or clopidogrel) for 12 months.

5. A. This gentleman has a HAS-BLED score of more than 3, therefore putting him at high risk of bleeding. He also has high ischaemic risk with a new proximal LAD stent and significant bystander disease. Therefore, based on the information given he should receive triple therapy for 1–4 weeks followed by dual therapy (single antiplatelet plus anticoagulation) for 11 months

6. D. For non-cardiac surgery that cannot be postponed it is recommended that peri-operative cessation of the P2Y12 inhibitor may be reasonable 1 month after PCI if the risk and consequences of a recurrent ischaemic event (e.g. stent thrombosis) was felt to be less severe than the risk of bleeding on DAPT. Various factors including stent type, extent of stenting etc. need to be considered (most contemporary drug eluting stents facilitate 1 month of DAPT).

7. D. In unstable NSTE-ACS (ongoing ischaemia or haemodynamic instability) patients requiring CABG, surgery should be performed urgently irrespective of antiplatelet therapy.

8. B. In stable patients without critical anatomy or high-risk features, postponing surgery for at least 3 days after discontinuation of ticagrelor, at least 5 days after clopidogrel, and at least 7 days after prasugrel should be considered.

9. E. In the context of ACS multiple anticoagulants and platelet inhibitors are likely to be used. A bleeding complication from femoral artery access is likely to increase overall morbidity/mortality significantly. Careful ultrasound guided access via the femoral artery may be equivalent but right radial artery access is the best route. Minimal safety data exists for distal radial artery access. The ulnar artery can be used but is not the first choice (more difficult to access and more painful). Brachial artery complications include lower arm ischaemia and potential compartment syndrome.

10. C. Bivalirudin is associated with a significantly higher rate of acute stent thrombosis (HEAT-PPCI). Fondaparinux is associated with thrombotic events when used procedurally (OASIS 6). Cangrelor is not an anticoagulant. Enoxaparin is used in some countries intravenously (France) but never subcutaneously as its onset of action is too slow.

Shahzad A, Kemp I, Mars C, Wilson K, Roome C, Cooper R, Andron M, Appleby C, Fisher M, Khand A, Kunadian B, Mills JD, Morris JL, Morrison WL, Munir S, Palmer ND, Perry RA, Ramsdale DR, Velavan P, Stables RH; HEAT-PPCI trial investigators. Unfractionated heparin versus bivalirudin in primary percutaneous coronary intervention (HEAT-PPCI): an open-label, single centre, randomised controlled trial. Lancet. 2014 Nov 22;384(9957):1849–58. doi: 10.1016/S0140-6736(14)60924-7. Epub 2014 Jul 4. Erratum in: Lancet. 2014 Nov 22;384(9957):1848. PMID: 25002178.

Yusuf S, Mehta SR, Chrolavicius S, Afzal R, Pogue J, Granger CB, Budaj A, Peters RJ, Bassand JP, Wallentin L, Joyner C, Fox KA; OASIS-6 Trial Group. Effects of fondaparinux on mortality and reinfarction in patients with acute ST-segment elevation myocardial infarction: the OASIS-6 randomized trial. JAMA. 2006 Apr 5;295(13):1519–30. doi: 10.1001/jama.295.13.joc60038. Epub 2006 Mar 14. PMID: 16537725.

11. C. Minimal evidence of the use of clarithromycin in ACS exists. Whilst research is ongoing predicting vulnerable plaques is not yet possible and treatment of non-flow limiting vulnerable plaque has no evidence. Longer term treatment with antiplatelet drugs does reduce further ACS events, especially in the first three months. Typically, it is thin capped fibro atheromas that are seen to rupture and cause an ACS

12. D. This is a typical presentation of SCAD, and a somewhat subacute presentation in a younger woman with no coronary risk factors. This patient is unlikely to have significant coronary atheroma. The presentation does not sound like an aortic dissection, but she should have an echocardiogram prior to invasive imaging of her coronaries.

13. B. This man has a GRACE score over 140, his risk of MI / death is considerable. After some initial investigations a coronary angiogram and discussion of his options would be a reasonable course of action. Coronary CT is not indicated here, this is an unstable patient rather than a patient with stable angina.

14. D. The patient has a high bleeding risk (age, renal failure and need for anticoagulation treatment) together with considerable co-morbidity. Glycoprotein IIb/IIIa inhibitor therapy and surgery are not optimal. Combining ticagrelor and DOAC / warfarin would lead to a very high bleeding risk. The use of a BMS vs specific drug eluting stent (with the option of short DAPT) provides no real advantage in terms of bleeding risks and will lead to a much higher rate of re-stenosis. A short period of aspirin together with clopidogrel and anticoagulant and a specific DES that allows reduced antiplatelet therapy is the optimal choice. This minimizes bleeding risk and provides effective treatment for his ischaemic heart disease. He is likely to have recurrent ischaemia on antiplatelet therapy alone.

15. D. No evidence for acute CABG in this setting. Fast and efficient revascularization is paramount here. Multiple RCTs suggest full revascularization in STEMI improves morbidity/mortality and should be done within 45 days. The benefit of primary PCI extends beyond 6 hours.

16. C. CABG has no role in STEMI with cardiogenic shock (the only exception would be a VSD or papillary muscle rupture). Treating the LAD occlusion is the most important step. Full revascularization (with a CTO) during the index procedure is associated with increased complication and no benefit. It would be very unlucky to present with both cardiogenic shock due to an anterior infarct together with an aortic dissection. However, an acute echo is extremely useful to assess the patient and rule out the rare presentation of an aortic dissection that involves the LMS. Left ventricular support with an Impella device or ECMO has no absolute randomized evidence although this is mostly due to the difficulty of performing an RCT in this situation.

17. D. There are some characteristic features that point towards SCAD: sudden stepdown in vessel calibre, pruning of side septal branches, and patient characteristics.

18. B. Medical therapy may be chosen in stable and lower risk patients or those in whom invasive treatment carries unacceptable risk. Patients with ongoing unstable clinical symptoms should be offered early or immediate coronary angiography. Young patients often have a good indication for early invasive investigation; a risk score alone should never dictate management. The rate of stroke is actually very low, considerably less than 1%

19. E. Long-term heparin infusion is associated with bleeding complications and heparin-induced thrombocytopenia (HITT). Prehospital or pre cath lab glycoprotein inhibitors are not recommended due to very high bleeding rates that often outweigh any advantage. The GRACE score is well proven to predict mortality and guide the speed and type of investigation. OASIS 6 indicated increased ischaemic complications with fondaparinux peri-procedurally.

20. B. IVUS should be considered to optimise treatment of left main lesions (ESC guidelines Class IIA. For left main disease of low/intermediate anatomical complexity, the EXCEL trial demonstrated no significant difference between PCI and CABG with respect to death/stroke/MI at 5 years. Pressure wire analysis is useful and indicated in assessing left main lesions of indeterminate significance. DAPT strategy is generally similar to non-left main interventions, although prolongation of DAPT therapy (due to higher ischaemic risk) should be considered if bleeding risk low.

chapter

2.2

CHRONIC CORONARY SYNDROME

QUESTIONS

1. A 41-year-old lady presents to cardiology clinic reporting a 3-month history of sharp chest pain both at rest and on exertion. She takes ramipril for blood pressure control and atorvastatin for hypercholesterolaemia. She also takes salbutamol inhalers occasionally when she exercises. She tells you that her younger brother recently died of a massive heart attack. On examination she is tachycardic at a heart rate of 110 bpm, and she is overweight with a BMI of 40. You decide to investigate her symptoms with a coronary CTA.

In patients with angina and suspected coronary artery disease which of the following does NOT preclude investigation with coronary CTA?

A. Irregular tachycardia
B. Inability to breath hold
C. Extensive calcification
D. Significant obesity
E. Asthma

2. A 78-year-old diabetic male patient is seen in rapid access chest pain clinic with a 6-month history of exertional squeezing chest tightness and breathlessness. He reports that he is now struggling with stairs and hills. His GP started him on aspirin and a statin, and provided him with a GTN spray, which he uses whenever he exercises. He gets no symptoms at rest.

Which of the following investigations is a class 1 indication for investigating patients with angina and/or dyspnoea with suspected chronic coronary syndrome?

A. Ambulatory ECG monitoring in patients with suspected vasospastic angina
B. Resting transthoracic echocardiogram
C. Non-stress cardiac MRI
D. Carotid artery ultrasound to detect plaque
E. Chest CT for patients with atypical presentation, signs and symptoms of heart failure, or suspicion of pulmonary disease

3. The patient in Q2 has an echocardiogram which shows normal left ventricular function with no obvious regional wall motion abnormalities. He is now also taking isosorbide mononitrate 60 mg bd and amlodipine 10mg od but remains very symptomatic with angina. He tells you that his friend recently had a CT scan to investigate 'similar heart troubles'.

In patients with angina and suspected chronic coronary syndrome which of the following statements is false?

A. Functional imaging for myocardial ischaemia is recommended if coronary CTA has shown CAD of uncertain functional significance or is not diagnostic X
B. Non-invasive functional imaging for myocardial ischaemia or coronary CTA is recommended as the initial test to diagnose CAD in symptomatic patients in whom obstructive CAD cannot be excluded by clinical assessment alone X
C. Coronary calcium detection by CT is not recommended to identify individuals with obstructive CAD. X
D. Coronary CTA is recommended to diagnose CAD in patients with a high clinical likelihood of coronary disease and ongoing symptoms despite medical therapy
E. It is recommended that selection of the initial non-invasive diagnostic test is done based on the clinical likelihood of CAD and patient characteristics that influence test performance and local expertise.

4. A 69-year-old male undergoes stress echocardiography for angina. This shows significant inducible ischaemia and hence he is listed for invasive coronary angiography, which demonstrates significant multi-vessel coronary disease. The patients is anxious about his prognosis and risk of acute cardiac events and after having done some research online he wishes to discuss this with you.

Which if the following defines high event risk for the respective investigations in patients with chronic coronary syndrome?

A. Area of ischaemia ≥5% of the left ventricle on myocardial SPECT or PET perfusion imaging
B. ≥2 of 16 segments with stress perfusion defects or ≥2 dobutamine-induced dysfunctional segments on cardiac MRI
C. FFR ≤0.9, iwFR ≤0.90 on invasive functional testing
D. Three-vessel disease with proximal stenoses, or left main disease on invasive angiography
E. ≥2 of 16 segments with stress-induced hypokinesia or akinesia on stress echocardiography

5. A 70 year-old lady who is being treated for angina by her GP is found to have moderate coronary artery disease on invasive angiography, with negative pressure wire studies. Her symptoms are presently well-controlled on nicorandil and bisoprolol, and she is able to get back to all her regular activities. She enquires about what changes she needs to make regarding her dietary intake in order to 'help keep her heart healthy'.

Which of the following ESC guidelines lifestyle recommendations is correct for patients with chronic coronary syndrome and angina?

A. Diet high in vegetables and fruits, limiting saturated fat to <15% total intake
B. Limit alcohol to <150 g/week
C. Maintain a healthy weight <20 kg/m^2, or reduce weight through recommended energy intake and increased physical activity
D. 60–120 minutes of moderate physical activity most days, but even irregular exercise is beneficial
E. Use pharmacological strategies to help patients quit smoking

6. Prior to her diagnosis of angina the above lady had been leading a fairly sedentary lifestyle. She enquires about what sort of levels of exercise as well as general lifestyle modifications would be recommended in her case.

Which of the following statements concerning lifestyle management in patients with angina is incorrect?

A. Exercise-based cardiac rehabilitation is recommended as an effective means for patients with chronic coronary syndrome to achieve a healthy lifestyle and manage risk factors
B. Cognitive behavioural interventions are not recommended in helping individuals achieve a healthy lifestyle
C. Improvement of lifestyle factors in addition to appropriate pharmacological management is recommended
D. Psychological interventions are recommended to improve symptoms of depression in patients with chronic coronary syndrome
E. Annual influenza vaccination is recommended for patients with chronic coronary syndromes, especially in the elderly

7. An 82-year-old male with previous history of stroke and hypertension presents to cardiology clinic with a 4-month history of exertional chest discomfort. He takes clopidogrel 75 mg od as well as ramipril 5 mg od. Cardiovascular examination shows normal heart sounds, with a blood pressure of 145/82 mmHg and resting heart rate of 51 bpm. His GP enquires about which medication to start to manage his stable angina.

Which of the following would be an appropriate first-line antianginal therapy in this patient?

A. Amlodipine
B. Bisoprolol
C. Long-acting nitrates
D. Ranolazine
E. Diltiazem

8. Mrs Smith is a 69-year-old lady who had two drug-eluting stents fitted to her right coronary artery for exertional angina persisting despite multiple anti-anginal medications. She is an ex heavy smoker and has no other comorbidities except for hypercholesterolaemia.

Which of the following statements is incorrect regarding antithrombotic therapy post PCI in patients with chronic coronary syndrome?

A. Aspirin 75–100mg daily is recommended following stenting
B. Prasugrel or ticagrelor may be considered in specific high-risk situations of elective stenting if dual antiplatelets cannot be used because of aspirin intolerance
C. Clopidogrel 75 mg daily following appropriate loading is recommended, in addition to aspirin, for 12 months following elective coronary stenting, in patients without risk of life-threatening bleeding
D. When oral anticoagulation is initiated in a patient with stable CAD and AF, a NOAC is preferable to warfarin
E. Long-term OAC therapy is recommended in patients with AF and a CHA_2DS_2-VASc score ≥2 in males and ≥3 in females

9. An 84-year-old male patient has ongoing angina despite taking isosorbide mononitrate 60mg bd, amlodipine 10mg od and ranolazine 500mg bd. He undergoes coronary angioplasty to the circumflex artery with a drug-eluting stent, following positive pressure wire studies. His past medical history includes hypertension, atrial fibrillation, prostate cancer, and a previous perforated duodenal ulcer for which he required emergency surgery 18 months ago.

Which of the following statements is incorrect regarding antithrombotic therapy in post-PCI patients with AF (requiring long term anticoagulation)?

A. Triple therapy with aspirin, clopidogrel and an OAC for ≥4 weeks should be considered when the risk of stent thrombosis outweighs the bleeding risk, with the total duration (≤6 months) decided according to risk assessment

B. The use of ticagrelor or prasugrel is not recommended as part of triple antithrombotic therapy with aspirin and an OAC

C. After uncomplicated PCI for NSTE-ACS, triple therapy for 4 weeks with aspirin, clopidogrel, and an OAC, followed by continuation of clopidogrel and an OAC to 1 year is recommended as the default strategy, provided ischaemic risk is not high

D. In patients with an indication for warfarin in combination with aspirin and/or clopidogrel, the dose-intensity of warfarin should be carefully regulated with a target INR in the range of 2.0–2.5.

E. Dual therapy with an OAC and either ticagrelor or prasugrel may be considered as an alternative to triple therapy with an OAC, aspirin, and clopidogrel in patients with moderate or high risk of stent thrombosis.

10. A 38-year-old male had recent percutaneous coronary angioplasty for angina. He is hypertensive and diabetic on insulin and has a strong family history of heart disease. His latest lipid profile on atorvastatin 80 mg od showed a total cholesterol of 5.9 and LDL 2.6. A recent transthoracic echocardiogram showed mild left ventricular impairment.

When considering event prevention in this patient with chronic coronary syndrome which of the following statements is incorrect?

A. Statins are recommended in all patients with chronic coronary syndrome

B. ACE inhibitors are recommended in this patient as he has other conditions such as hypertension as well as diabetes

C. If this patient's goal is not achieved with the maximum tolerated dose of statin, ezetimibe may be added to the lipid-lowering regime

D. In young patients with CCS, early initiation of PCSK9 inhibitors is recommended.

E. A beta-blocker would be recommended in this patient as he has LV dysfunction demonstrated on his echocardiogram.

11. A 70-year-old female is being investigated for exertional chest pain and breathlessness. Her resting ECG shows a left bundle-branch block whilst an echocardiogram shows an impaired left ventricle with estimated ejection fraction of 32%. This was not previously known. She is started on furosemide, ramipril, and spironolactone. On follow-up she reports ongoing exertional angina. Whilst she is awaiting coronary angiography you decide to start her on antianginal therapy.

Which if the following is a contraindication for using ivabradine in patients with chronic coronary syndromes and new onset heart failure?

A. Heart rate 75 bpm
B. Sinus rhythm
C. LVEF ≤35%
D. Concurrent treatment with beta-blocker
E. Pacemaker dependency

12. A 68 year-old male with angina and previous coronary angiography showing moderate coronary disease only has been stable for the last 2 years on medical therapy with bisoprolol and amlodipine. He is able to play golf and go for long walks without trouble and does not use his GTN spray. He enquires whether he needs further tests in future as routine.

In asymptomatic patients with a long-standing diagnosis of chronic coronary syndrome which of the following is recommended as follow up strategy?

A. Coronary CT as routine follow-up for patients with established CAD
B. Invasive coronary angiography for risk stratification
C. A periodic visit to a cardiovascular healthcare professional to reassess any potential change in the risk status of patients
D. Invasive coronary angiography (with FFR when necessary) in patients with mild or no symptoms receiving medical treatment in whom non-invasive risk stratification indicates a low or moderate risk
E. Routine exercise treadmill test for risk stratification

13. A 58-year-old lady with long-standing diabetes has an invasive coronary angiogram which excludes flow-limiting disease, with negative pressure wire studies. Medical history includes smoking and a BMI of 36. She is suspected to have microvascular angina. On follow-up she continues to report stable exertional angina, and she is keen on further tests.

Which of the following is NOT recommended in patients with stable angina with microvascular angina where significant obstructive epicardial disease has been excluded?

A. Guidewire-based CFR
B. Myocardial perfusion scan
C. Transthoracic Doppler of the LAD
D. PET scanning
E. Cardiac MRI

14. A 49-year-old male, who is previously fit and well, is referred to you by his GP as his brother aged 52 recently had a heart attack and is awaiting coronary artery bypass surgery for severe multi-vessel disease. The patient denies any chest pain but admits to living a fairly sedentary lifestyle.

Which of the following is an incorrect statement in screening asymptomatic patients for CAD?

A. It is recommended that patients aged <50 years with a family history of premature CVD in first-degree relative are screened using a validated score.
B. Individuals aged <50 years with familial hypercholesterolaemia should be screened using a validated score.
C. Assessment of coronary calcium score with CT may be considered as a risk modifier in the cardiovascular risk assessment of asymptomatic patients
D. ABI may be considered as a risk modifier in cardiovascular risk assessment
E. An exercise ECG is of no value in asymptomatic adults

15. A 60-year-old diabetic male has multiple stents to his left anterior descending artery and right coronary artery for angina. Following revascularization, he remains symptomatic and can hardly manage 200 metres before getting chest discomfort and breathlessness. He takes aspirin 75 mg od, atorvastatin 80 mg od, metformin 1 g bd, isosorbide mononitrate 60 mg bd, bisoprolol 10 mg od, amlodipine 10 mg od, and ranolazine 750 mg bd. He is desperate for 'some sort of intervention' as his lifestyle is being significantly impacted by his angina.

Which of the following is not recommended in patients with debilitating angina refractory to optimal medical and revascularization strategies?

A. Trans myocardial laser revascularization
B. Spinal cord stimulation
C. Coronary sinus reducer device
D. Enhanced external counter pulsation
E. Referral to a refractory angina specialist centre

16. A 60-year-old man presents to your outpatient clinic with chest pain that is precipitated by exertion (particularly in cold weather), that improves with rest. The pain occurs about once a day, when he takes the dog for a walk.

Which answer is most correct?

A. Anti anginal medication and reassurance that angiography is unnecessary if his symptoms are resolved
B. Direct referral to invasive angiography
C. Referral for CT coronary angiography and further discussion
D. Start anti anginal medication and refer for either perfusion imaging or CT coronary angiography followed by a discussion on indication for invasive angiography
E. No further investigation or treatment. Advising that neither medical therapy or invasive treatment changes the risk of death or heart attack

17. A 55-year-old lady reports central heavy chest pain radiating to her jaw and both arms. These episodes come on at rest and are not related to exertion, food, or cold weather. She is seen in the rapid access chest pain clinic. A transthoracic echocardiogram is normal. No significant atheroma is seen on CT coronary angiography.

Which of the following recommendations are appropriate?

A. Reassurance and discharge from chest pain clinic
B. A beta-blocker should be initiated
C. Ambulatory ECG monitoring should be arranged to look for an underlying arrhythmia
D. Invasive coronary angiography with intracoronary acetylcholine provocation testing should be considered
E. None of the above

18. Mr Jones is a 68-year-old man who suffers from CCS class 3 angina. He has diabetes, hypertension, and hypercholesterolaemia. Left ventricular function is normal. He is currently on aspirin 75mg od, bisoprolol 5mg od, atorvastatin 40mg od, metformin 1g bd, and rampiril 2.5mg od. His blood pressure is 135/80 mmHg and his heart rate is 60 bpm.

Which of the following anti-anginal medications would you recommend whilst he awaits coronary angiography?

A. Isosorbide mononitrate 60 mg od
B. Ranolazine 375 mg bd
C. Amlodipine 5 mg od
D. Ivabradine 5 mg bd
E. Nicorandil 10 mg bd

19. Mr Jones (from Q18) undergoes coronary angiography. This shows a 70% stenosis in his proximal LAD artery, a 90% stenosis in his posterior descending artery (PDA) and an 80% stenosis in his first obtuse marginal (OM) artery. He is now asymptomatic.

Which of the following recommendations are correct?

A. Continue medical therapy. Revascularization not indicated as now asymptomatic
B. He should have PCI to his LAD artery
C. He should have PCI to his posterior descending artery
D. He should be referred for coronary artery bypass grafting
E. He should have an assessment for ischaemia

20. Mr Jones (from Q18 and Q19) has multi-vessel PCI with three drug eluting stents.

Which of the following recommendations are correct?

A. Aspirin long term, clopidogrel 1 year
B. Aspirin long term, clopidogrel 1 month
C. Consider PCSK9 inhibitor if LDL-C> 3.0mmol/L despite maximum statin therapy
D. Consider Colchicine 0.5mg bd
E. Consider SGLT2 inhibitor

chapter

2.2

CHRONIC CORONARY SYNDROME

ANSWERS

1. E. Asthma in itself is not a contraindication to having a coronary CTA; if the patient has previously experienced bronchospasm with beta-blockers then optimal heart rate may be achieved using ivabradine or rate-limiting calcium antagonists.

2. A. Other appropriate investigations include coronary CT angiography, stress echocardiography, stress perfusion cardiac MRI, myocardial perfusion scintigraphy, and invasive coronary angiography.

3. D. Invasive coronary angiography is recommended to diagnose (and potentially treat) CAD in patients with high clinical likelihood, severe symptoms refractory to medical therapy or typical angina at low level of exercise, and clinical evaluation that indicates high events risk.

4. D. Significant left main or proximal three-vessel coronary artery disease carries high prognostic risk as a result of the large myocardial territory at risk. ESC guidelines define high event risk for the following investigations as below:

- area of ischaemia ≥ 10% of the left ventricle myocardial on SPECT or PET perfusion imaging
- ≥2 of 16 segments with stress perfusion defects or ≥3 dobutamine-induced dysfunctional segments on cardiac MRI
- FFR ≤0.8, iwFR ≤0.89 on invasive functional testing
- ≥3 of 16 segments with stress-induced hypokinesia or akinesia on stress echocardiography

5. E. The use of pharmacological as well as behavioural strategies is encouraged in order to help patients quit smoking; passive smoking is also discouraged. Saturated fat intake is limited to ≤10% of total intake, while alcohol is limited to <100 g/week or 15 g/day. In terms of physical activity the recommended exercise is 30–60 min of moderate activity most days.

6. B. Evidence shows that decisions are usually not deliberate, but rather automatic and influenced by environment. A recent meta-analysis looking at 10 randomized controlled trials involving a total population of 1949 patients has demonstrated that integrated motivational interviewing and cognitive behaviour therapy had a significant effect in increasing physical activity levels in community-dwelling adults.

7. A. According to current ESC guidelines, first-step anti-anginal drugs in patients with chronic coronary syndrome include beta-blockers or calcium channel blockers. As this patient is bradycardic, amlodipine is more appropriate than bisoprolol or other rate-limiting medication. Long-acting nitrates, ranolazine, ivabradine, and nicorandil are second-line agents.

8. C. ISAR-SAFE was a large double-blinded randomized study of 4005 patients, which confirmed that a 12-month course of DAPT did not afford any benefit over a 6-month course with respect to ischaemic endpoints. Likewise, the net clinical benefit (composite of death, MI, stent thrombosis, stroke, and TIMI major bleeding) was neutral. Thus, systematic use of dual antiplatelet therapy beyond 6 months is not justified for all patients but should be decided based on the individual risk profile of the patient.

9. C. Recent ESC guidelines 2020 recommend that in AF patients (requiring long-term anticoagulation) undergoing PCI for NSTE-ACS, the default strategy is up to 1 week of triple therapy (in hospital) for patients without high ischaemic risk.

10. D. A combination with a PCSK9 inhibitor is recommended only for patients at very high risk who do not achieve their goal on the maximum tolerated dose of statin and ezetimibe.

The UK NICE guidelines suggest that in those with a history of a heart event or coronary heart disease, ischaemic stroke, or peripheral arterial disease—patients at high risk of further CVD must have LDL-C concentrations persistently above 4.0 mmol/L.

11. E. Ivabradine is a hyperpolarization-activated cyclic nucleotide-gated (HCN) channel blocker which works by lowering the heart rate and is licensed for use in patients with chronic stable angina. Its use is contraindicated in patients where heart rate is maintained exclusively by their pacemaker.

12. C. A periodic follow-up with a cardiovascular healthcare professional is recommended (class I indication) in order to reassess any potential change in the risk status of patients. This would entail clinical evaluation of lifestyle-modification measures, adherence to targets of cardiovascular risk factor prevention, and the development of comorbidities that may affect treatment and outcomes.

13. B. Proposed mechanisms in microvascular angina include endothelial dysfunction, myocardial ischaemia, and abnormal autonomic control. Imaging modalities such as PET scanning and cardiac MRI, as well as invasive and non-invasive assessment of coronary flow reserve (CFR) using transthoracic doppler, have been shown to be useful in quantitative assessments of coronary microvascular function.

14. E. In asymptomatic adults (including sedentary adults considering starting a vigorous exercise programme), an exercise ECG may be considered (class IIb indication) for cardiovascular risk assessment, particularly when attention is paid to non-ECG makers such as functional exercise capacity.

15. A. There is no evidence to support trans myocardial laser revascularization for the treatment of chronic refractory angina.

16. D. It is important to exclude left main stem or proximal three-vessel disease with whichever imaging modality is available in your local centre. Communication is central to the successful treatment of stable angina.

17. D. She may have vasospastic angina. A 12-lead ECG or ambulatory monitoring during symptoms may show significant ST segment change. Invasive coronary angiography with intracoronary acetylcholine provocation may induce coronary spasm in susceptible individuals.

18. C. Guidelines recommend combining a beta-blocker with a dihydropyridine calcium channel blocker as first-line anti-anginal therapy.

19. E. The angiogram suggests potentially significant three-vessel disease, but it is unclear whether one, two, or all the lesions are ischaemic based on angiographic appearances alone. Ischaemia testing (e.g. invasive pressure wire assessment) would help delineate the burden and distribution of ischaemia to inform a discussion on revascularization. Revascularization should be offered for ongoing symptoms or prognostically important disease. Medical therapy may be appropriate for this patient if he is truly asymptomatic (based on the ISCHAEMIA trial) but the implications of a conservative strategy need to be discussed in full (risk of Type 1 spontaneous MI with medical therapy).

20. E. The recommendation DAPT strategy post elective PCI for stable angina is aspirin long term and clopidogrel for 6 months. PCSK9 inhibitors should be considered if LDL levels remain high despite optimal doses (or intolerance) of other lipid-lowering therapy. For secondary prevention, the UK NICE guidelines approve the use of PCSK9 inhibitors if LDL-C levels are above 4 mmol/L. Low dose colchicine 0.5 mg od has been shown to reduce cardiovascular events in patients with chronic coronary syndromes (LoDoCo Trial). SGLT2 inhibitors are recommended in patients with diabetes and cardiovascular disease.

14/20

chapter

2.3 CARDIAC CATHETERIZATION

QUESTIONS

1. A 56-year-old man is admitted with chest pain and a troponin T of 157 ng/L. He undergoes coronary angiography which demonstrates moderate diffuse atheroma in the distal left circumflex. He is diagnosed with an NSTEMI. A decision is made to manage medically and no PCI is performed. He undergoes an echocardiogram which shows normal left ventricular systolic function. The patient asks when he can recommence driving his car for personal use. He holds a Group 1 Licence and does not hold a HGV (heavy goods vehicle) licence.

Based on UK DVLA (Driver and Vehicle Licensing Agency) guidelines, what would be the most appropriate advice?

A. Four weeks after the MI
B. One week after the MI
C. He requires a stress test and a repeat echocardiogram, and he can only drive if his ejection fraction is >40%
D. He must relinquish his licence indefinitely
E. He may return to driving once discharged from hospital

2. While working in the Cath lab, you note that the typical distance between the operator and the centre of the patient is 0.5 metres. You are concerned about radiation scatter and therefore attach extra tubing to the catheter to increase this distance to 0.75 metres.

What impact would this have on radiation exposure?

A. No impact on exposure
B. Reduce radiation exposure by a factor of 2
C. Reduce radiation exposure by a factor of 4
D. Reduce radiation exposure by a factor of 6
E. Reduce radiation exposure by a factor of 8

3. When performing angiography, which of the following is incorrect regarding the left coronary artery.

A. Judkins left catheter (e.g. JL4) is usually used to engage the left coronary ostium when using the femoral access route

B. A JL3.5 is frequently used first line to engage the left coronary ostium when using radial access

C. A JL5 or JL6 catheter may be required if the aorta is dilated

D. The secondary curve of the Judkins left catheter normally engages the left main stem ostium

E. The left anterior oblique (LAO) cranial view is usually a good view for assessing the left main stem ostium

4. A 56-year-old gentleman is reviewed by the heart team. He has been referred to the cardiology outpatient's department with a 3-month history of shortness of breath and leg swelling. He underwent an echocardiogram and was found to have an ejection fraction of 30%. He subsequently had an invasive coronary angiogram which demonstrated severe three vessel disease and a CMR which showed viable myocardium.

Which of the following is TRUE regarding his management?

A. In terms of revascularization, PCI should be considered first line to manage his coronary artery disease as this has been shown to confer a survival benefit

B. In terms of revascularization, CABG is favoured if there is an acceptable surgical risk

C. An ICD should be offered upfront on diagnosing severe left ventricular failure

D. An ACE inhibitor, beta-blocker and mineralocorticoid receptor antagonist should be offered upfront on diagnosing severe left ventricular failure

E. Cardiac Resynchronization Therapy (CRT) should be offered upfront on diagnosing severe left ventricular dysfunction with an ejection fraction less than 35% if the QRS duration is over 130 ms

5. **The intensive care consultant calls about a 46-year-old man admitted to the ITU generally unwell with chest discomfort and profound hypotension. He has a history of diabetes and smokes. His ECG demonstrated a pre-existing right bundle branch block. His Troponin T level is 2166 ng/L. A focused echocardiogram performed by the intensive care doctor demonstrated severe global left ventricular dysfunction and he is now being managed for suspected cardiogenic shock. He has been commenced on dobutamine and noradrenaline. The ITU consultant seeks your advice on the best course of action.**

   Which of the following is true regarding the management of this patient?

   A. Suggest immediate invasive angiography and emergency complete revascularization treating all diseased coronary arteries
   B. Suggest immediate invasive angiography, emergency complete revascularization treating all diseased coronary arteries, and insertion of an intra-aortic balloon pump to maintain blood pressure and reduce inotropic requirements
   C. Suggest immediate invasive angiography and emergency culprit vessel only revascularization in the first instance
   D. Suggest immediate invasive angiography and emergency culprit vessel only revascularization in the first instance and insertion of an intra-aortic balloon pump to maintain blood pressure and reduce inotropic requirements
   E. Emergency coronary angiography is not indicated as there is no history of ST elevation

6. **A 66-year-old man is admitted to CCU and treated for ACS. He has a previous medical history of hypertension, type 2 diabetes, and mild rheumatoid arthritis. He undergoes an angiogram which demonstrates three-vessel disease including left main stem disease and an intermediate SYNTAX score of 26.**

   Which of the following statements is correct?

   A. As the SYNTAX score has been used, the heart team is not required to decide on a revascularization strategy
   B. In terms of treatment of choice, CABG is favoured
   C. In terms of treatment of choice, PCI is favoured
   D. In terms of treatment of choice, CABG or PCI are both acceptable
   E. The SYNTAX II score should *not* be used in this situation

7. A 67-year-old gentleman with a background of angina pectoris is admitted for elective PCI to his right coronary artery. He has a previous medical history of AF and is taking warfarin with a recent INR of 2.1.

Which of the following is true regarding his management?

A. A bare metal stent should be considered to facilitate short duration of dual antiplatelets
B. A potent $P2Y_{12}$ inhibitor, i.e. ticagrelor or prasugrel, should be considered post PCI in addition to warfarin
C. A dose of 70–100 units/kg of unfractionated heparin should be used during PCI with a view to achieving an ACT of ≥250 seconds
D. A glycoprotein IIb/IIIa inhibitor should be considered during PCI to reduce the risk of clot formation
E. Cangrelor should be used during PCI in view of concomitant warfarin

8. A 75-year-old gentleman with a history of stable chest pain undergoes a coronary angiogram which demonstrated an intermediate stenosis in the mid left anterior descending artery (LAD). His current medical treatment includes amlodipine and bisoprolol. He tells you that he had his cholesterol check three months ago and it was normal.

Which of the following is TRUE regarding this management?

A. FFR or iFR measurement using a pressure wire should be considered first line to assess the haemodynamic significance of intermediate-grade stenosis
B. In view of the clinical history of chest pain, direct stenting of the LAD is indicated
C. PCI is currently not indicated and a third anti-anginal medication should be prescribed with follow up to re-evaluate symptoms before considering an invasive treatment strategy
D. As the mid LAD is involved, CABG should be considered on prognostic grounds
E. A statin is not indicated in view of his normal cholesterol

9. Which of the following are TRUE regarding intracoronary imaging?

A. Optical coherence tomography (OCT) should be considered to assess the severity of stenosis within an unprotected left main stem
B. Intravascular ultrasound (IVUS) should be considered to assess the severity of stenosis within an unprotected left main stem
C. IVUS of the left main stem can be technically challenging due to the requirement to administer contrast during image acquisition
D. IVUS should be preferred over OCT for stent assessment due to superior image resolution
E. OCT should not be used in the assessment of coronary calcium due to poor tissue characterization

10. A 64-year-old gentleman is transferred directly to the cath lab having presented with severe central chest pain and associated anterior ST segment elevation. He is found to have an occluded LAD with thrombus observed.

Which of the following is incorrect regarding the management of this patient?

A Primary PCI is recommended over fibrinolysis if performed by an experienced team within 120 minutes of first medical contact

B. Primary PCI should be considered in patients presenting with less than 12 hours of chest pain and persistent ST elevation or new LBBB

C. Following successful fibrinolysis, transfer to the cath lab should be considered within 24 hours

D. Following unsuccessful fibrinolysis, urgent transfer to the cath lab should be considered

E Aspiration thrombectomy should be performed routinely to remove thrombus and prevent no-reflow

11. Which of the following is not a potential indication for an intra-aortic balloon pump (IABP)?

A. Cardiogenic shock

B. Mechanical complication of myocardial infarction, e.g. VSD

C. Support in high-risk PCI Bridge to CABG/transplant

D. Acute severe mitral regurgitation with associated shock

E. Acute severe aortic regurgitation with associated shock

12. Which of the following is incorrect regarding no reflow?

A. May occur after ballooning or stent deployment

B. Occurs in the presence of a patent coronary lumen and is a reflection of microvascular obstruction, which may be appreciated by abnormal myocardial blush

C. Associated with thrombotic lesions, e.g. STEMI

D. The management options include intracoronary nitrate, adenosine, verapamil, or sodium nitroprusside

E Injection into distal vessel via a microcathether, aspiration or dual lumen catheter should be avoided due to distal microvascular obstruction

13. A 80-year-old gentleman is admitted to CCU for an urgent angiogram and PCI having presented with a NSTEMI with associated deep ST depression. Due to significant subclavian tortuosity, he undergoes PCI to his proximal LAD via the right femoral route. The femoral sheath was removed in the lab post procedure and his ACT was documented as 120 seconds. Approximately 80 minutes after this procedure, the nursing staff become concerned when the patient reports to be feeling generally unwell and his blood pressure has dropped significantly to 80/50 mmHg with a heart rate of 110 bpm.

Which of the following management strategies would be considered to be the LEAST appropriate?

A. An ECG
B. A focused echocardiogram
C. An urgent femoral ultrasound scan of the groin once the patient is stabilized
D. An urgent CT scan to assess the femoral artery once the patient is stabilized
E. An advanced life support (ALS) approach using a full A to E assessment with thorough examination

14. A 60-year-old gentleman is referred by the renal team with chest pain on exertion. He has a history of polycystic kidney disease and CKD stage 4 with an eGFR of 18 ml/min/1.73 m^2 but has never required renal replacement therapy. He has also recently been diagnosed with type 2 diabetes and hypertension. Following an outpatient invasive angiogram, his case was reviewed by the Heart Team who felt that PCI should be considered as he had non-prognostic coronary disease. He was therefore admitted for elective PCI to his RCA using rotational atherectomy and shockwave intravascular lithotripsy (IVL).

Which of the following statements is incorrect concerning this case?

A. Contrast-induced nephropathy (CIN) is an important consideration in this case, and it usually manifests as deteriorating renal function 48–72 hours post-exposure
B. Pre-hydration is important in this patient due to his reduced eGFR
C. The minimum volume of low- or iso-osmolar contrast media should be used
D. Traditionally it has been recommended to withhold metformin for 48 hours after elective angiography or PCI
E. If there is deterioration of renal function, N-acetylcysteine is an essential treatment in order to limit deterioration caused by contrast-induced nephropathy

15. A 60-year-old gentleman is admitted with insidious right-sided heart failure. Following review of his echocardiogram at the MDT, he is referred for a right heart cath study as the differential diagnosis included both restrictive cardiomyopathy and constrictive pericarditis.

Which of the following would best support a diagnosis of restrictive cardiomyopathy as opposed to constrictive pericarditis?

A. A separation of right ventricular end diastolic pressure and left ventricular end diastolic pressure of <5 mmHg
B. A previous history of cardiac surgery
C. A previous history of tuberculosis
D. Ventricular pressure tracing showing ventricular concordance of the RV and LV pressure with respiration, i.e. concordant right ventricle and left ventricle systolic pressure tracings with respiration
E. Ventricular pressure tracing showing equalization of right ventricular and left ventricular end diastolic pressure manifesting as the 'square root' or 'dip and plateau' sign on the tracing

16. A 67-year-old gentleman is admitted for an angiogram and potential PCI having previously presented to the Rapid Access Chest Pain Clinic with typical angina symptoms. He underwent a CT coronary angiogram, which showed a dominant RCA with a significant stenosis in the posterior descending artery (PDA) branch just distal to the bifurcation. He continues to have chest pain despite two antianginal medications.

Which view would be the best to visualize the stenosis of the PDA artery.

A. Right anterior oblique view
B. Left anterior oblique view
C. Left anterior oblique view with cranial angulation
D. Right anterior oblique view with caudal angulation
E. Left anterior oblique view with caudal angulation

17. An 88-year-old lady is admitted with a NSTEMI. She has a previous medical history of hypertension and CKD stage 4 with an eGFR of 17 ml/min/1.73 m^2.

Which of the following should be used WITH CAUTION prior to angiography?

A. Fondaparinux
B. Aspirin
C. Unfractionated heparin
D. Ticagrelor
E. Bisoprolol

18. A 56-year-old gentleman is admitted with ACS. He has a medical history of hypertension and hypercholesterolaemia. He undergoes PCI with a third-generation drug eluting stent. He is commenced on aspirin and prasugrel.

How long should he continue dual antiplatelet therapy?

A. 1 month
B. 3 months
C. 6 months
D. 12 months
E. >12 months

19. A 92-year-old lady is admitted with chest pain and diagnosed with NSTEMI. She has a previous medical history of hypertension and a previous upper GI bleed. She has an echocardiogram which shows preserved LV systolic function.

Which of the following statements is TRUE?

A. A proton pump inhibitor should be considered
B. Prasugrel 60 mg loading and 10 mg daily should be considered
C. An invasive management strategy via coronary angiography should be avoided with preference for medical management
D. A glycoprotein IIb/IIIa inhibitor should be considered
E. A mineralocorticoid receptor antagonist should be considered

20. A 50-year-old lady is brought to the catheter lab for PCI having been diagnosed with a non-ST-segment elevation acute coronary syndrome (NSTE-ACS). She has a previous medical history of AF and normally takes apixaban 5 mg twice daily. Whilst on the ward prior to coming to the cath lab, she has been prescribed aspirin, clopidogrel, and apixaban.

Which of the following statements is incorrect?

A. During PCI, additional parenteral anticoagulation is recommended irrespective of the timing of the last dose of apixaban
B. PCI must be postponed and rescheduled for when the patient has been off her apixaban for a minimum period of 24 hours
C. Periprocedural dual antiplatelet therapy administration consisting of aspirin and clopidogrel up to 1 week is recommended
D. Following discharge, dual antithrombotic therapy is recommended as one strategy using apixaban 5 mg twice daily and clopidogrel 75 mg daily
E. Discontinuation of all antiplatelet agents is recommended in patients treated with an oral anticoagulant after 12 months

chapter 2.3

CARDIAC CATHETERIZATION

ANSWERS

1. A. According to the DVLA, driving may resume one week after ACS if successful percutaneous coronary intervention (PCI) is performed and there is no other urgent (within 4 weeks of acute event) revascularization planned, left ventricular ejection fraction is at least 40% before hospital discharge, and there is no other disqualifying condition. If not treated by successful PCI or any of the above are not met, driving may resume only after 4 weeks from the acute event, provided there is no other disqualifying condition.

2. B. This question is related to the inverse-square law of radiation ($1/x^2$) which means that doubling the distance from the radiation source reduces the radiation dose by a factor of 4. Therefore, using the inverse square law by increasing the distance between the operator and patient from 0.5 m to 0.75 m, the operator can decrease radiation exposure by approximately a half.

3. D. If access is via the right radial artery, the steeper angle of approach usually mandates using a shorter JL3.5 catheter. Longer catheters, e.g. JL5, are frequently required if the aorta is dilated therefore prior knowledge of aortic dimensions should be reviewed before starting the procedure if a previous echocardiogram has been performed. The primary (distal) curve engages and the secondary curve stabilizes on the opposite aortic wall. The left anterior oblique (LAO) cranial view is often the best view for assessing the left main stem ostium.

4. B. According to ESC guidelines, if there is extensive CAD, ejection fraction ≤35% and viable myocardium, CABG is favoured if the surgical risk is acceptable. ICD, CRT, and mineralocorticoid receptor antagonists are normally not started first line on diagnosing severe left ventricular systolic dysfunction before initiating an ACE inhibitor and beta-blocker and then re-evaluating.

5. C. The SHOCK trial showed that in patients with cardiogenic shock caused by acute myocardial infarction, emergency revascularization with PCI or CABG improved long-term survival when compared with initial intensive medical therapy. ESC guidelines recommend that emergency coronary angiography is indicated in acute heart failure or cardiogenic shock complicating ACS. CULPRIT-SHOCK trial showed that a strategy with PCI of the culprit lesion only with possible staged revascularization had a lower 30-day risk of the composite of all-cause mortality or severe renal failure compared with immediate multivessel PCI. ESC guidelines on myocardial revascularization (2018) recommend culprit lesion-only PCI as the default strategy in patients with AMI with cardiogenic shock. While initial studies with IABP were promising, the IABP-SHOCK II study demonstrated that routine use of intra-aortic balloon pumps in such cases is not associated with improved outcomes. The ESC guidelines on myocardial revascularization (2018) do not recommend the routine use of IABP in cardiogenic shock secondary to ACS.

6. B. The heart team has an important role when deciding on a revascularization strategy. Patient factors such as the patient's status and co-morbidities should be used in combination with the SYNTAX score to help guide decisions. The SYNTAX score II combines clinical variables (age, creatinine clearance, LVEF, left main disease, gender, COPD, PVD) with the anatomical SYNTAX score, providing expected 4-year mortality for both CABG and PCI. CABG is usually favoured in diabetic patients with complex three-vessel disease, especially left main and with intermediate or high SYNTAX scores (>22).

7. C. ESC guidelines on myocardial revascularization (2018) recommend drug eluting stents first line (class 1 level A recommendation) meaning that bare metal stents have now been phased out in many centres. These guidelines also recommend only considering glycoprotein IIb/IIIa in specific bailout situations including high intra-procedural thrombus burden, slow flow, or no flow with closure of stented coronary segment. Combining a potent P2Y12 inhibitor with an anticoagulant will increase bleeding risk. Cangrelor is an IV P2Y12 inhibitor which may be considered in patients who have not received an oral P2Y12 inhibitor.

8. A. ESC guidelines on myocardial revascularization (2018) recommend FFR or iFR first line in the assessment of the haemodynamic significance of intermediate-grade stenosis (class 1 level A recommendation). These guidelines also recommend that FFR-guided PCI should be considered in patients with multi-vessel disease under-going PCI (class IIa level B recommendation). As there is chest pain despite two anti-anginal medications, invasive management should be considered if indicated. There is no history of left main stem, proximal LAD, or three-vessel disease so there is no indication to consider CABG. Statin therapy is recommended for secondary prevention.

9. B. The ESC guidelines on myocardial revascularization (2018) recommend that IVUS should be considered to assess the severity of unprotected left main stem lesions (class IIa level B recommendation). These guidelines also recommend that IVUS or OCT should be used for stent optimization in selected patients (class IIa level B recommendation). OCT has good image resolution and can be used to evaluate stent characteristics and coronary calcium.

10. E. The ESC guidelines on myocardial revascularization (2018) do not recommend the routine use of aspiration thrombectomy. This is because the TOTAL trial showed no improvement in outcome but an increase in stroke rate with routine manual thrombectomy (0.7% in the thrombectomy arm vs 0.3% in the PCI only arm).

11. E. Moderate to severe aortic regurgitation is a contraindication to the use of IABP. Other contraindications include severe peripheral vascular disease, severe thrombocytopaenia, active haemorrhage, and a porcelain aorta.

12. E. Injection into distal vessels via a microcathether, aspiration, or dual lumen catheter using intracoronary nitrate, adenosine, verapamil, or sodium nitroprusside is preferred. According to ESC guidelines, glycoprotein IIb/IIIa drugs can also be considered in the treatment of no reflow.

13. C. After a thorough examination, if a femoral haemorrhage is suspected, an urgent CT scan to assess the femoral artery and exclude retroperitoneal haemorrhage should be considered, once the patient is stabilized. An ECG helps to exclude acute ischaemia and a focused echo helps to exclude important complications such as cardiac tamponade. Femoral ultrasound can be useful if a pseudoaneurysm is considered. However, in this situation, as there is haemodynamic instability, a large retroperitoneal bleed should be considered meaning that a CT scan would be more appropriate than an ultrasound. An A to E approach should be used in all situations in which significant haemodynamic instability is suspected.

14. E. There is a significant paucity of evidence to guide best practice in the prevention and managment of contrast-induced nephropathy. ESC guidelines on myocardial revascularization state that the minimum volume of use of low- or iso-osmolar contrast media should be used in patients with moderate-to-severe CKD. While N-acetylcysteine has been used in the past, there is limited clinical evidence to support its use. Its routine use has therefore fallen out of favour and it is not considered to be an essential treatment to limit deterioration caused by contrast-induced nephropathy.

15. D. Option D is the best answer as concordance would be seen in restrictive cardiomyopathy. The other features point towards a diagnosis of constrictive pericarditis. In constrictive pericarditis, the ventricular pressure trace would show ventricular discordance meaning that the peak RV pressure rises and peak LV pressure drops during inspiration. There can, however, be an increase in and equalization of end-diastolic pressures, pulmonary capillary wedge pressures in constrictive pericarditis, restrictive cardiomyopathy, and cardiac tamponade. However, in constrictive pericarditis, there is ventricular interdependence resulting in discordance of right and left ventricular pressures seen during simultaneous right and left heart catheterization making this a more sensitive sign. Risk factors for constrictive pericarditis include previous pericarditis, cardiac surgery, radiation therapy, and tuberculosis.

16. C. The left anterior oblique view is favourable to evaluate the right coronary ostium, proximal, and mid right coronary artery. The right anterior oblique view is favourable to evaluate mid RCA and branches to the RV. The left anterior oblique view with cranial angulation enables superior visualization of the distal RCA and facilitates evaluation of the bifurcation into the posterior LV branch and PDA.

17. A. Fondaparinux should be avoided if eGFR is less than 20 ml/min/1.73 m^2. For ticagrelor, a loading dose of 180 mg orally, followed by a maintenance dose of 90 mg twice daily can be used with no specific dose adjustment in CKD patients.

18. D. According to 2020 ESC guidelines, following PCI for non-ST-segment elevation acute coronary syndrome (NSTE-ACS), dual antiplatelet therapy consisting of a potent P2Y12 receptor inhibitor in addition to aspirin is generally recommended for 12 months. In patients with NSTE-ACS and stent implantation who are at high risk of bleeding (e.g. PRECISE-DAPT ≥25), discontinuation of P2Y12 receptor inhibitor therapy after 3–6 months should be considered. In patients at very high risk of bleeding, defined as a recent bleeding episode in the past month or planned, not deferrable surgery in the near future, 1 month of aspirin and clopidogrel should be considered.

19. A. According to ESC guidelines, concomitant use of a proton pump inhibitor is recommended in patients receiving antiplatelets and anticoagulants who are at risk of gastrointestinal bleeding in order to reduce the risk of gastric bleeds. In patients aged ≥75 years, prasugrel should only be used with caution and at a dose of 5 mg od if treatment is deemed necessary. It is recommended to apply the same diagnostic strategies in older patients as for younger patients. Glycoprotein IIb/IIIa inhibitor may only be considered in specific bailout situations including high intra-procedural thrombus burden, slow flow, or no flow with closure of stented coronary segment. Following ACS, MRAs are recommended in patients with heart failure with reduced LVEF (<40%) in order to reduce all-cause and cardiovascular mortality and cardiovascular morbidity.

20. B. According to ESC 2020 guidelines for acute coronary syndromes in patients presenting without persistent ST-segment elevation, uninterrupted therapeutic anticoagulation with vitamin A antagonist (VKA) or NOAC should be considered during the periprocedural phase. Also, during

PCI, additional parenteral anticoagulation is recommended irrespective of the timing of the last dose of NOAC and if INR is <2.5 in VKA treated patients. Periprocedural dual antiplatelet therapy administration consisting of aspirin and clopidogrel up to 1 week is recommended. Following the procedure, dual antithrombotic therapy is recommended as the default strategy using NOAC at the recommended dose for stroke prevention and a single antiplatelet, preferably clopidogrel. While it may seem counterintuitive, ESC guidelines state that discontinuation of the antiplatelet is recommended in patients treated with an oral anticoagulant after 12 months.

chapter 3

VALVULAR HEART DISEASE

chapter

3.1

VALVULAR HEART DISEASE

QUESTIONS

1. A 56-year-old male patient is identified to have to have severe aortic regurgitation through a trileaflet aortic valve. He is clinically asymptomatic and otherwise well. There is no family history of aortopathy.

Which of the following would be an indication for aortic valve surgery?

A. Tubular ascending aorta measuring 48 mm.
B. Ejection fraction 56%
C. Left ventricular end diastolic dimension of 55 mm
D. Left ventricular end systolic dimension of 53 mm
E. Systemic hypertension

2. A 39-year-old female patient is listed for mitral valve repair. Her main presentation is of breathlessness and reduced exercise tolerance.

In what circumstance may coronary artery disease be assessed by CT coronary angiography?

A. Mild left ventricular dysfunction in the absence of chest pain
B. Presence of an atypical story for ischaemic chest pain
C. Previously successful PCI with no ongoing symptoms
D. Treated hypertension
E. Pre-menopausal status and absence of ischaemic symptoms and risk factors

3. A 28-year-old male intravenous drug user presents with tricuspid valve endocarditis and severe tricuspid regurgitation. He has no prior medical problems. Prior to his presentation, his exercise tolerance was good and he did not suffer from chest pain. Following heart team discussion, it is agreed that he should proceed to tricuspid valve repair.

Which of the following non-invasive tests are appropriate to assess for coronary artery disease?

A. CT coronary angiography
B. Exercise tolerance test
C. Dobutamine stress echocardiography
D. Myocardial perfusion scanning
E. Exercise echocardiography

4. Quantitative markers of severe primary mitral regurgitation include:

A. Vena contracta ≥6 mm
B. E wave dominant inflow > 1.2 m/s
C. Effective regurgitant orifice area (EROA) ≥30 mm^2
D. A regurgitant volume of > 45 ml/beat
E. Systolic hepatic vein reversal

5. Which of the following is the most common aetiology of aortic regurgitation in the Western population?

A. Rheumatic heart disease
B. Infective endocarditis
C. Degenerative valve disease
D. Aortic dissection
E. Aortic root dilatation

6. A 75-year-old male patient of normal stature is seen in clinic with reduced exercise tolerance and exertional chest pains. His GP identified an ejection systolic murmur. Transthoracic echocardiography identified a calcified trileaflet aortic valve with peak velocity of 3.0 m/s and a mean gradient of 31 mmHg. The valve area as calculated by the continuity equation was 0.8 cm^2. The ejection fraction is 40% and indexed stroke volume 30 ml/m^2.

What would be the next recommended test to assess to assess whether the aortic stenosis is severe or not?

A. Exercise tolerance test
B. CT calcium score assessment of the aortic valve
C. Transoesophageal echocardiography with planimetry assessment of the aortic valve
D. Cardiac MRI
E. Dobutamine echocardiography

7. You are reviewing an 82-year-old female patient in clinic. She has been referred for assessment due to an ejection systolic murmur radiating to the carotids. She has a background history of treated hyperthyroidism and hypertension. An echocardiogram has identified a peak aortic velocity of 3.5 m/s. Her mean gradient is 33 mmHg. The aortic valve area is 0.8 cm^2. The report highlights that her indexed stroke volume is reduced, but the ejection fraction is normal.

What term best describes her aortic pathology?

A. Low flow, low gradient aortic stenosis with reduced ejection fraction
B. High gradient aortic stenosis
C. Low flow, low gradient aortic stenosis with preserved ejection fraction
D. Normal flow, low gradient aortic stenosis with preserved ejection fraction
E. Pseudosevere aortic stenosis

8. A 72-year-old lady is followed up in the cardiology clinic. She was recently an inpatient with a lower respiratory tract infection. During her admission she was noted to have an ejection systolic murmur and an outpatient echocardiogram has identified severe aortic stenosis with peak velocity of 4.2 m/s and an aortic valve area of 0.8 cm^2. She has recovered well post her admission and has returned to her previous performance status. Prior to admission she was independent and did not feel limited by shortness of breath or chest pains. There is no history of syncope.

Which of the following findings would be an indication to refer her for surgical aortic valve replacement?

A. Left ventricular ejection fraction 58%
B. Abnormal exercise tolerance test with symptoms on exercise
C. Exercise tolerance test with 10–20mmHg increase in systolic blood pressure on exercise
D. A need for elective inguinal hernia repair
E. A normal NT proBNP level

9. A 54-year-old male presents with angina from symptomatic aortic stenosis with a peak velocity of 4.3 m/s. Coronary angiography has revealed unobstructed coronary arteries. His EuroSCORE II is <4% and he is otherwise well.

How should he be managed?

A. Monitoring at 6 months for new symptoms of heart failure or syncope
B. Surgical aortic valve replacement (SAVR)
C. Exercise test
D. Medical therapy
E. Transcatheter aortic valve implantation

10. A 70-year-old male presents to the emergency department with a 50-minute history of acute chest pain. An ECG demonstrates T wave changes in leads II, III, aVF and an initial diagnosis of non-ST-elevation ACS is made. Arrangements for percutaneous coronary angiography are made. Previous medical history includes a mechanical aortic valve, hypertension well controlled with losartan, and mild left ventricular impairment. He was otherwise wise well and active. Regular medication includes warfarin, losartan, and bisoprolol. He is a non-smoker and consumes one glass of wine with his evening meal each day. His weight is 83 kg. He undergoes an uncomplicated PCI to his right coronary artery with a drug eluting stent. There is mild distal LAD atheroma. The mid circumflex has moderate disease (60%).

Following his PCI, what antithrombotic strategy should be chosen?

A. One week of triple therapy (aspirin, clopidogrel, and warfarin) followed by dual therapy with clopidogrel and warfarin, followed by warfarin alone after 12 months.
B. Six months of clopidogrel and warfarin followed by warfarin alone after 6 months.
C. Six months of triple therapy, followed by six months of dual therapy, followed by warfarin alone.
D. Switch to DOAC and give a month triple therapy, then clopidogrel and DOAC to 12 months, then DOAC only.
E. Six months of triple therapy, then continue warfarin and clopidogrel lifelong.

11. A 68-year-old female with known atrial fibrillation attends for review. Previous echocardiography has shown a left ventricle of normal size and function and moderate mitral regurgitation. Valve leaflets were mobile. She is otherwise well with no other medical history and is asymptomatic from her arrhythmia. She has been established on warfarin. However, she wishes to discuss the need for an anticoagulant and possible alternatives to warfarin.

Which one of the following statements is correct?

A. Monotherapy with aspirin will suffice.
B. A non-vitamin K antagonist oral anticoagulant (NOAC) is contraindicated due to mitral valve disease. She should continue warfarin.
C. She is low risk and may discontinue anticoagulation.
D. She should be referred for left atrial appendage occlusion.
E. A NOAC may be offered as an alternative to warfarin post appropriate counselling.

12. A 48-year-old Egyptian male presents with exertional breathlessness and chest pain. He is an ex-smoker. He works as a barber and prior to his current presentation was well. A transthoracic echocardiogram demonstrates severe mitral stenosis with a mitral valve area of 1.4 cm^2 on planimetry. His overall ventricular function demonstrates mild impairment. He is in sinus rhythm. He proceeds to have coronary angiography. This demonstrates three-vessel disease with severe narrowing and calcification of the left main stem.

How should he be managed?

A. Percutaneous coronary intervention as first line and reassess symptoms post revascularization
B. Exercise stress echocardiography
C. Combined, or in short time frame, percutaneous coronary intervention and percutaneous mitral commissurotomy
D. Coronary artery bypass grafting and mitral valve surgery
E. Coronary artery bypass grafting and percutaneous mitral commissurotomy

13. An asymptomatic 68-year-old man had an echocardiogram after his GP found a heart murmur. He was found to have severe primary mitral regurgitation.

Which of the following is not an indication for consideration for surgery in this man?

A. Left ventricular ejection fraction 55%
B. Left ventricular ejection fraction 45%
C. LVESD 50 mm
D. LVEDD 61 mm
E. New AF

14. An asymptomatic 70-year-old woman with low surgical risk is being followed up in clinic for severe aortic stenosis.

Which of the following would prompt surgical referral?

A. A rise in blood pressure on exercising
B. Severe valve calcification and a rate of Vmax progression of 0.3 m/s/year
C. LVEF 58%
D. New AF
E. Elevated BNP levels to 1.5 × corrected normal range

15. A 45-year-old woman was referred for echocardiogram after her brother was found to have a bicuspid aortic valve. She had a trileaflet aortic valve with a central jet of aortic regurgitation. The pressure half-time was recorded as 400 ms. She had no symptoms. Her only past medical history of note is hypertension.

Which of the following statements is true?

A. Her children should have a screening echocardiogram
B. She should have a repeat echocardiogram in 6 months
C. She should be considered for aortic root surgery if her ascending aortic diameter is 48 mm
D. She should have surgery if her LVEDD is 55 mm
E. Presence of holodiastolic flow reversal in the descending aorta would question the accuracy of the pressure half-time measurement

16. A 73-year-old man was seen in clinic for follow-up of his known for valvular heart disease. His echocardiogram showed a calcified bicuspid aortic valve with a mean pressure drop of 45 mmHg, mitral regurgitation with a dense continuous wave doppler signal of the regurgitant jet with a vena contracta of 8mm and tricuspid regurgitation that was reported as severe. His aortic root measured 45 mm. He reported he felt short of breath on exertion.

Which of the following statements is false?

A. The aortic stenosis gradient may be underestimated due to the mitral regurgitation
B. Even in the absence of signs of right heart failure, TV repair should be considered if he has surgery on his aortic valve
C. He would require a coronary angiogram pre-surgery given his age
D. There will be diastolic pulmonary vein flow reversal
E. If he has surgery for his aortic valve, replacement of his aortic root should be considered

17. A 83-year-old lady was admitted with shortness of breath on minimal exertion. Her echo showed a calcified aortic valve with a Vmax of 3.3 m/s and a mean gradient of 33 mmHg. The area was calculated as 0.8 cm^2. Her LVEF by Simpson's biplane is recorded as 35%.

Which of the following statements is true?

A. A flow status of SVi 25 ml/m^2 makes severe aortic stenosis unlikely
B. The next step in management should be a CT for calcium score
C. A low dose dobutamine stress echo is inappropriate given she has dyspnoea on minimal exertion
D. A deep transgastric transoesophageal echocardiogram (TOE) would give a better Doppler trace for calculation of velocity and gradient.
E. None of the above

18. A 70-year-old man is being followed up for known mitral regurgitation and is seen in outpatient clinic, where he denies any symptoms. His most recent echo report states 'The mitral valve leaflets are slightly thickened. There is prolapse of the anterior leaflet with a jet of posteriorly directed regurgitation which reaches the back of a dilated atrium. The Doppler signal is dense.'

Which of the following statements is correct?

A. The report describes a Carpentier Type 3 mechanism of mitral regurgitation
B. A dominant E wave of 1.5 m/s would support this being severe mitral regurgitation
C. An LV end diastolic dimension of 58 mm would be an indication for surgery
D. A TVI mitral/TVI aortic of 1.2 would support this being severe mitral regurgitation
E. None of the above

19. Regarding the tricuspid valve, what is the most common aetiology of pathological tricuspid regurgitation?

A. Secondary to right ventricular dysfunction.
B. Ebstein's anomaly
C. Carcinoid syndrome
D. Myxomatous disease
E. Infective endocarditis

20. A 29-year-old female presents with breathlessness and palpitations. Echocardiography demonstrates tricuspid regurgitation and right ventricular basal dimensions of 4.1 cm and tricuspid annular plane systolic excursion (TAPSE) of 1.6 cm.

Which of the following is the best test for assessing right ventricular (RV) size and function?

A. RV global longitudinal strain
B. TOE including detailed assessment of the atrial septum
C. Cardiac catheterization
D. Cardiac MRI
E. Assessment of fractional area change on transthoracic echocardiogram

21. A 52-year-old male presents with severe mitral regurgitation and left ventricular dilatation due to mitral valve prolapse. Assessment of the tricuspid valve reveals moderate tricuspid regurgitation. The tricuspid annulus measures 41 mm. The tricuspid regurgitation is thought to be secondary to the mitral valve disease. The patient is referred for mitral valve surgery.

How should the tricuspid regurgitation be managed?

A. Tricuspid valve replacement
B. Tricuspid valve repair with ring annuloplasty
C. Surgical treatment of mitral valve disease: consider tricuspid valve surgery at a later point if developing right heart failure symptoms
D. Surgical treatment of mitral valve disease and ongoing diuretic therapy
E. Repeat echocardiography prior to mitral valve surgery; for tricuspid valve surgery if worsening dilatation

22. A well 72-year-old male is followed up in clinic. He had a mechanical aortic valve replacement 6 years previously with a Carbomedics valve. He has had a thromboembolic stroke 2 years ago with some residual right arm weakness. His valve is functioning well and left ventricular ejection fraction is reported at 51%.

What should his target INR be?

A. 2.0
B. 2.5
C. 3.0
D. 3.5
E. 4.0

23. A patient with a previous mechanical aortic valve replacement presents with an episode of dysphasia. Cerebral imaging confirms the presence of a thromboembolic infarct. Transthoracic echocardiography reveals the presence of a 7 mm × 6 mm thrombus on the aortic valve. The patient has recently missed some doses of anticoagulation. The patient is otherwise well.

What is the next step in management of this case of mechanical prosthetic well obstruction?

A. Surgery to aortic valve
B. Valve in valve TAVI
C. Fibrinolysis
D. Valve fluoroscopy
E. Optimization of anticoagulation

24. A 75-year-old male is seen by the general surgeons for an elective cholecystectomy. Perioperative assessment identifies an ejection systolic murmur which is evaluated by transthoracic echocardiography. This reveals severe aortic stenosis. He is otherwise asymptomatic. He would like his hernia repaired.

How should his aortic stenosis be managed with regard to his non-cardiac surgery?

A. Proceed with non-cardiac surgery
B. Surgical aortic valve replacement prior to non-cardiac surgery
C. Proceed with non-cardiac surgery with strict monitoring
D. Balloon aortic valvuloplasty prior to non-cardiac surgery and reassess for definitive management
E. Transcatheter aortic valve implantation

chapter 3.1

VALVULAR HEART DISEASE

ANSWERS

1. D. Indications for surgery in aortic regurgitation include: Symptomatic patients, asymptomatic patients with resting LV ejection fraction ≤ 50% (or ≤55% if low risk for surgery), undergoing CABG or surgery of the ascending aorta or of another valve, symptomatic patients with resting ejection fraction >50% with severe LV dilatation : LV end-systolic diameter >50 mm (or LVESD >25 mm/m^2 in patients with small body size)

2. E. CT angiography should be considered as an alternative to coronary angiography before valve surgery in patients with severe VHD and low probability of CAD, or in whom conventional coronary angiography is technically not feasible or who are at high risk. Coronary angiography is recommended before valve surgery in patients with severe VHD and any of the following:

- History of cardiovascular disease
- Suspected myocardial ischaemia
- LV systolic dysfunction
- In men >40 years of age and postmenopausal women
- One or more cardiovascular risk factors

3. A. He is under 40 and has no risk factors for coronary artery disease and so CTCA can be used if pre-test probability of CAD is low. The use of stress tests to detect CAD associated with severe valvular disease is discouraged.

4. B. Markers of severe MR are a vena contracta ≥ 7mm, systolic pulmonary, (rather than hepatic) vein reversal, E wave dominance > 1.2 m/s. The values stated for EROA and RV are applicable for secondary MR under certain circumstance and not for primary MR.

5. C. Degenerative aortic valve disease is the most common cause.

6. E. This patient has low gradient, low flow aortic stenosis. The SVi <35 ml/m^2 and the reduced ejection fraction has highlighted this. The next test advocated by the ESC would be a dobutamine echocardiogram. If flow reserve is present then this will either lead to an increase in aortic valve area to > 1.0 cm^2 which would give a diagnosis of pseudosevere AS or evidence of criteria that would allow true severe AS to be diagnosed.

7. C. This is an example of low flow (SVi <35ml/m^2), low gradient (<40mmHg) aortic stenosis with preserved ejection fraction. This is most commonly encountered in the elderly with a history of hypertension and left ventricular hypertrophy. There is a place for multislice CT in providing a calcium score for the aortic valve. Scores of greater than 1,600 in females and 3,000 in males suggest that the patient is highly likely have severe aortic stenosis.

8. B. The best indication for surgical aortic valve replacement in an asymptomatic patient would be the identification of symptoms on exercise tolerance testing. Patients can often adapt to their limitations if they are developing slowly and exercise testing is an objective way of revealing the situation. Guidance only advocates surgery if the blood pressure falls on exercise. Surgery is indicated if the ejection fraction is less than 50% provided this is not due to an alternative cause. Non-cardiac surgery can be performed safely in patients with asymptomatic aortic stenosis.

9. B. This patient has severe, high-gradient aortic stenosis. Factors favouring SAVR include the low EuroSCORE II and his age

10. A. The patient has a mechanical aortic valve and coronary disease that required treatment with coronary intervention. Wafarin must therefore be continued. The 2023 ESC Guidelines for the management of Acute Coronary Syndromes recommends that in ACS patients in whom warfarin is mandated, there should be up to a one week period of triple therapy before switching to warfarin and a single antiplatelet, preferably clopidogrel.

11. E. The NOACs are suitable for use in atrial fibrillation associated with valvular heart disease with the exception of moderate and severe mitral stenosis.

12. D. He has severe mitral stenosis and coronary disease. The coronary disease described would be best treated by CABG. Concomitant coronary artery disease requiring bypass surgery is a contraindication for percutaneous mitral commissurotomy.

13. D. Indications for surgery in asymptomatic primary severe mitral regurgitation are:

- LVEF≤60%
- LVESD ≥40mm
- new AF
- SPAP >50 mmHg
- LA volume ≥60 ml/m^2 BSA

14. B. Indications for surgery in asymptomatic aortic stenosis from exercise tests are symptoms on exercise clearly related to aortic stenosis or a decrease in blood pressure below baseline on exercising. LVEF <50% not due to another cause should also prompt referral for SAVR. Other reasons to consider SAVR in asymptomatic patients with severe AS and low surgical risk are Vmax >5 m/s; mean gradient ≥60 mmHg; severe valve calcification and a rate of Vmax progression ≥ 0.3 m/s/year; markedly elevated BNP levels (>threefold age- and sex-corrected normal ranges) without other explanations; severe pulmonary hypertension (systolic pulmonary artery pressure at rest >60 mmHg confirmed by invasive measurement) without other explanation.

15. E. There is no information in the question to suggest her children should have a screening echocardiogram. A pressure half time of 400 ms suggests moderate aortic regurgitation, and the ESC guidelines suggest yearly clinical review with echocardiograms every 2 years. She does not require surgery as she does not have severe aortic regurgitation from the information provided; if she did, LVEDD >65 mm and progressive dilation could be an indication for surgery. Given that she does not require aortic valve surgery no intervention is needed on her root when it is 48 mm. Holodiastolic flow reversal in the descending aorta suggests severe aortic regurgitation, which would be inconsistent with the pressure half-time measurement reported.

16. D. The echo findings suggest severe aortic stenosis. This is despite the fact that the aortic stenosis may be underestimated due to the mitral regurgitation. If he had surgery given the TR is moderate concurrent TV repair should be considered. As he is over 40 years of age he should have a coronary angiogram before valve surgery. Surgery for the aortic root should be considered if it is ≥45 mm if he is having surgery on the aortic valve, particularly in the presence of a bicuspid valve. Given that he has severe mitral regurgitation, he may have systolic pulmonary vein flow reversal.

17. E. The aortic stenosis is low gradient by Vmax and mean gradient, but may still be severe given the valve area is calculated as 0.8 cm^2 (in the context of impaired LV ejection fraction). The next steps should be to exclude measurement errors, and then define the flow states. This is likely to be low (SVi <35 ml/m^2). Given that she has an LVEF of 35% a low dose dobutamine stress echo would be appropriate to further assess the severity of the aortic stenosis.

18. B. The Carpentier classification is:

i. Type 1: normal leaflet motion
ii. Type 2: leaflet prolapse
iii. Type 3: restricted leaflet mobility.

This question therefore describes Carpentier type 2.

A dominant E wave ≥1.2 m/s would support this being severe mitral regurgitation, so this is correct. TVI mitral/TVI aortic needs to be greater than 1.4 to support severe MR. It is the left ventricular end systolic dimension which is important in determining need for surgery in asymptomatic mitral regurgitation, not the end diastolic dimension.

19. A. Pathological tricuspid regurgitation is most commonly due to right ventricular dysfunction occurring following pressure and/or volume overload in the presence of normal valve leaflets. Other causes, in addition to those in the question include: rheumatic heart disease, endomyocardial fibrosis, congenitally dysplastic valves, drug induced valve disease, thoracic trauma, and iatrogenic damage.

20. D. Cardiac MRI is seen as the gold standard for assessing RV volumes and function. In experienced hands 3D echocardiographic assessment can achieve results comparable to MRI. Assessment of fractional area change is less reliable than cardiac MRI. Whilst the presentation may be linked to an atrial septal defect which may be evaluated by a TOE the question is seeking the optimum test to assess RV size and function.

21. B. In secondary tricuspid valve regurgitation tricuspid repair should be performed when the patient is undergoing left sided surgery either if the tricuspid regurgitation is severe, or if the tricuspid regurgitation is mild or moderate and there is tricuspid annular dilatation of 40 mm or greater or recent right heart failure. Reoperation at a later date after mitral valve surgery confers a higher risk.

22. C. The ESC recommends median target values for INR rather than ranges with a mechanical prothesis. The rationale is that this avoids a situation whereby the extreme values of the range are considered as valid targets. The target is based on patient factors and the thrombogenicity of the prosthesis. Patient factors include: a mitral or tricuspid valve replacement, mitral stenosis of any degree, previous thromboembolism, atrial fibrillation, and left ventricular ejection fraction of < 35%. The thrombogenicity of the valve is categorized as low, medium, or high (Table 3.1.A1). Low thrombogenicity valves include Carbomedics, Medtronic Hall, ATS, Medtronic Open-Pivot, St Jude Medical, On-X and Sorin Bicarbon; medium thrombogenicity are other bileaflet valves with insufficient data; high thrombogenicity include Lillehei-Kaster, Omniscience, Starr-Edwards (ball-cage), Bjork-Shiley, and other tilting-disc valves. A summary of target INR is shown in Table 3.1.A1.

Table 3.1.A1

Prothesis thrombogenicity	**Patient-related risk factors**	
	None	**≥1 Risk factor**
Low	2.5	3.0
Medium	3.0	3.5
High	3.5	4.0

23. E. This is a case of left sided non-obstructive mechanical prosthetic thrombosis. The diagnosis can be confirmed by transthoracic or transoesophageal echocardiography, cinefluoroscopy or CT scanning. Surgery is indicated in the setting of thromboembolism with a large thrombus measuring greater than 10 mm. Fibrinolysis may be indicated if surgery is high risk. In this patient as the thrombus is less than 10 mm initial management is to optimize anticoagulation and then follow up. If thrombus is still present and there are recurrent thromboembolic events then surgery (or fibrinolysis) should be performed. If the size of the thrombus is decreasing, follow-up can be continued. Of those patients with a large thrombus but no thromboembolic complications optimization of anticoagulation is again advised with intervention reserved for those with a persistent thrombus or thromboembolic complications. Patients with smaller amounts of thrombus and no complications are managed in the same way as patients with a small thrombus and thromboembolism.

24. A. The patient is asymptomatic from his aortic stenosis. The approach should then be determined post an assessment of risk of cardiac complications of the procedure he is listed for. A cholecystectomy is an intermediate risk procedure and this asymptomatic patient can proceed with non-cardiac surgery. If the patient was symptomatic from aortic stenosis and a non-cardiac elective operation desired, then the aortic stenosis should be treated first if the patient is low risk for aortic valve replacement. If high risk then non-cardiac surgery can proceed under strict monitoring only if the procedure is strictly needed.

chapter 3.2

INFECTIVE ENDOCARDITIS

QUESTIONS

1. **A 72-year-old male patient with a background history of bioprosthetic aortic valve replacement for severe degenerative aortic stenosis presents for routine review 5 years after surgery. He enquires about the risk of infective endocarditis and need for prophylactic antibiotic treatment.**

   In which of the following scenarios should antibiotic prophylaxis be considered?

   A. Urinary catheterization X
   B. Adjustment of removable dentures X
   C. Treatment of superficial caries under local anaesthetic
   D. Subgingival ultrasonic dental scaling
   E. None of the above

2. **A 34-year-old female patient with a background history of recurrent miscarriages and unprovoked deep vein thrombosis presents with a posterior circulation stroke. As part of her work up, she undergoes a transthoracic echocardiogram showing a sessile, broad based 6 mm lesion on the basal portion of the posterior mitral valve leaflet, associated with leaflet thickening.**

   Which of the following investigations is most likely to yield a unifying diagnosis?

   A. Three sets of blood cultures
   B. Transoesophageal echocardiogram (TOE)
   C. Full blood count
   D. Anti-nuclear antibodies (ANA)
   E. Antiphospholipid antibodies

3. A 44-year-old patient with a background history of hypertension was admitted with aortic valve infective endocarditis. He is known to have a hypermobile 1.5-cm mobile vegetation associated with severe aortic regurgitation and is currently undergoing IV antibiotic therapy with a view to aortic valve replacement. He is haemodynamically stable and inflammatory markers are improving.

Which of the following investigations would be most appropriate prior to surgery?

A. Invasive coronary angiography
B. Dobutamine stress echocardiogram
C. Cardiac CT
D. Exercise tolerance test
E. None of the above

4. A 45-year-old patient presents to the orthopaedic team with back pain and sepsis. An MRI of the lumbar spine shows multilevel discitis with associated abscess formation. All three sets of blood cultures taken prior to administration of broad-spectrum antibiotics show *Staphylococcus aureus* **and a transthoracic echocardiogram is non-diagnostic.**

Which of the following statements is correct?

A. Transthoracic echocardiography is not indicated unless there are specific signs pointing towards a diagnosis of infective endocarditis
B. Addition of gentamicin is not recommended in native valve infective endocarditis caused by methicillin-susceptible staphylococci
C. Left-sided *S. aureus* native valve infective endocarditis has better prognosis than right-sided native valve infective endocarditis
D. Eradication of the primary source of infection is always necessary prior to cardiac surgical intervention for infective endocarditis
E. Co-trimoxazole monotherapy is an appropriate treatment option for native valve *S. aureus* endocarditis

5. A 58-year-old male patient presents to hospital with a 2-week history of malaise, fever, and shortness of breath. Clinical examination reveals a new aortic regurgitant murmur, splinter haemorrhages, and finger clubbing. Inflammatory markers are significantly elevated and blood cultures show a group G streptococcus. A transthoracic echocardiogram demonstrates an aortic valve vegetation consistent with infective endocarditis.

Which of the following clinical features is not an indication for surgical management of infective endocarditis?

A. Severe aortic regurgitation and elevated left ventricular end diastolic pressure
B. 12-mm vegetation with moderate aortic regurgitation
C. Positive blood cultures 7 days after commencement of appropriate antibiotic therapy
D. 12-mm vegetation and evidence of splenic emboli despite antibiotic therapy
E. Evidence of aortic root abscess

6. **A 55-year-old woman with a history of atrial fibrillation and mitral valve repair is receiving IV benzylpenicillin and gentamicin for *Streptococcus pneumoniae* mitral valve infective endocarditis. Three days into treatment she remains febrile and complains of a headache, followed by drowsiness and subtle left arm weakness.**

Which of the following statements is correct?

A. Cardiac surgery is not recommended after an ischaemic stroke
B. Cardiac surgery should be postponed >3 months after a haemorrhagic stroke
C. Mycotic aneurysms are only rarely found within the cerebral vasculature
D. Escalation of antibiotic therapy to ceftriaxone may be required
E. ^{18}F-FDG PET/CT imaging can be helpful in diagnosing metastatic brain infections

7. **A 55-year-old patient with a history of metallic aortic valve replacement for a bicuspid aortic valve presents to hospital with a 3-week history of fever and malaise. Inflammatory markers are mildly elevated and cardiac auscultation reveals a diastolic murmur. Transthoracic echocardiography confirms significant paravalvular aortic regurgitation.**

Which of the following is incorrect?

A. Use of radiolabelled leucocyte SPECT/CT may be indicated
B. 3D echocardiography is a gold standard technique to detect perivalvular extension of infection
C. High degree AV block is associated with worse prognosis
D. A negative TOE does not exclude the diagnosis of infective endocarditis
E. Rifampicin should be delayed in staphylococcal infections until day 3–5 of effective antibiotic therapy

8. **A 28-year-old patient is receiving antibiotic treatment for streptococcal mitral valve endocarditis associated with severe mitral regurgitation and a 20 mm hypermobile vegetation. He has completed 4 weeks of IV antibiotic therapy and is currently being prepared for surgery.**

Which of the following statements is correct?

A. Day 1 of effective antibiotic therapy is determined by the first day when the patient received a full dose of a given antibiotic regimen.
B. The post-operative antibiotic regimen in native valve endocarditis requiring valve replacement during antibiotic therapy should be switched to one suitable for prosthetic valve endocarditis.
C. The intended duration of antibiotic therapy in surgically managed infective endocarditis should begin on day 1 of effective antibiotic therapy.
D. The duration of antibiotic treatment should be extended by 2 weeks from the date of surgery if valve cultures are positive.
E. Intraoperative TOE is unlikely to be necessary.

9. A 45-year-old patient with a history of severe aortic stenosis affecting a bicuspid valve and aortic dilatation underwent aortic root and valve replacement. He recovered well but developed low-grade fever and fatigue a few weeks later. He was admitted to hospital and found to have significantly elevated inflammatory markers. Clinical examination was unremarkable except for the presence of a few splinter haemorrhages. Although blood cultures grew coagulase-negative staphylococci in two sets, no extra-cardiac source of infection was found and a TOE showed non-specific post-operative changes only.

Which of the following would be the next investigation of choice?

A. CT thorax
B. ^{18}F-FDG PET/CT
C. Radio-labelled leucocyte SPECT/CT
D. USS chest wall
E. No further investigation required

10. A 76-year-old patient with a history of bi-ventricular pacemaker implantation for ischaemic cardiomyopathy and complete heart block presents with a tender and erythematous implant site associated with fever and malaise. Blood cultures grow *Staphylococcus epidermis*. Although TTE and TOE do not show evidence of endocarditis, ^{18}F-FDG-PET/CT reveals areas of increased uptake around the device pocket.

Which of the following is correct?

A. Device box extraction is sufficient to control the infection.
B. IV antibiotics should continue for 2 weeks if blood cultures are still positive after extraction.
C. Blood cultures should be negative for 24 hours prior to the procedure if a new device is to be re-implanted.
D. Surgical lead extraction is preferred to transvenous extraction.
E. A temporary externalised pacemaker is an appropriate option in pacing dependent patients while awaiting device reimplantation.

11. A 22-year-old patient who is an intravenous drug user presents to hospital with haemoptysis and fever. A CT pulmonary angiogram shows multiple septic pulmonary emboli with evidence of right heart strain, and an incomplete view of the left kidney suggests renal infarcts. He undergoes a transthoracic echocardiogram that reveals a 2.5-cm tricuspid valve vegetation with associated severe tricuspid regurgitation. Blood cultures show a heavy growth of *Staphylococcus aureus* and blood cultures remain positive fourteen days after initiation of antibiotic therapy.

Which of the following statements is correct?

A. TOE is not indicated
B. Tricuspid valvectomy without replacement is the treatment of choice in current intravenous drug users
C. Surgical management should be considered in severe tricuspid regurgitation associated with right heart failure
D. Tricuspid valve repair is associated with better outcomes than valve replacement
E. Pulmonary hypertension is a contraindication to surgical management

12. A 54-year-old lawyer who is currently undergoing antibiotic treatment for mitral valve endocarditis develops sudden onset right-sided hemiparesis with inattention and aphasia. A CT head scan performed within 1 hour of the event shows hyper-density in the left middle cerebral artery with early signs of infarction in the same territory. The National Institute of Health Stroke Scale (NIHSS) score is 22.

What is the most appropriate treatment strategy?

A. Intravenous alteplase administration.
B. Referral to a tertiary centre for mechanical thrombectomy.
C. Two-week course of aspirin 300 mg, followed by formal anticoagulation with a direct oral anticoagulant.
D. Aspirin 300 mg until definitive surgical management.
E. Immediate valve surgery.

13. A 76-year-old patient presents with fever and malaise three weeks after transurethral resection of the prostate. His inflammatory markers are significantly elevated and there is evidence of proteinuria and haematuria. A bedside echocardiogram suggests a 0.8cm aortic valve vegetation with associated aortic regurgitation. Three sets of blood cultures have been taken but results are pending.

Which of the following organisms is the most likely explanation for this presentation?

A. *Staphylococcus aureus*
B. *Enterococcus faecalis*
C. *Escherichia coli*
D. *Streptococcus gallolyticus* (formerly *S. bovis*)
E. *Enterococcus faecium*

14. A 45-year-old patient with a history of mitral valve replacement performed 4 years previously presents with several days' fever and shortness of breath. She had a recent dental extraction performed without antibiotic prophylaxis. On admission she is hypotensive and tachycardic with a loud pansystolic murmur and bilateral lung crepitations. Urinalysis reveals proteinuria and haematuria. Inflammatory markers are markedly elevated with evidence of an acute kidney injury. Three sets of blood cultures are taken.

According to 2023 ESC guidelines, what is the most appropriate antibiotic regimen?

A. Await blood culture results before commencing a targeted antibiotic regime.
B. Ceftriaxone monotherapy
C. Benzylpenicillin + gentamicin
D. Vancomycin + gentamicin + rifampicin
E. Ampicillin + flucloxacillin + gentamicin

15. A 55-year-old nurse is undergoing outpatient treatment for uncomplicated *Streptococcus viridans* aortic valve endocarditis and presents for review after three weeks of IV ceftriaxone. He denies fevers and feels well in himself, although CRP and WCC are increasing. An ECG performed in the ambulatory clinic shows sinus rhythm with a PR interval of 270 ms, QRS duration of 110 ms, and QT_c interval of 430 ms. Previous ECGs have been normal.

What is the most appropriate course of action?

A. Further routine review in 3 days
B. Routine outpatient transthoracic echocardiogram
C. Urgent outpatient transthoracic echocardiogram
D. Urgent outpatient TOE
E. Admit for inpatient management

16. A 72-year-old patient with a history of hypertension and diabetes presents with a history of fever and malaise. Her inflammatory markers are elevated and blood cultures grow *Streptococcus gallolyticus* (formerly *S. bovis*). An echocardiogram shows a 7-mm vegetation on the anterior mitral valve leaflet with mild mitral regurgitation. She has microcytic anaemia and admits to altered bowel habit over the past few months.

What is the most appropriate course of action?

A. Refer to gastroenterology for routine OP review
B. Faecal occult blood (FOB) testing
C. CT abdomen/pelvis
D. PET/CT abdomen/pelvis
E. Inpatient colonoscopy

17. A 33-year-old patient who works at a petting farm presents with a several month history of intermittent fevers, night sweats, and unintentional weight loss >5 kg. Her past medical history includes a bicuspid aortic valve and hospitalization for pneumonia associated with transaminitis 12 months previously. On examination she appears chronically unwell with finger clubbing, mild splenomegaly and a quiet ejection systolic murmur. An echocardiogram reveals two subtle echogenic lesions attached to the aortic valve leaflets.

Which of the following tests is most likely to yield a diagnosis?

A. Three sets of blood cultures
B. *Coxiella burnetti* serology
C. Beta-glucan antigen
D. *Legionella pneumophila* serology
E. *Bartonella henselae* serology

18. A 24-year-old female patient with residual moderate pulmonary regurgitation after tetralogy of Fallot repair is 32 weeks pregnant and the obstetrics team enquire about the need for antibiotic prophylaxis at the time of delivery.

Which of the following statements is correct?

A. Antibiotic prophylaxis is only required for Caesarean section delivery
B. Antibiotic prophylaxis is only required for normal vaginal delivery
C. Amoxicillin 2g IV is recommended 30–60 minutes prior to delivery
D. Clindamycin 600 mg IV can be considered in penicillin allergic patients
E. Antibiotic prophylaxis is not recommended

19. A 65-year-old patient with atrial fibrillation presents with a three-week history of fever and malaise. Her inflammatory markers are elevated and blood cultures show *Enterococcus faecalis*. Echocardiography reveals a 10 × 15 mm mobile echogenic lesion on the aortic valve, associated with moderate aortic stenosis and moderate aortic regurgitation.

Which of the following is correct?

A. Surgical management should be considered to prevent embolism in all patients with uncomplicated vegetations >10 mm in size
B. The risk of embolism is highest mid-way through antibiotic treatment as vegetation volume diminishes
C. Antiplatelet therapy reduces the risk of embolism in aortic valve endocarditis
D. Surgery to prevent embolism should be undertaken within the first few days of treatment
E. Atrial fibrillation is associated with a lower risk of embolism in the context of concurrent anticoagulant therapy

20. A 23-year-old intravenous drug user is admitted under the vascular team with an infected right femoral pseudoaneurysm. Venepuncture is difficult but two sets of blood cultures are obtained from the same puncture on admission, both of which grow coagulase-negative staphylococci. An echocardiogram and CT thorax are performed.

According to 2023 ESC guidelines for the investigation and management of infective endocarditis, which of the following are major diagnostic criteria for endocarditis?

A. Two sets of blood cultures positive for coagulase-negative staphylococci.
B. Aortic root abscess seen on computed tomography.
C. One set of blood cultures positive for *Staphylococcus aureus*.
D. Echocardiographic detection of new valvular regurgitation.
E. Predisposing condition (such as intravenous drug use).

chapter 3.2

INFECTIVE ENDOCARDITIS

ANSWERS

1. D. The 2023 ESC Guidelines for the management of infective endocarditis (IE) recommend that antibiotic prophylaxis should be considered for all patients with a high-risk cardiac condition who undergo high-risk procedures. High-risk patients include those with prosthetic valve replacements (including TAVI) and with any material used for cardiac valve repair, a prior history of infective endocarditis, cyanotic congenital heart disease (or non-cyanotic congenital heart disease with a history of defect repair involving prosthetic material), or patients with a ventricular assist device. High-risk procedures are those requiring manipulation of the gingival or periapical region of the teeth or perforation of the oral mucosa (such as root canal treatment or subgingival dental scaling). There is no compelling evidence that bacteraemia resulting from invasive respiratory tract procedures, gastrointestinal or genitourinary procedures (including vaginal and caesarean delivery), or dermatological or musculoskeletal procedures causes IE. However, due to an ageing population with increased co-morbidities and susceptibility to systemic infections, antibiotic prophylaxis may be considered in high-risk patients.

2. E. Vegetations seen on the echocardiogram in the context of this clinical history most likely represent Libman–Sacks endocarditis, which is thought to arise secondary to endothelial damage in the context of a hypercoaguable state, e.g. in association with concurrent malignancy, systemic lupus erythematosus (SLE), or antiphospholipid syndrome. This leads to local deposition of platelet thrombi and inflammatory molecules in the affected valves, causing leaflet thickening and the formation of broad-based, sessile vegetations which most commonly affect the coaptation line of the affected leaflets (but can extend throughout the leaflet or protrude to the other side). Infective endocarditis is unlikely in this scenario given the lack of clinical features or typical history, and blood cultures are likely to be negative. TOE would help determine the characteristic features of the vegetation. ANA (in particular anti-ds DNA antibody) are likely to be positive in SLE. However, recurrent miscarriages accompanied by unprovoked arterial and venous thromboembolic disease in this young patient point towards antiphospholipid syndrome, which would be best diagnosed with a positive assay for anti-phospholipid antibodies (ideally on two occasions 12 weeks apart).

3. C. The 2023 ESC Guidelines on the management of valvular disease recommend coronary angiography when considering valve replacement in men aged >40 years, post-menopausal women, and patients with at least one cardiovascular risk factor or a history of coronary artery disease. Exceptions arise when there are aortic vegetations that may be dislodged during cardiac catheterisation or when emergency surgery is necessary. In these situations, high-resolution CT may be used to rule out significant coronary artery disease in haemodynamically stable patients. Moreover, CT can be used to detect perivalvular complications with diagnostic accuracy similar to TOE. In aortic IE, CT can also facilitate surgical planning by defining the size, anatomy, and extent of calcification of the aortic valve, root and ascending aorta.

4. B. Transthoracic echocardiography should be considered in all patients with *S. aureus* bacteraemia since *S. aureus* infective endocarditis is very aggressive and carries poor prognosis, regardless of the presence or absence of clinical signs. Addition of gentamicin is not recommended in native valve infective endocarditis caused by methicillin-susceptible staphylococci, since clinical benefit has not been demonstrated and there is increased risk of renal toxicity. Gentamicin is, however, recommended in *S. aureus* prosthetic-valve infective endocarditis. Right-sided endocarditis carries a better prognosis than left-sided lesions. Eradication of the primary source of infection should be performed prior to cardiac surgery, unless this needs to be performed as an emergency. Co-trimoxazole plus clindamycin is an appropriate alternative to flucloxacillin in penicillin-allergic patients with native valve *S. aureus* endocarditis.

5. B. Surgical management aims to reduce the risk of peripheral emboli, treat resistant heart failure, and control the source of infection, and is indicated in patients with persistent vegetations >10 mm after one or more clinical or silent embolic events despite appropriate antibiotic treatment. Surgery may be considered in patients with large (>15 mm) isolated vegetations on the aortic or mitral valve, although this decision is more difficult and must be carefully individualized according to the probability of valve sparing surgery. Severe valve regurgitation with signs of heart failure, cardiogenic shock refractory to medical therapy and uncontrolled infection are all indications for surgical management.

6. D. 30% of *S. pneumoniae* endocarditis is associated with meningitis. Benzylpenicillin has poor blood–brain barrier penetration and should be replaced by ceftriaxone, or cefotaxime +/- vancomycin (according to bacterial sensitivities). The case for surgery is often strengthened following an embolic event (TIA or ischaemic stroke), provided the neurological prognosis is not judged to be too poor. Intracranial haemorrhage is generally associated with worse neurological prognosis and cardiac surgery should be postponed by 1 month. Mycotic aneurysms are present in 2–4% of infective endocarditis patients and most commonly found in the cerebral circulation. 18F-FDG tracer uptake is particularly high in healthy brain tissue which precludes detection of metastatic brain infections.

7. B. TOE is the investigation of choice in suspected prosthetic valve endocarditis. While 3D TOE is very useful in detecting perivalvular pathology, its use is currently considered supplementary to standard 2D imaging. The diagnostic accuracy of TOE in prosthetic valve endocarditis is less than in native valve endocarditis resulting from the degree of artefact related to prosthetic valves. A negative TOE does not exclude the diagnosis of endocarditis and should be repeated in 5–7 days (or even earlier in suspected *Staphylococcus aureus* endocarditis) when clinical suspicion is high. Abnormal activity around the site of valve implantation (in prostheses >3 months old) detected by 18F-FDG PET/CT or radiolabelled leucocyte SPECT/CT is a major criterion for the diagnosis of infective endocarditis. All degrees of AV block point towards perivalvular abscess formation and are associated with worse prognosis. Delayed administration of rifampicin reduces the likelihood of antagonistic reactions with other drugs relating to bacterial proliferation and production of rifampicin-resistant variants.

8. C. Day 1 of effective antibiotic therapy is most accurately determined by the date when previously positive blood cultures turn negative. In surgically managed endocarditis, the post-operative antibiotic regimen should remain the same (unless valve cultures are positive, in which case a full new course of antibiotics is required based upon culture sensitivities). Intraoperative TOE is recommended for all cases of IE requiring surgical management, as it can determine the exact location and extent of infection, guide surgery, assess the result, and help in early post-operative follow-up.

9. C. A CT thorax would be useful in assessing the presence of mediastinal collections but would be unable to identify infected tissue or prosthetic material. USS of the chest wall can identify chest wall collections, which can also be detected on physical examination. Both 18F-FDG PET/CT and radio-labelled leucocyte SPECT/CT are useful in detecting infection in the context of prosthetic material, although SPECT is able to distinguish between infected and inflamed tissues and therefore recommended in the early post-operative period (<3 months). Option E is incorrect since the diagnosis of prosthetic valve endocarditis remains possible.

10. E. Differentiating between local device infection and cardiac device related endocarditis is difficult and mis-diagnosis leads to increased mortality. Removal of the entire system is therefore recommended, even if infection is seemingly restricted to pocket infection. The course of IV antibiotics should be prolonged (4–6 weeks) in device-related endocarditis, both before and after device extraction. However, if blood cultures are persistently positive after lead extraction, antibiotic therapy should continue for at least 4 weeks. Device re-implantation, if indicated, should be performed at a sight distant from the previous generator, and delayed as long as possible once signs and symptoms of infection have abated. Blood cultures should be negative for at least 72 hours prior to device re-implantation. Transvenous extraction is the first-line treatment option, unless surgery is required for another indication (e.g. tricuspid valve repair/replacement for IE), and should be performed in a cardiothoracic centre. An externalised pacemaker is the safest option in pacing-dependent patients, allowing early mobilisation and reduced risk of pacing related adverse events.

11. C. Transthoracic echocardiography is a good imaging modality in this setting due to the anterior location of the tricuspid valve. However, the presence of systemic emboli suggests a left-sided lesion and TOE should be considered. Surgical management should generally be avoided in infective endocarditis in intravenous drug users due to the high risk of recurrence, but should be considered in patients with large persistent vegetations despite recurrent embolism, severe tricuspid regurgitation with or without right heart failure and poor response to diuretic therapy, or persistent bacteraemia after at least 1 week of appropriate antibiotic therapy. Tricuspid valve repair should be considered instead of valve replacement, when possible, though replacement is more commonly performed than valve repair and outcomes of the two techniques are comparable. Tricuspid valvectomy without valve replacement can be considered in extreme circumstances, but is associated with severe post-operative right heart failure. Pulmonary hypertension is associated with worse outcomes but is not a contraindication to surgery.

12. B. This patient has sustained a total anterior circulation ischaemic stroke, presumably as a complication of mitral valve infective endocarditis. His NIHSS score is high and the onset of symptoms was very recent. Intravenous thrombolysis is contraindicated in ischaemic stroke associated with infective endocarditis (due to the increased risk of haemorrhage) but mechanical thrombectomy should be considered in the absence of any other contraindication. Option C would be the standard therapy for ischaemic stroke in a patient with indications for anticoagulation (e.g. AF), but anticoagulant or antiplatelet therapies do not reduce the risk of further embolism in infective endocarditis. While early surgery is recommended in patients with ischaemic stroke, acute cerebral ischaemia takes priority here and any further decisions regarding valve surgery require expert neurology/neurosurgical assessment to assess the probability of neurological recovery.

13. B. Enterococcal bacteraemia is associated with urological instrumentation and 90% of enterococcal endocarditis is caused by *Enterococcus faecalis*.

14. E. The history suggests late prosthetic valve endocarditis with evidence of sepsis, heart failure and glomerulonephritis. Prompt antibiotic therapy is required before results of blood cultures are available. The history of recent dental extraction makes oral streptococci the most likely culprit and options B and C would be appropriate if this is confirmed. However, in the context of suspected late prosthetic valve endocarditis (>12 months post implant) and absence of a known organism, an empirical antibiotic regime including ampicillin in combination with ceftriaxone or flucloxacillin and gentamicin is most appropriate.

15. E. Development of first-degree heart block in patients with aortic valve endocarditis suggests the development of a perivalvular abscess (that is also signalled by the increase in inflammatory markers). Suspected complicated aortic valve endocarditis should be managed in the in-patient setting and the patient should have a TOE to rule out perivalvular complications.

16. E. *Streptococcus gallolyticus* (formerly *S. bovis*) infection in association with microcytic anaemia and altered bowel habit is highly suggestive of co-existing colonic malignancy. Routine outpatient review would be likely to delay diagnosis and treatment, and FOB testing is not recommended in this setting. Cross-sectional imaging (CT or 18F-FDG PET/CT) is useful to detect large tumours, but colonoscopy is the gold standard investigation for suspected bowel cancer.

17. B. The most likely diagnosis is chronic Q fever endocarditis caused by *Coxiella burnetti* acquired through exposure to farm animals in the course of her work. In this context, hospitalisation the previous year most likely represents acute Q fever, which usually presents with self-limiting malaise, fever, and flu-like symptoms (sometimes developing into pneumonia or hepatitis) 2–5 weeks after exposure. Chronic Q fever presents months (or even years) after exposure and clinical presentation is often non-specific with constitutional symptoms, congestive cardiac failure or valve dysfunction. Echocardiographic features are often subtle (and can be missed in 50% of cases) and serological testing is the gold standard. The organism is intra-cellular and blood cultures (Option A) are unlikely to achieve diagnosis. Beta glucan (Option C) can be used to detect fungal infection, but presentation would usually be more acute and less likely in an immunocompetent patient. *Legionella* endocarditis (Option D) is uncommon and presents more acutely, often in association with pneumonia. *Bartonella* endocarditis (Option E) follows exposure to cats and is associated with disseminated skin and bone lesions, and lymphadenopathy. *Bartonella* antibody testing has been withdrawn as a UK Health Security Agency (UKHSA) service.

18. E. Antibiotic prophylaxis is only recommended for high-risk dental procedures (those requiring manipulation of the gingival or periapical region of the teeth, or perforation of the oral mucosa) in patients at high risk of developing infective endocarditis (those with prosthetic valve replacements [including TAVI] or with any material used for cardiac valve repair, a prior history of infective endocarditis, cyanotic congenital heart disease [or non-cyanotic congenital heart disease with a history of defect repair involving prosthetic material]) and in patients with ventricular assist devices as destination therapy.

19. D. Surgery to prevent embolism should be undertaken within the first few days of treatment when risk of embolism is highest. Neither antiplatelet or anticoagulant therapies reduce the risk of embolism in patients with infective endocarditis. Age, diabetes, atrial fibrillation, vegetation length, previous embolism, and *Staphylococcus aureus* endocarditis are six factors associated with increased embolic risk. Surgical management should be considered in all patients with a vegetation >10 mm in size and one or more clinical/radiological embolic events, and in all patients with an aortic or mitral vegetation >15 mm in size (particularly if valve sparing treatment is feasible).

20. B. The 2023 ESC guidelines include advanced imaging techniques within the definition of infective endocarditis major diagnostic criteria – namely, the presence of definite peri-valvular lesions on cardiac CT and abnormal activity around the site of prosthetic valve implantation detected by 18F-FDG PET/CT (in valves >3 months' old) or radio-labelled leukocyte SPECT/CT. For typical microorganisms (such as *Streptococcus viridans*, *Staphylococcus aureus*, HACEK, enterococci or

Streptococcus gallolyticus (formerly *S. bovis*)), two separate blood cultures are required to fulfil a major criterion. For other microorganisms, persistent bacteraemia needs to be confirmed by ≥2 positive blood cultures drawn >12 hours apart, all of 3 or a majority of ≥4 separate blood cultures (with first and last samples drawn ≥1 hour apart). In this case, two blood cultures taken at the same time are not considered as a major criterion (Option B). New valve regurgitation is not a major criterion (unless in the context of perforated valve leaflet, aneurysm, or prosthetic valve dehiscence), and intravenous drug use is a minor criterion.

chapter 4

RHYTHM DISORDERS

chapter

4.1

THE ELECTROCARDIOGRAM

QUESTIONS

1. A 68-year-old gentleman is seen in cardiology outpatients after a routine ECG was found to be abnormal. He has a background of hypercholesterolaemia for which he takes a statin. On questioning, he reports an episode of syncope several months ago after standing for a prolonged period of time on a hot day. An echocardiogram has been performed which was unremarkable. His ECG is shown (Figure 4.1.1).

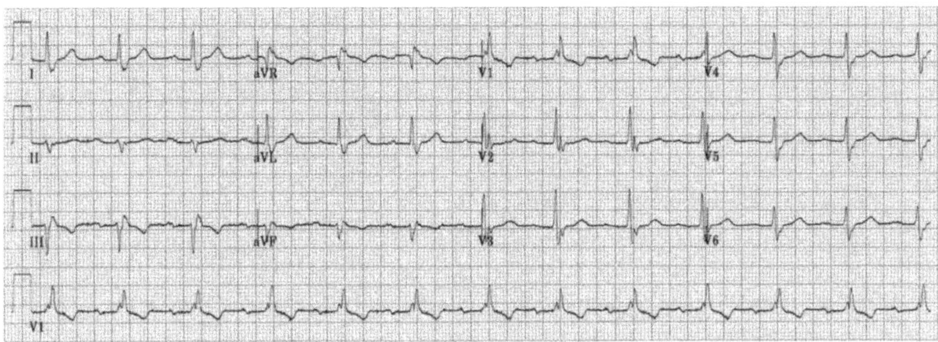

Figure 4.1.1

The patient undergoes an electrophysiology study. Which of the following findings would be considered an indication for cardiac pacing?

A. HV interval <35 ms

B. Left lateral accessory pathway

C. Wenckebach phenomenon

D. HV interval >70 ms

E. AH interval >150 ms

2. A 57-year-old gentleman presents to the Emergency Department with chest pain which came on 1 hour ago. He has previously been under the care of a cardiologist for 'heart failure' but has never had a coronary angiogram. An old clinic letter provided by his wife states that he had left-bundle branch block (LBBB) on an ECG several years ago. His current ECG is shown in Figure 4.1.2.

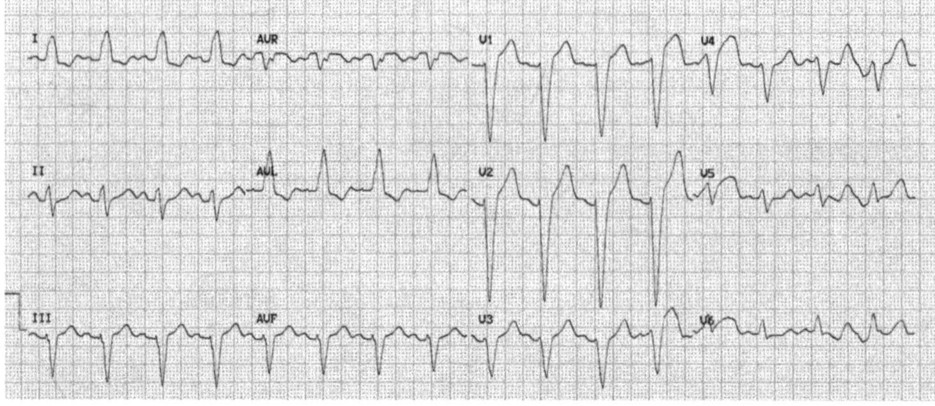

Figure 4.1.2

Which of the following is true?

A. Sgarbossa's criteria have high sensitivity and specificity for diagnosing myocardial infarction
B. Concordant ST elevation >1 mm is likely to represent acute myocardial infarction
C. Discordant ST elevation >1 mm is likely to represent acute myocardial infarction
D. A negative troponin on presentation excludes myocardial infarction
E. The ST segment cannot be interpreted in the context of pre-existing LBBB

3. A 47-year-old gentleman presents to the Emergency Department with lower limb cellulitis. He has a routine ECG on admission and you are asked to review it as it is found to be abnormal (Figure 4.1.3).

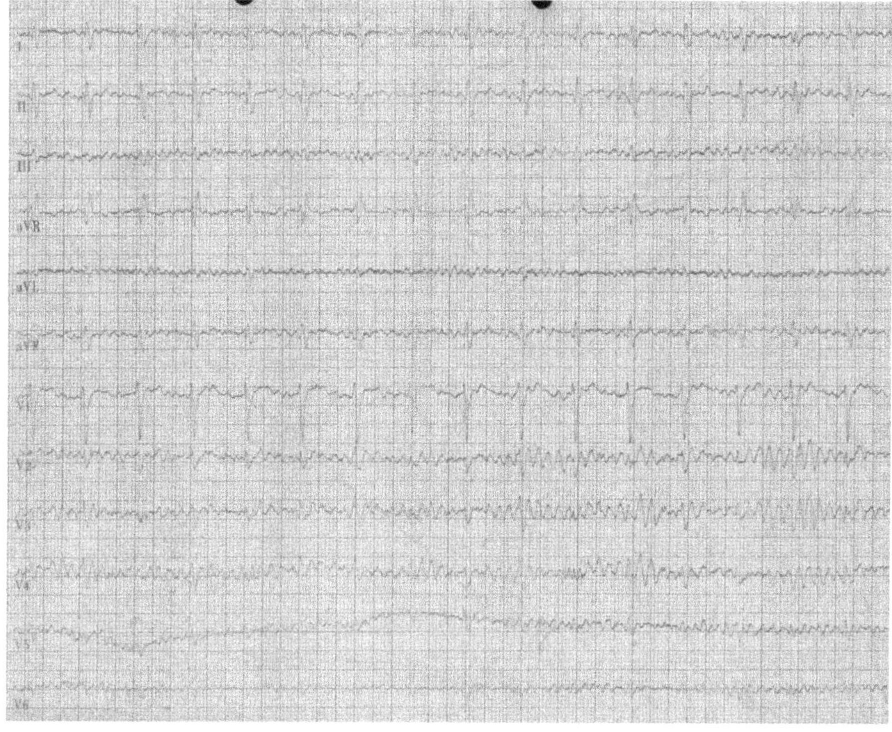

Figure 4.1.3

Which of the following is not a possible explanation for the ECG appearances?

A. Patient tremor
B. Seizure
C. Heterotopic heart transplant
D. Electromagnetic interference
E. Atrial fibrillation

4. A 26-year-old female presents to the Emergency Department with palpitations and dizziness. The tachycardia terminates spontaneously in the department, without any treatment. The ECGs of the tachycardia and sinus rhythm are shown in Figures 4.1.4 and 4.1.5.

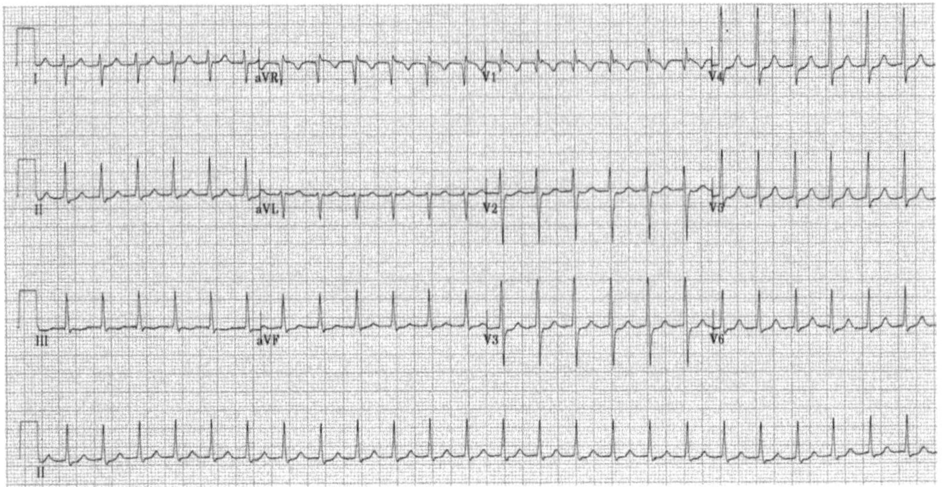

Figure 4.1.4

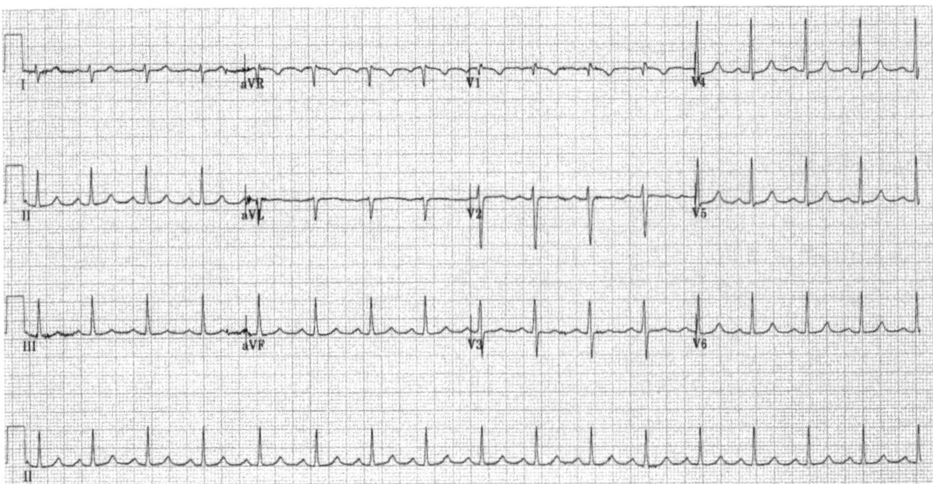

Figure 4.1.5

Which is the most likely diagnosis?

A. Typical AVNRT
B. Antidromic AVRT
C. Atypical AVNRT
D. Ventricular tachycardia
E. Sinus tachycardia

5. A 67-year-old gentleman with a history of heart failure and ischaemic heart disease presents to the Emergency Department with an episode of palpitations. He is on optimal medical therapy for heart failure and reports no chest pain. He has an echocardiogram which shows an LV ejection fraction of 30%. He reports having an implantable loop recorder and you organize a download which shows the following (Figure 4.1.6). He is admitted for cardiac monitoring and further investigation.

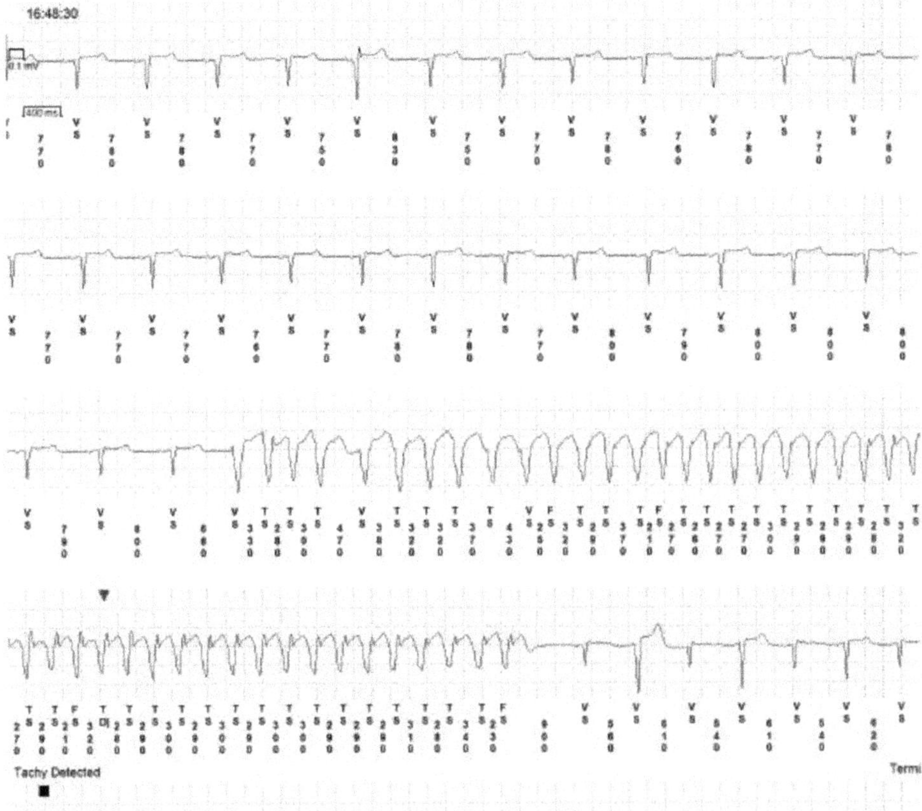

Figure 4.1.6

Which of the following statements is true?

A. An rSr' pattern in V1 where r>r' is more suggestive of VT than SVT with aberrancy
B. VT with a LBBB-like pattern and negative complexes in the inferior leads is likely to be of RVOT origin
C. Fascicular VT is the most common VT in patients with a structurally normal heart
D. An ICD is not indicated
E. Amiodarone will reduce the risk of death

6. You are asked to review the ECGs (Figure 4.1.7) of a 19-year-old male patient who presented to ED with a cough and fever. He has no known medical co-morbidities.

Initial ECG:

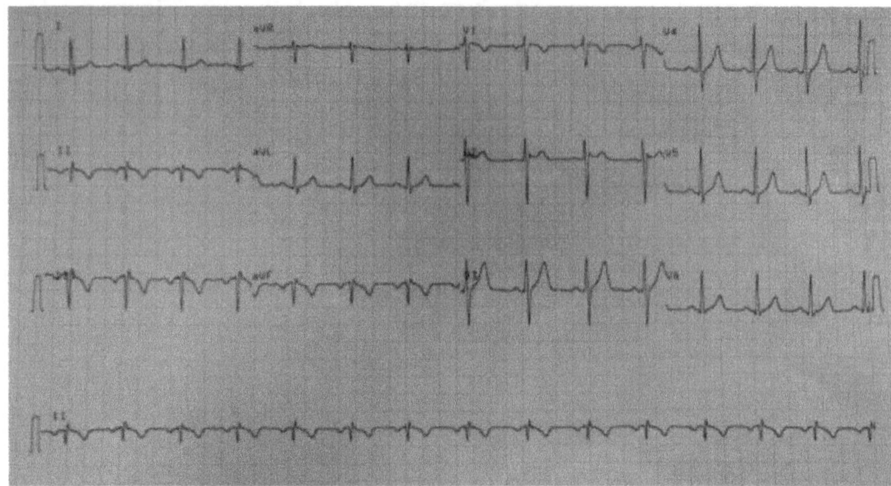

Figure 4.1.7

Repeat ECG after 30 minutes Figure 4.1.8:

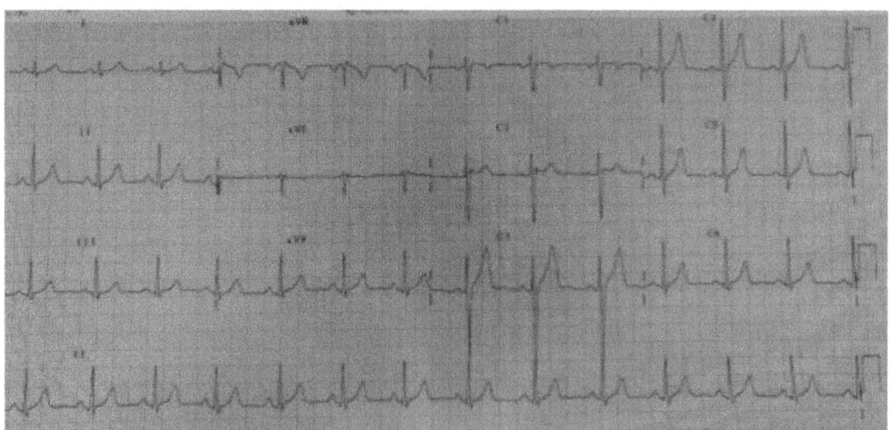

Figure 4.1.8

Which of the following is the most likely diagnosis?

A. Previous inferior myocardial infarction
B. Brugada syndrome
C. Wolff–Parkinson–White syndrome
D. Myocardial ischaemia
E. Lead placement error

7. A 76-year-old lady presents to the Emergency Department with breathlessness. Her ECG is shown in Figure 4.1.9

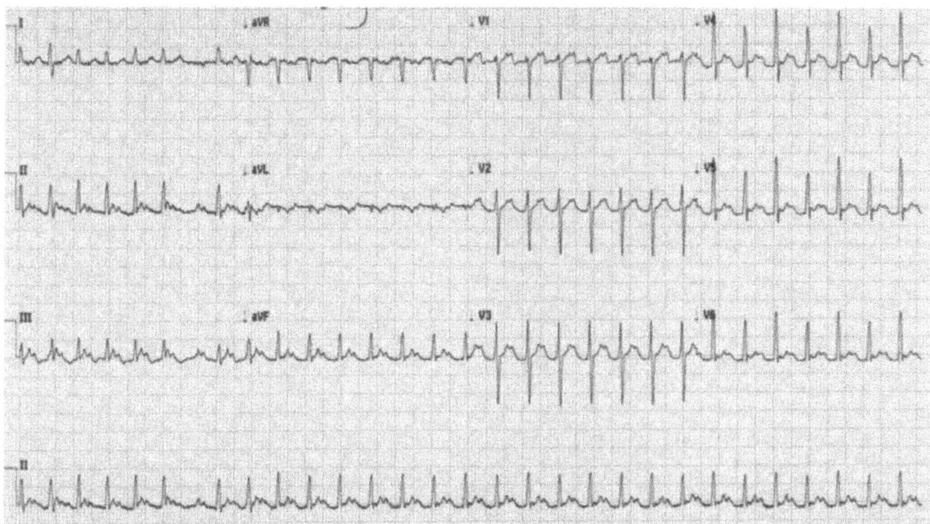

Figure 4.1.9

Which of the following is the most likely diagnosis?

A. Typical AVNRT
B. Orthodromic AVRT
C. Antidromic AVRT
D. Atrial tachycardia
E. Atrial fibrillation

8. A 81-year-old gentleman presents to the Emergency Department after a fall. His ECG is shown in Figure 4.1.10:

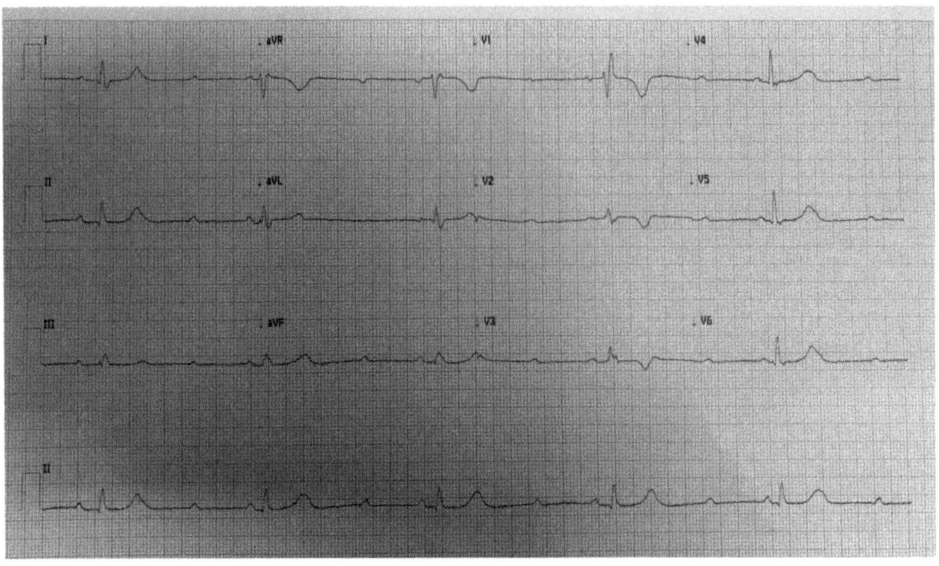

Figure 4.1.10

What is the best description of this ECG?

A. 2:1 AV block
B. Third-degree (complete) heart block
C. High grade AV block
D. Second-degree heart block Mobitz type 1
E. Bifascicular block

9. A 51-year-old gentleman is seen in the cardiology clinic with breathlessness. His ECG is shown in Figure 4.1.11:

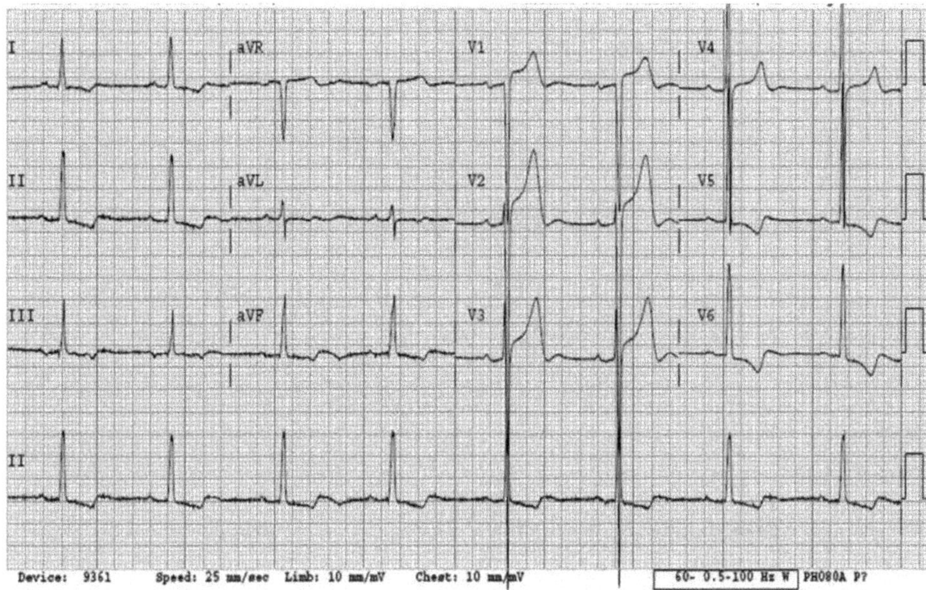

Figure 4.1.11

Which of the following is true?

A. The Romhilt–Estes Score has a high sensitivity and specificity for diagnosing left ventricular hypertrophy

B. The ECG appearances are associated with an increased risk of future cardiovascular events

C. Genetic testing should be performed

D. The ECG appearance is pathognomonic for hypertrophic cardiomyopathy

E. A cardiac CT is the first-line imaging test

10. A 62-year-old gentleman presents to the Emergency Department with central chest pain for the last 2 hours. He has a background of hypertension and was a previous smoker. On arrival his oxygen saturations are 99% on room air, HR 90 bpm, and BP 80/50 mmHg. His ECG is shown in Figure 4.1.12

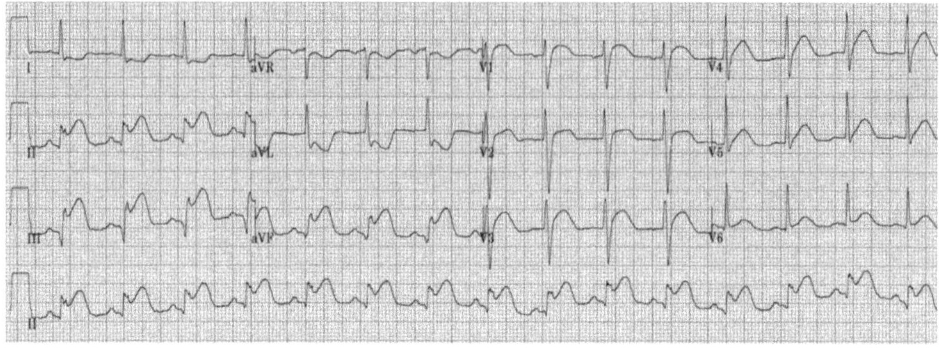

Figure 4.1.12

Which of the following is true?

A. Right-sided ECG leads (V1R-V6R) may be helpful

B. The appearances are diagnostic of an occluded right coronary artery

C. A bolus of furosemide should be given

D. If the patient develops complete heart block, a permanent pacemaker is urgently required

E. The most likely diagnosis is acute occlusion of the left anterior descending artery

11. A 29-year-old gentleman presented to the A&E department with a broken toe. He has no past medical history. He is a pilot. A routine resting ECG performed (Figure 4.1.13) demonstrated the following findings.

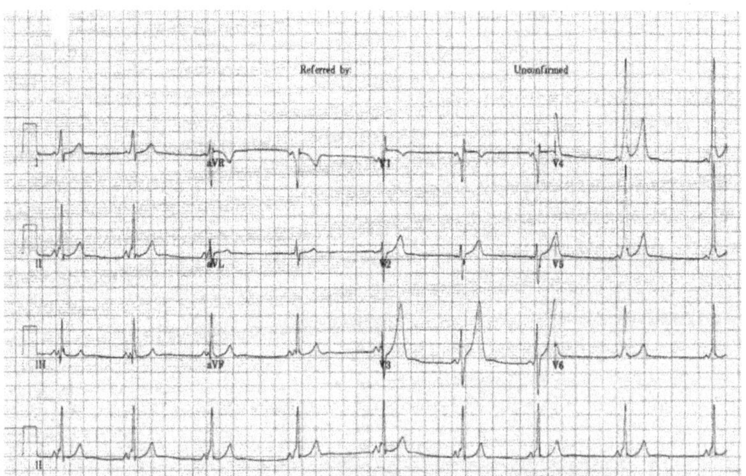

Figure 4.1.13

What is the appropriate next step in management?

A. Electrophysiology study for risk stratification
B. Catheter ablation
C. Ambulatory ECG Monitoring
D. Outpatient follow-up
E. Exercise test

12. A 65-year-old male with a history of hypertension, presented to A&E with palpitations and dizziness. His blood pressure was 70/48 mmHg and he was breathless (Figure 4.1.14).

What is the most appropriate immediate step in his management?

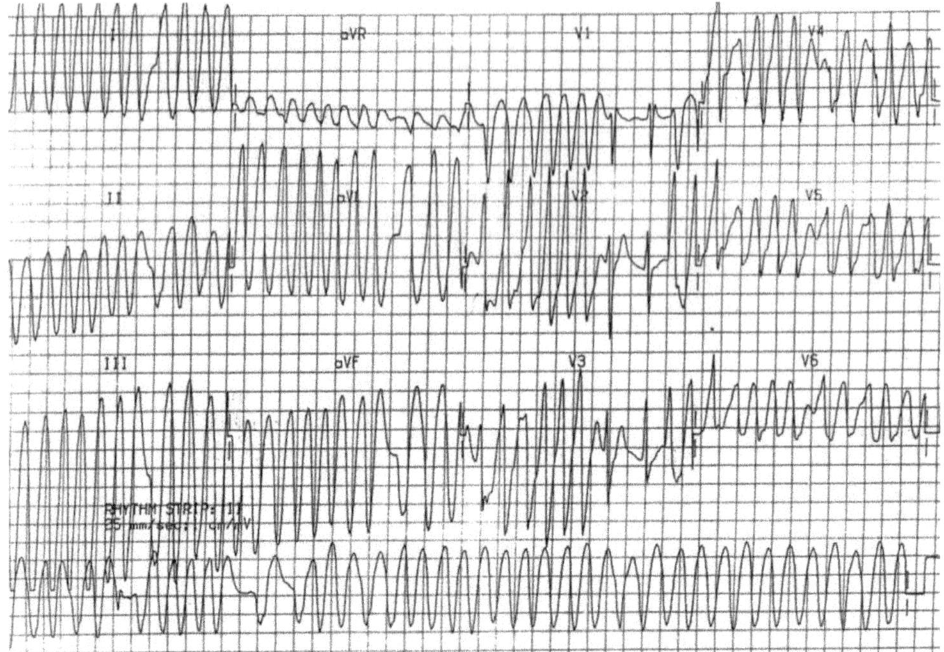

Figure 4.1.14

A. Synchronized DC cardioversion
B. IV adenosine
C. Vagal manoeuvres
D. IV amiodarone
E. IV flecainide

13. What is the most likely diagnosis from the ECG in question 12?

A. AF with aberrancy
B. Ventricular tachycardia
C. AF with pre-excitation
D. Orthodromic AVNRT
E. Antidromic AVNRT

14. A 55-year-old male presented to his A&E intoxicated with alcohol and with pyrexia. He has no known medical history. An ECG was performed (Figure 4.1.15).

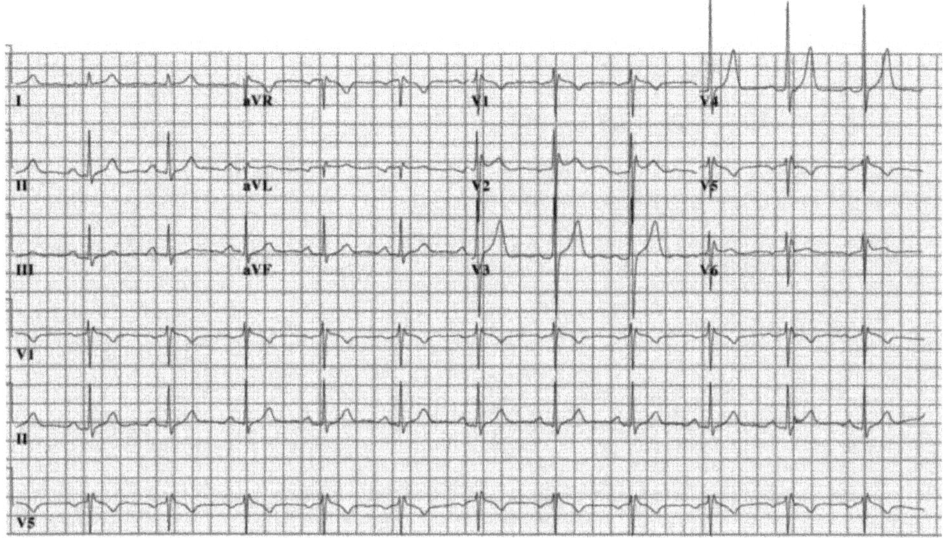

Figure 4.1.15

What does this likely demonstrate?

A. Pericarditis
B. Brugada Type 1 pattern
C. Brugada Type 2 pattern
D. Brugada Type 3 pattern
E. Non-ST elevation myocardial infarction

15. A 34-year-old male was referred to a cardiologist due to a history of recurrent, unexplained syncope. He has no past medical history or family history of sudden cardiac death. A 12-lead ECG demonstrated the following findings (Figure 4.1.16).

What is the definitive management for this patient?

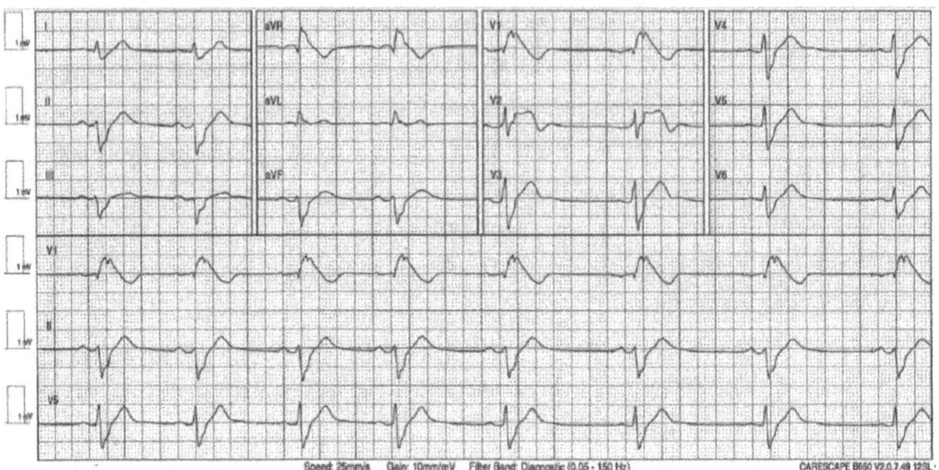

Figure 4.1.16

A. Implantable cardioverter defibrillator
B. Ajmaline challenge
C. Electrophysiology study
D. Ambulatory ECG monitoring
E. Implantable loop recorder device

16. An Emergency Department doctor contacts you as he has an 82-year-old patient who is unconscious and he has noticed a prolonged QT interval on the ECG of the patient. He wants to know what factors might lead to a prolonged QT.

Of the following, what is not a known cause of prolongation of the QT interval?

A. Hypokalaemia
B. Hypothermia
C. Raised intracranial pressure
D. Hypocalcaemia
E. Hypermagnesemia

17. A 40-year-old female patient presents with pyrexia and increasingly sharp, intermittent chest pain over a period of 2 weeks and has become increasingly breathless on exertion. She has a background of CKD stage 3 and alcohol excess. Troponin is 0.3 ng/ml [0.04–0.39 ng/ml] and CRP is 16 mg/L [<3.0 mg/L]. An ECG is performed (Figure 4.1.17).

What is the most appropriate management?

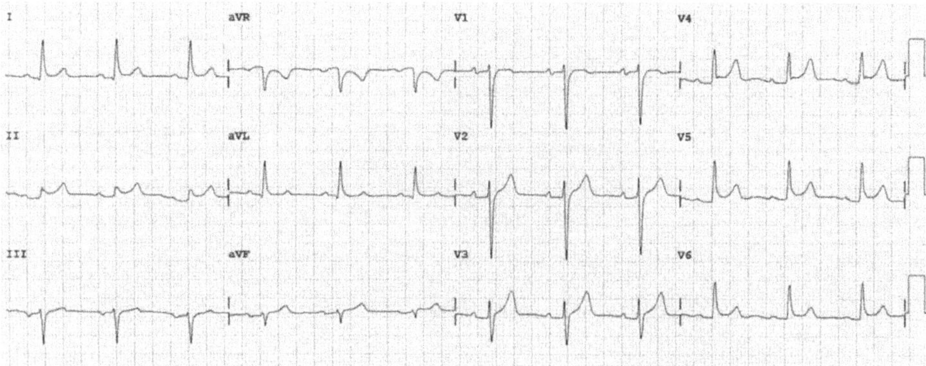

Figure 4.1.17

A. Outpatient management with Ibuprofen
B. Outpatient management with colchicine
C. Admission for further management
D. Primary PCI
E. Discharge without further follow up

18. An 83-year-old lady with a history of polypharmacy, and multiple comorbidities including CKD and AF, presents with unsteadiness and nausea. Her digoxin level is 3.0 nmol/L (therapeutic range 1.0–2.6 nmol/L) (Figure 4.1.18).

What is the most appropriate management?

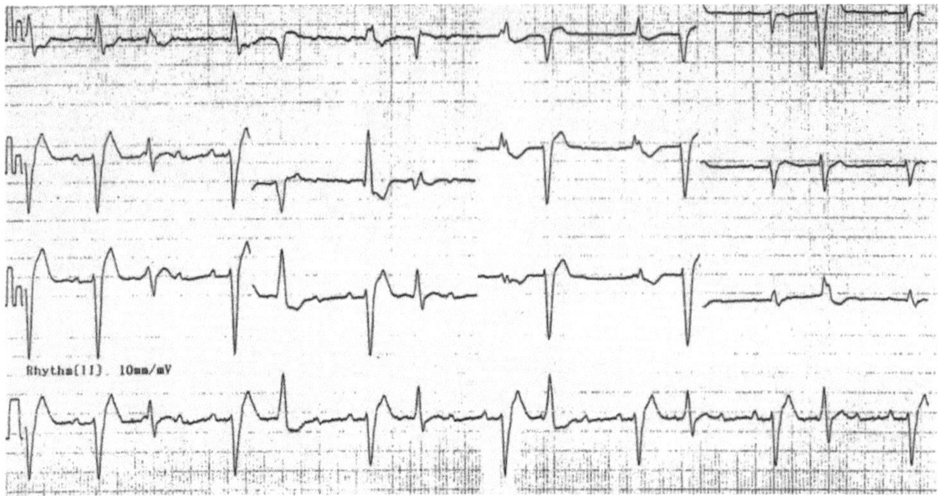

Figure 4.1.18

A. Continue current digoxin dose
B. Prescribe digoxin specific antibody fragments
C. Reduce the dose
D. Stop the digoxin and restart the medication at the same dose when the levels are therapeutic again
E. Stop the digoxin and consider restarting digoxin at a lower dose when levels are therapeutic again

19 This intracardiac electrogram (EGM) (Figure 4.1.19) trace demonstrates which of the following findings?

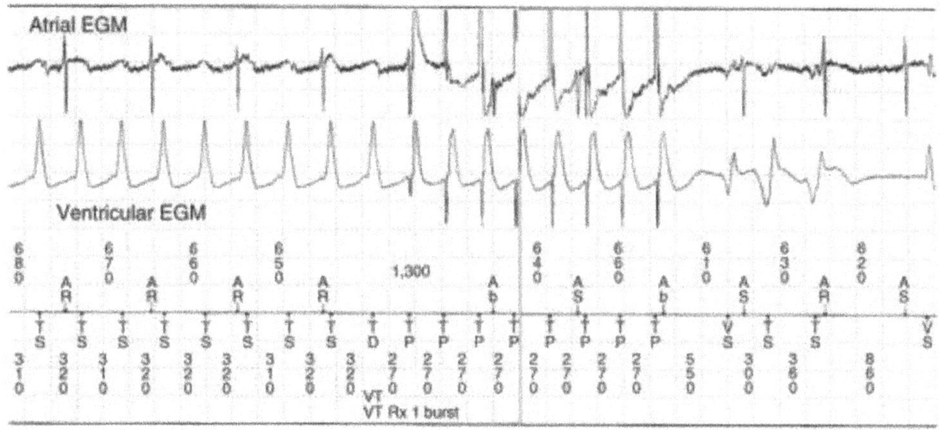

Figure 4.1.19

EGM, electrogram; AR, atrial event in refractory period; Ab, atrial far-field; AS, atrial sensed event; TS, ventricular tachycardia sensed event; TD, ventricular tachycardia detected; TP, antitachycardia pace; VS, ventricular sensed event. (Marker Channel Abbreviations for Medtronic [slightly different for other vendors].)

A. Ventricular tachycardia with an inappropriate shock
B. Ventricular tachycardia with an appropriate shock
C. Ventricular tachycardia with inappropriate ATP delivery
D. Ventricular tachycardia with appropriate ATP delivery
E. Atrial fibrillation with a rapid ventricular response

20. An emergency dual chamber pacemaker was inserted for an 84-year-old gentleman who presented with intermittent complete heart block, with frequent ventricular ectopics. Below is his ECG (Figure 4.1.20) and device trace post implantation (Figure 4.1.21 and Figure 4.1.22).

What is the most likely diagnosis?

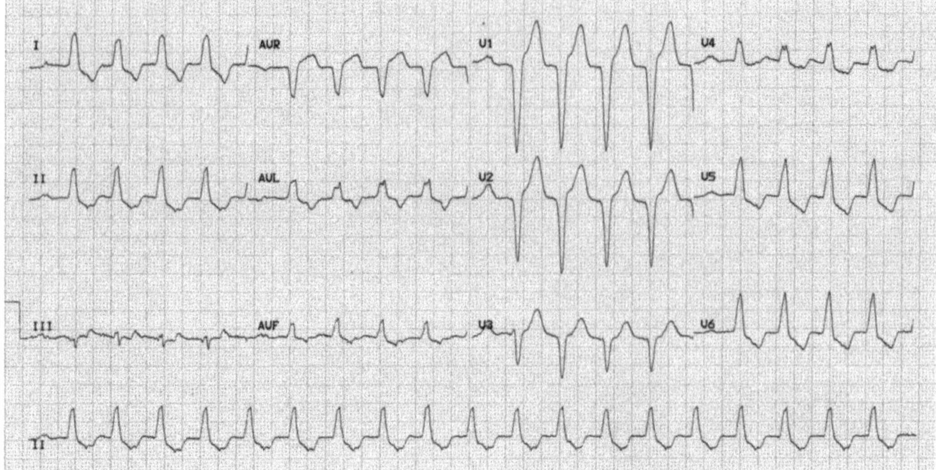

Figure 4.1.20

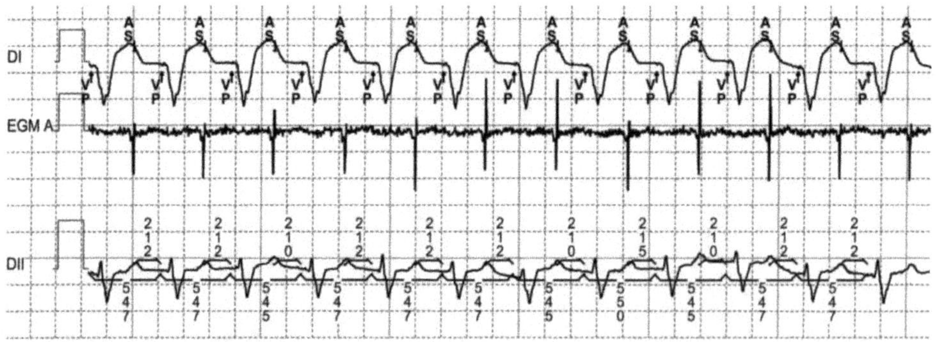

Figure 4.1.21

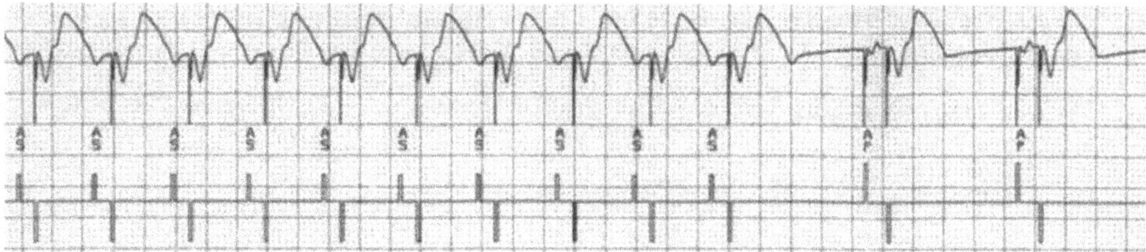

Figure 4.1.22

A. Ventricular tachycardia
B. Atrial flutter with 1:1 conduction
C. Pacemaker-mediated tachycardia
D. Atrial tachycardia with 1:1 conduction
E. Atrial fibrillation with aberrant conduction

21. A 72-year-old female presents to A&E with worsening peripheral oedema and confusion.

What type of implanted cardiac device does she have (Figure 4.1.23)?

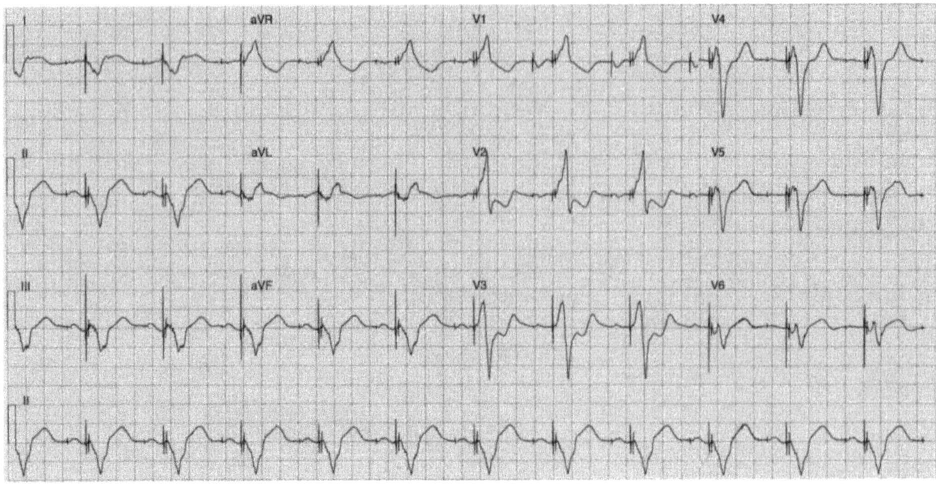

Figure 4.1.23

A. CRT device
B. Dual chamber pacemaker
C. Single chamber pacemaker
D. Single chamber ICD
E. Dual chamber ICD

22. A 24-year-old lady with a family history of sudden death and syncope was placed on telemetry (Figure 4.1.24).

What will reduce her risk of sudden death?

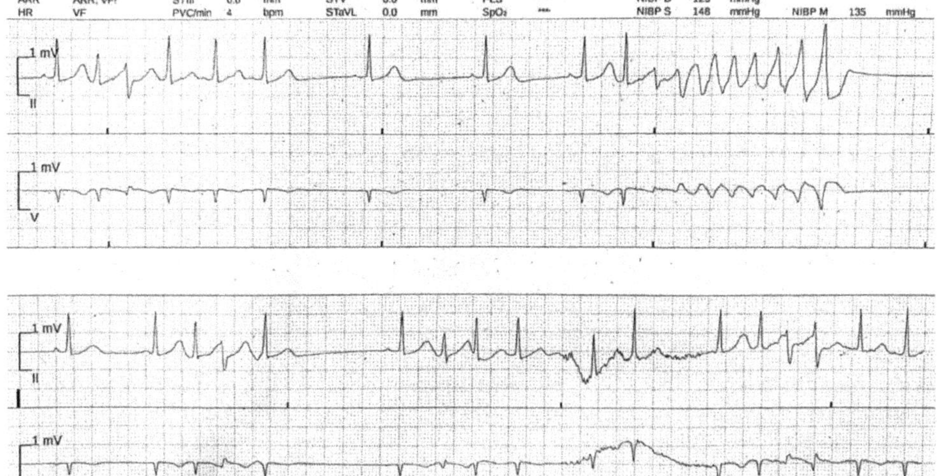

Figure 4.1.24

A. ICD implantation
B. Verapamil
C. Beta-blockers
D. Amiodarone
E. EPS with ablation

23. A 23-year-old patient has found out their sister has been diagnosed with ARVC.

What is the typical pattern of inheritance in ARVC?

A. Autosomal recessive
B. Autosomal dominant
C. X-linked recessive
D. Mitochondrial
E. X-linked dominant

chapter 4.1

THE ELECTROCARDIOGRAM

ANSWERS

1. D. While the episode of syncope sounds vasovagal, the ECG raises the suspicion of cardiac syncope caused by atrioventricular block. There is right bundle branch block and left anterior hemiblock. There is also a prolonged PR interval which suggests either delayed conduction in the AV node, or disease in the last remaining fascicle. An electrophysiology study allows measurement of the HV interval. A prolonged HV interval (>70 ms) suggests disease in the His-Purkinje system. In combination with the ECG findings and episode of syncope, this would be a class I indication for cardiac pacing. Figure 4.1.1 was taken (with permission) from https://litfl.com/trifascicular-block-ecg-library/

2. B. Sgarbossa's criteria (Table 4.1.1) has a high specificity (98%) but low sensitivity (20%) for diagnosing acute myocardial infarction in the context of left bundle branch block (Tabas et al 2008). The diagnostic criteria are shown in Table 4.1.A1. Concordant ST elevation >1 mm scores 5 points and therefore meets the criteria. Discordant ST elevation >1 mm alone scores 2 points and is insufficient to meet criteria. Figure 4.1.2 was taken (with permission) from https://litfl.com/left-bundle-branch-block-lbbb-ecg-library/

Table 4.1.A1 Sgarbossa's criteria for assisting with diagnosis of myocardial infarction in pre-existing left bundle branch block (score of >3 more likely to represent myocardial infarction)

Criteria	Points
ST elevation ≥1mm in a lead with a positive QRS complex (concordance)	5
Concordant ST depression ≥1mm in lead V1, V2 or V3	3
ST elevation ≥5mm in a lead with a negative (discordant) QRS complex	2

3. E. The ECG shows a regular ventricular rate at 100 bpm with fibrillatory activity between beats. It is from a patient with a heterotopic heart transplant (or 'piggyback heart') which is when the cardiac graft is connected in parallel to the native heart. In this case, the native heart is in ventricular fibrillation, while the graft heart is in sinus rhythm. This appearance could also be found with coarse artefact, such as patient tremor, seizure activity or electromagnetic interference. Given that the ventricular complexes are regular, atrial fibrillation is not a possible cause.

4. A. This is a narrow complex tachycardia with pseudo R-waves in V1-V2 and pseudo S-waves in the inferior leads. These are features of typical AVNRT (slow–fast) and represent retrograde P-waves that are just visible at the terminal portion of the QRS. Importantly, these deflections are not seen on the sinus rhythm ECG. Antidromic AVRT typically causes a broad complex tachycardia. Atypical AVNRT (fast–slow) is less common than typical AVRT, and the retrograde p-waves are usually found later after the QRS. While some ventricular tachycardias (e.g. fascicular VT) can have relatively narrow QRS complexes, it is unlikely in this case as the axis and morphology of the QRS complexes are the same in tachycardia and in sinus rhythm. Figure 4.1.4 was taken (with permission) from https://litfl.com/wp-content/uploads/ 2019/06/AVNRT-slow-fast-ECG-Libr ary-001.jpeg

5. A. The 'typical' appearance in RBBB is when the r' is larger than the r. If the converse is seen in the context of a RBBB-pattern broad complex tachycardia, it is suggestive of VT, rather than SVT with RBBB. RVOT VT classically results in a LBBB-pattern broad complex tachycardia with an inferior axis (positive in inferior leads). Fascicular VT is the second most common VT in a structurally normal heart, after RVOT VT. In this case, although the VT duration is short (<30 s), there is an indication for a primary prevention ICD given the patient has an LVEF<35% on optimal heart failure therapy. Although amiodarone reduces the incidence of ventricular arrhythmias and ICD shocks in patients with previous myocardial infarction and heart failure, it has not been conclusively shown to reduce mortality. Figure 4.1.5 was taken (with permission) from https://litfl.com/wp-content/uplo ads/2018/08/Typical-AVNRT-resolved-2.jpg

6. E. There is a marked difference in the appearance in the limb leads between the initial and repeat ECGs. The initial ECG shows a positive p-wave and T-wave in lead aVR, lead axis deviation, and an atypical inverted appearance of all the inferior leads. The most likely explanation is a lead placement error.

7. D. This is a narrow complex tachycardia with visible p-waves at the terminal portion of the t-wave. There is one p-wave which is not conducted to the ventricle and this makes atrial tachycardia the most likely diagnosis. While intermittent infra-Hisian block can occur in AVNRT, the p-waves in typical AVNRT occur retrogradely (negative in inferior leads) and are usually buried within the QRS or seen very shortly afterwards. The re-entry circuit in AVRT involves both the atria and ventricles, and you would not expect to see a non-conducted p-wave with immediate resumption of the tachycardia.

8. C. This ECG shows 3:1 AV block. Two P-waves are clearly seen before each QRS, however there is a further P-wave buried in the terminal portion of the T-wave (best seen in V3 and V6) which fits temporally with regular sinus activity. High grade AV block is defined as ≥2 consecutive P-waves that do not conduct to the ventricle with evidence of some atrioventricular conduction (i.e. 3:1 block, 4:1 block etc). While this is a type of 2nd degree AV block, it could be due to either Mobitz 1 (block within the AV node) or Mobitz 2 (block below the AV node) block.

9. B. The ECG shows left ventricular hypertrophy (LVH) by voltage criteria. This is a non-specific finding with multiple possible underlying causes including hypertensive heart disease, aortic stenosis, and hypertrophic cardiomyopathy. There are multiple voltage criteria for LVH, including the Romhilt–Estes Score; however, they all have a relatively low sensitivity and specific for true LVH seen on imaging. LVH by voltage criteria on ECG is an independent risk factor for future cardiovascular events, even if there is no LVH on imaging. The first line imaging test here would be an echocardiogram. Figure 4.1.11 was taken (with permission) from https://litfl.com/left-ventricular-hypertrophy-lvh-ecg-library/

10. A. This ECG shows inferior ST elevation. There is also ST elevation in V1 which, in combination with hypotension, raises the suspicion of right ventricular infarction. This can be confirmed with right-sided precordial leads (V1R–V6R). RV infarction often requires fluid resuscitation to treat hypotension. While acute occlusion of the right coronary artery (RCA) is the most likely cause here, the ECG is not diagnostic of this. In 15–20% of patients there is left coronary dominance with the circumflex artery supplying the inferior wall of the left ventricle. Furthermore, 5–10% of patients presenting with STEMI do not have occlusive coronary disease on angiography. Other possible causes include coronary vasospasm, coronary dissection, and myocarditis. Complete heart block in the context of an inferior MI is usually resolves spontaneously and only requires permanent pacing in around 10% of cases.

11. A. This ECG has some of the classical features of a pre-excitation syndrome as characterized by a PR interval <120 ms, a delta wave and QRS prolongation >110 ms. The most likely form of pre-excitation syndrome in this case is Wolf–Parkinson–White Syndrome. A dominant R-wave in V1 would suggest a 'Type A' WPW and is associated with a left sided accessory pathway. However, this ECG a dominant S-wave in V1 suggests a 'Type B' WPW.

For a patient with asymptomatic pre-excitation, who has a high risk occupation or is a competitive athlete, should have an EPS for risk stratification +/- catheter ablation (Figure 4.1.A1).

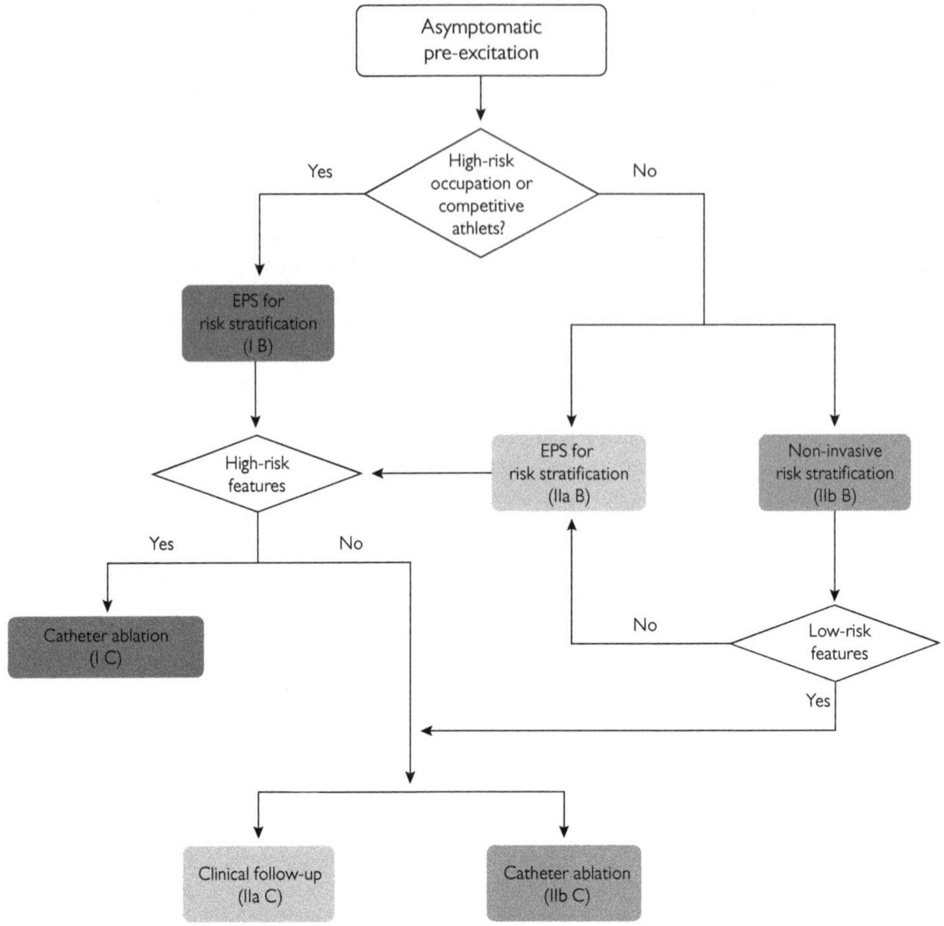

Figure 4.1.A1 Reproduced from Brugada J, Katritsis DG, Arbelo E, et al; ESC Scientific Document Group. 2019 ESC Guidelines for the management of patients with supraventricular tachycardiaThe Task Force for the management of patients with supraventricular tachycardia of the European Society of Cardiology (ESC). Eur Heart J. 2020 Feb 1;41(5):655–720. doi: 10.1093/eurheartj/ehz467. © European Society of Cardiology. With permission from Oxford University Press.

12. A. This case is discussed below in the related explainer for question 13. Figure 4.1.14 was taken (with permission) from https://litfl.com/pre-excitation-syndromes-ecg-library/

13. C. The ECG demonstrates fast, irregularly conducted QRS complexes with a rate of up to 300 bpm, with a broad morphology. Rapidly conducted AF with aberrancy is a possible diagnosis; however, the rate is unlikely to be so high if it is truly conducted via the AV node. In addition, the QRS morphology is not typical of a bundle branch block morphology. In this case, there is a compromised patient with very short R-R intervals and AF with pre-excitation should be high on the differential list. There are two narrow complexes in V1–V3, where the atrial impulses are conducted via the AV node rather than an accessory pathway. This rhythm is difficult to distinguish from polymorphic VT; however, it does not demonstrate the typical twisting morphology of torsade's de pointes. AV-node blocking manoeuvres and drugs, such as adenosine, would be ineffective as conduction is via an alternative pathway. Negatively ionotropic medications, such as calcium channel blockers and beta blockers, may worsen haemodynamic so should be avoided. Intravenous flecainide can be effective in slowing conduction down an accessory pathway; however, in such a compromised patient confronted with such an ECG, prompt DC cardioversion is the main priority.

14. C. Three types of Brugada pattern are recognized. This ECG demonstrates findings consistent with a type 2 pattern. There is >= 2mm J point elevation, >= 1mm of ST segment elevation and a saddle back appearance, followed by a positive or biphasic T-wave. Whilst type 1 pattern is considered a diagnostic pattern, types 2 and 3 are suggestive of the disease. These ECG findings, could be confused with pericarditis, however the lack of PR depression, and as Brugada ECG changes are more commonly unmasked in pyrexia and alcohol use, suggest this case is a Brugada type 2 pattern. Figure 4.1.15 was taken (with permission) from https://commons.wikimedia.org/ wiki/File:Brugada_syndrome_type2_example1_(CardioNetworks_ECGpedia).png

15. A. This ECG demonstrates typical features of Brugada Type 1 (Figure 4.1.A2). It is characterized by prominent coved ST-segment elevation displaying J-point amplitude or ST-segment elevation ≥2mm, followed by a negative T-wave. Type 1 pattern is considered a diagnostic pattern of the disease. After identifying the type 1 pattern, one should search for the clinical criteria for the disease, of which syncope is one—thereby giving this patient a diagnosis of Brugada Syndrome (BrS). Once diagnosis is made, the next step is to risk stratify such patients for risk of SCD or VF. To date, the only proven effective treatment for the prevention of SCD in BrS is an ICD. In a patient with a spontaneous Type 1 Brugada ECG pattern, who is symptomatic with likely arrhythmogenic syncope there is a class I indication for an ICD.

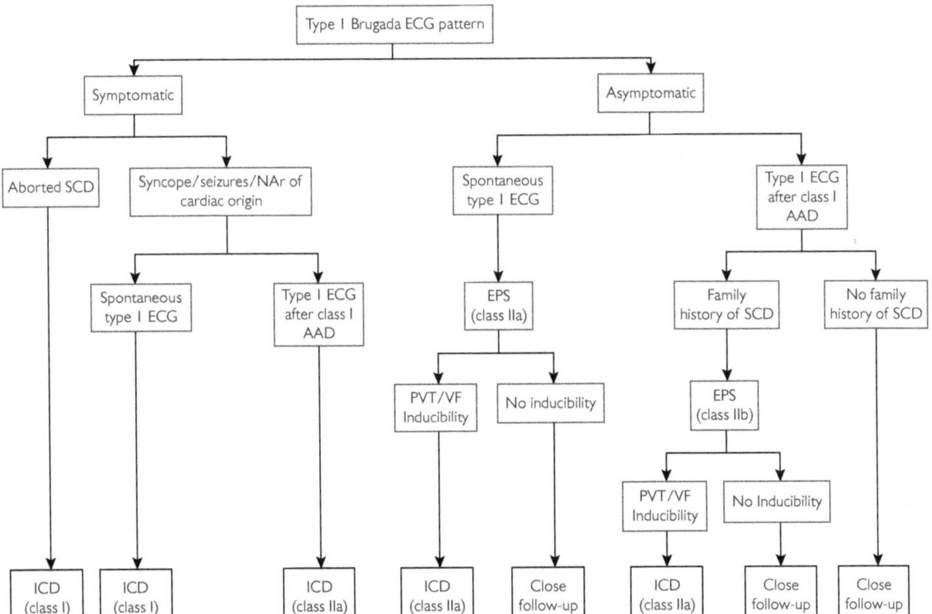

Figure 4.1.A2 Brugada J. Management of patients with a Brugada ECG pattern. E-journal of the ESC Council for Cardiology Practice. 2009 Mar;17:7. (24). Available from:www.escardio.org/Journals/E-Journal-of-Cardiology-Practice/Volume-7/Management-of-patients-with-a-Brugada-ECG-pattern.

16. E. There are several causes of a prolonged QT interval. A corrected QT value of >440 ms in men and >460 ms in women is considered abnormal. Common medications causing prolongation are antiarrhythmic medications (e.g. amiodarone and sotalol), certain antibiotics (e.g. erythromycin), and some antipsychotics and the antidepressant citalopram (see https://www.crediblemeds.org/ for a comprehensive list). Physiological states such as raised intracranial pressure and hypothermia can also cause it. Electrolyte disturbances of hypokalaemia, hypocalcaemia, and hypomagnesemia are other important causes.

17. C. The patient presents with typical pericarditic chest pain and ECG findings consistent with acute pericarditis. The precordial and limb leads demonstrate widespread concave ST elevation and associated PR depression. Lead aVR shows reciprocal ST segment depression. Elevation of inflammatory markers are additional supporting features. The subacute onset and pyrexia are poor prognostic markers and ESC guidelines suggest admission and aetiology search in such cases. Without these higher risk features, option B would be appropriate drug management in view of the history of CKD.

18. E. The patient has non-specific symptoms of digoxin toxicity with nausea, and a raised digoxin level. Her ECG is typical of this, in that she has a tachyarrhythmia occurring alongside sinus or AV node suppression. In this case, she has an underlying atrial tachycardia, 4:1 AV block, and frequent premature ventricular contractions (PVCs). Severe toxicity can cause ventricular tachyarrhythmia. The presentation is not life-threatening, and therefore digoxin specific antibody fragments are not indicated. It is likely that her CKD has contributed to the digoxin toxicity, and therefore it would be appropriate to wait for her arrhythmia and digoxin level to normalize, before either adjusting the digoxin dose accordingly, or considering an alternative anti-arrhythmic medication. Figure 4.1.18 was taken (with permission) from https://litfl.com/digoxin-toxicity-ecg-library/

19. D. Figure 4.1.19 is an EGM of a dual chamber ICD, demonstrating ventricular tachycardia. The atrial and ventricular marker channels demonstrate AV dissociation, with V>A. The cycle length (CL) of the VT is 320 ms (approximately 190 bpm) and is sensed by the device (TS) at the beginning of the EGM. It is detected (TD) by the device and eight beats of anti-tachycardia pacing is delivered (TP) at a shorter, i.e. faster, CL of 270 ms. There is successful termination of the arrhythmia after delivery of ATP. https://thoracickey.com/clinical-management-of-patients-with-implantable-cardioverter-defibrillators/

20. C. There is a regular, broad complex tachycardia with no discernible P-waves, at a rate of approximately 120 bpm. There are no clear pacing spikes; however, it may not always be possible to see pacing spikes, particularly if a bipolar lead is implanted. There is no extreme axis or concordance, which makes VT less likely. AF with aberrant conduction is also unlikely as the rhythm is very regular. As the rate is not particularly fast, it could be the upper tracking rate of the pacemaker, indicating a possible pacemaker mediated tachycardia. The device interrogation reveals, a persistent and stable tachycardia with consecutive AS–VP cycles at the maximum rate of 110 bpm. This, alongside the high percentage of ventricular pacing with atrial sensing at high rate suggests episodes of pacemaker-mediated tachycardia, which can be initiated by a PVC, and as this patient had frequent VEs, this is the likely mechanism initiating the tachycardia.

Placing a magnet on the device during the pacemaker-mediated tachycardia will change the pacemaker's mode to DOO, whereby intrinsic P-waves and R-waves are ignored. This will result in the termination of tachycardia by suspending the pacemaker's sensing function, as demonstrated below.

21. A. This ECG demonstrates a rate of 72 bpm with A–V sequential pacing throughout. The QRS complexes are prolonged with a north–west axis. The ventricular pacing consists of two spikes approximately 20–40ms apart (referred to as the LV–RV offset), with a tall R-wave in V1 indicating predominantly LV pacing. The negative vector in the QRS complex in leads II, III, aVF, and V2–V6 suggest an inferior apical LV lead position. This ECG demonstrated biventricular pacing consistent with a CRT device. Figure 4.1.23 was taken (with permission) from http://jhcedecg.blogspot.com/2014/06/ecg-of-week-2nd-june-2014- interpretation.html

22. A. This telemetry trace demonstrates short-coupled Torsade's de Pointes, which a rare form of polymorphic VT of unclear aetiology. It is characterized by a very short-coupled interval of the first PVC initiating the tachycardia. Typically, the tachycardia is non-uniform but organized electrical activity with progressive changes in morphology, amplitude, and polarity. It can deteriorate to VF and if it had done so here, intravenous verapamil is one of the only medications that can suppress the arrhythmia in the acute setting. In the long term, verapamil does not reduce the risk of sudden cardiac death, therefore ICD implantation is strongly recommended. In cases of recurrent episodes, EPS with ablation targeting the culprit PVC should be considered.

23. B. ARVC is mostly inherited in an autosomal dominant fashion, with a genetic trait caused by mutations in genes encoding for desmosomal proteins (plakoglobin): desmoplakin, plakophilin-2, demoglein-2, and desmocollin-2. Few cases are due to mutations in non-desmosomal genes. The most common mutant gene is *PKP2* (10–45%), followed by *DSP* (10–15%), *DSG2* (7–10%), and *DSC2* (2%). Even rarer recessive forms associated with a cutaneous phenotype of palmar and plantar hyperkeratosis, such as Carvajal syndrome and Naxos disease, are also recognized. Interestingly, unlike other cardiomyopathies, genotype forms a major criterion in the establishment of the ARVC diagnosis (Corrado et al. Eur Heart J, 2020).

Corrado D, Van Tintelen PJ, McKenna WJ, et al. Arrhythmogenic right ventricular cardiomyopathy: Evaluation of the current diagnostic criteria and differential diagnosis. Eur Heart J, **41,** (14), 1414–27b (2020). https://doi.org/10.1093/eurheartj/ehz669

17/23

chapter

4.2

TRANSIENT LOSS OF CONSCIOUSNESS

QUESTIONS

1. **A 70-year-old man was referred to your clinic having suffered two syncopal episodes in the last 4 months. The first occurred whilst he was shaving and was brief with a quick recovery. The second occurred when he returned home after attending a funeral and was reversing his car into the garage. Again, the episode was brief with quick recovery. His 12-lead ECG was normal and physical examination was unremarkable.**

   Which one of the following tests is the most likely to be useful here?

   A. Ambulatory ECG monitor (Holter)
   B. CT coronary angiogram
   C. Tilt table test with carotid sinus massage
   D. Echocardiogram
   E. Ambulatory blood pressure monitor

2. **A 55-year-old male accountant was previously diagnosed with cough syncope 4 years ago. He had been symptom free until a recent lower respiratory tract infection for which he was treated, and his cough resolved. However, during this illness and over a 2-day period he suffered two syncopal episodes whilst standing.**

   According to UK DVLA guidance, which of the following recommendations are correct?

   A. As his lower respiratory tract infection resolved after treatment he can drive
   B. As his episodes of syncope were explained and from a standing position, he may drive
   C. He should refrain from driving for 3 months
   D. He should refrain from driving for 6 months
   E. He should refrain from driving for 12 months

3. A 26-year-old woman presents with 4 episodes of sudden onset presyncope and 2 episodes of syncope in the last 18 months. She reports palpitations prior to the onset of dizziness and/or syncope. This is her 12-lead ECG (Figure 4.2.1):

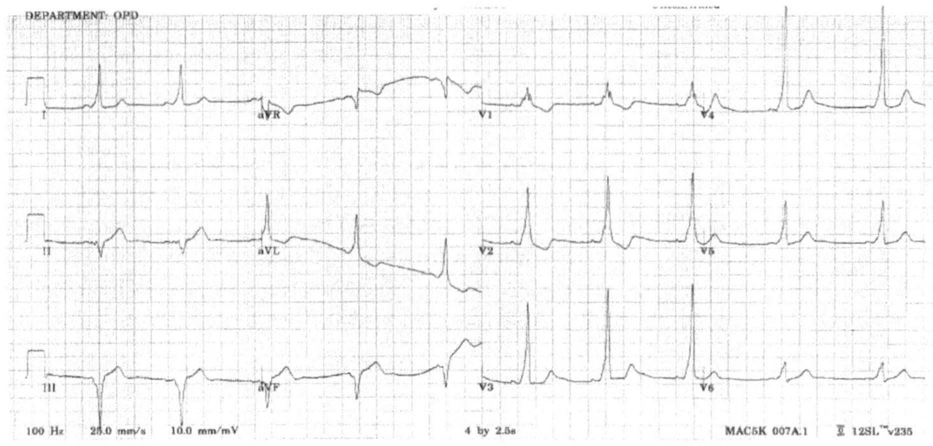

Figure 4.2.1

Which of the following tests would you recommend investigating further with in the first instance?

A. Ajmaline challenge
B. Tilt table test
C. Electrophysiological study +/– ablation
D. 7-day event recorder
E. Exercise tolerance test

4. A 42-year-old woman who was previously diagnosed with vasovagal syncope presents to the emergency department having experienced a series of four syncopal episodes in 3 hours. She had returned home from work early because she had been feeling generally unwell and recalls a prodromal warning before the first two. She vomited after her second event and then went to bed, and the third occurred after getting out of bed. She does not recall her fourth but awoke back on the bed. She was not sure how she got there but was aware of a thumping feeling in her heart before vomiting again. Her BP is 95/60 mmHg. Her ECG shows normal sinus rhythm and physical examination was otherwise unremarkable.

What would you recommend?

A. Implantable loop recorder implantation
B. Refer back to her syncope team for further investigation
C. Admit for inpatient investigation
D. Offer reassurance and reiteration of conservative advice
E. Seek a neurological opinion

5. A 55-year-old woman has presented with dizzy spells and one episode of near syncope. She has a history of hypertension, anxiety, migraines, back pain, and is currently being treated for cellulitis. Her ECG shows sinus rhythm with a QTc of 510 ms.

Which of her following medications is the LEAST likely to contribute to her QTc prolongation?

A. Sumatriptan
B. Clarithromycin
C. Citalopram
D. Indapamide
E. Amitriptyline

6. A 25-year-old female student attends the Emergency Department after having suffered a syncopal episode whilst interval training at the gym one evening. She felt dizzy beforehand and the episode was brief with an uncomplicated recovery. She describes feeling dehydrated, had skipped lunch that day, and has no previous history of fainting. She reports her maternal aunt died of a heart attack in her late '30s and there is history of a cousin who may also have died young of unclear cause.

What is NOT an appropriate next stage investigation?

A. Exercise tolerance test
B. Echocardiogram
C. Implantable loop recorder
D. Tilt table test
E. 12-lead ECG

7. You are asked to review a 25-year-old female patient who is 32 weeks pregnant. Over the last 3 weeks she has been dizzy and lightheaded and had a number of episodes of transient loss of consciousness. More recently she remembers waking up in the morning, sitting on the table to have her breakfast, and collapsing for a few seconds. These episodes tend to happen when she is standing but occasionally sitting as well. She remembers she used to faint as a child. There is no significant family history. Both echocardiogram and ECG are normal.

What would be the most appropriate next step?

A. Implantable loop recorder
B. Ambulatory ECG monitor (Holter)
C. Tilt table test
D. Reassure and discharge
E. Start midodrine

8. A 19-year-old patient attends the Emergency Department after suffering a syncopal episode in the bathroom following a hot shower. She is known to be hypotensive at her baseline. She had felt lightheaded during her shower and remembers leaving the shower cubical. Her parents heard her fall. When they gained entry to the bathroom, they found her wedged in a seated position between the cubicle and the wash basin. She was stiff. Her arms were jerking, and she was later found to have been incontinent. She was left in that position as paramedics were called. The jerking was reported as lasting for 15 seconds. Her mother was concerned that she could not find a pulse. She became alert after another 2 minutes although she was initially disorientated and later wanted to sleep. Her 12-lead ECG with the paramedics was normal. She has fainted once before as a child.

Which would be the most appropriate investigation in the first instance?

A. Implantable loop recorder
B. Electroencephalogram (EEG)
C. MRI head
D. Tilt table test
E. None of the above

9. A 64-year-old woman has been referred by her GP to clinic because of recurrent syncope and presyncope on standing up and after prolonged standing. She has a history of depression and migraine. Her tilt test trace is shown in Figure 4.2.2.

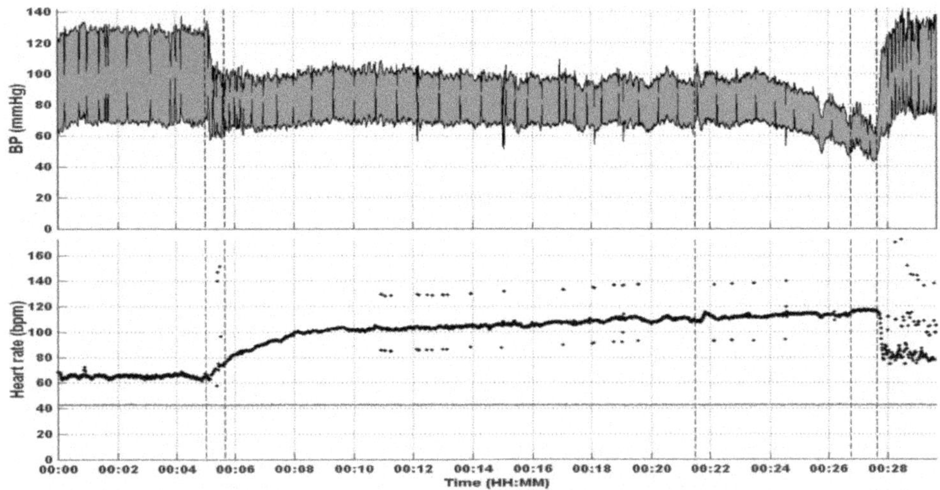

Figure 4.2.2

Which of the following would you NOT recommend?

A. Grade two thigh high compression tights
B. Abdominal binders
C. Fludrocortisone
D. Midodrine
E. Pacemaker

10. A 39-year-old fit and healthy man has a history of frequent childhood syncope with 2 minutes of prodromal warning. The episodes are usually triggered by heat and prolonged standing. Four months ago, after a late-night workout session at his gym and a hot shower, he felt sick and sweaty, and sat down before he had a 40-second episode of loss of consciousness associated with jerking movements of his limbs. His tilt test showed a 27-second pause with an anoxic response.

Which of the following options would be the most appropriate in his management?

A. Discharge as diagnosis of vasovagal syncope confirmed
B. Tell patient to avoid exercise
C. Refer for an exercise test
D. Refer for consideration of pacemaker implant
E. Recommend conservative advice, and consider implantable loop recorder if recurrent symptoms

11. A 34-year-old man has a history of multiple episodes of loss of consciousness throughout his life and a tendency to postural dizziness. He presents to the emergency department with extreme dizziness and nausea in the context of a tooth abscess. There is no significant family history in first degree relatives, but he mentions that his cousin died in his sleep at a young age. On arrival his blood pressure is 95/60 mmHg. On standing up in the Emergency Department he collapses. His ECG is shown In Figure 4.2.3.

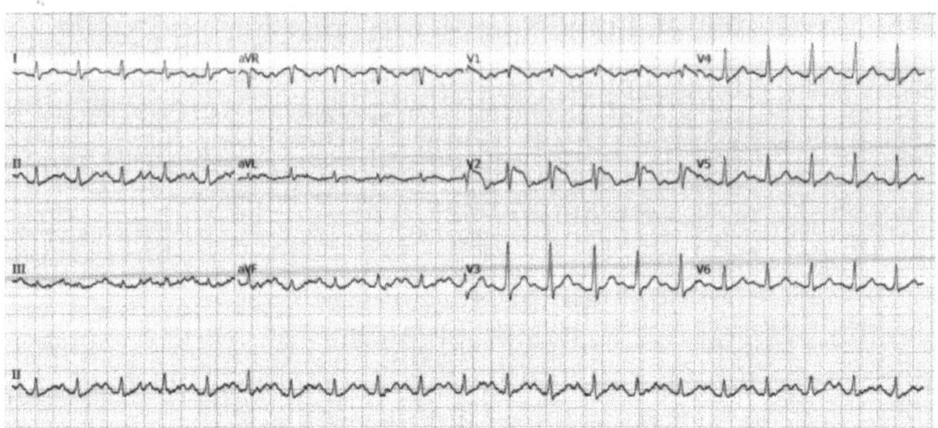

Figure 4.2.3

What would be the most appropriate next step in management?

A. Carotid sinus massage
B. Cardiac MRI
C. Coronary angiogram
D. Electrophysiological study with a VT stimulation test followed by electrophysiology opinion
E. Discharge with reassurance as likely diagnosis of dehydration and postural hypotension

12. A 30-year-old woman suffers a brief collapse after jumping out of bed to see to her crying toddler at night. Both she and her toddler were suffering from a cold at the time. She has a history of postural symptoms but no syncope since she was a teenager. Her previous events were always preceded by a prodromal warning and usually triggered by hot environs. Unfortunately, she hit her head on the edge of a dresser as she fell and required medical attention.

She is reliant on her car because of having recently moved to a rural address. You are asked about her ability to drive. In line with UK DVLA guidance, which of the following options is correct?

A. She cannot drive for 3 months
B. She can drive normally
C. She should return her Licence to DVLA indefinitely
D. She should await the result of a Holter and echo before return to driving
E. She should inform DVLA should she have a second syncope within 3 months

13. Which of the following statements are NOT usual in the presentation of psychogenic pseudo syncope?

A. Eyes open during syncope
B. Laying immobile for 15–30mins
C. Multiple presentations per day or week
D. No identifiable triggers
E. No pallor or sweating noted by observers prior or during events

14. A 26-year-old has returned to the cardiology clinic after his tilt test. The result is reported as having replicated his usual syncopal and presyncopal symptoms with a mixed cardioinhibitory and vasodepressor response (VASIS 1). He has been asked to make a number of lifestyle changes which he finds intrusive. He has heard that sometimes pacemakers are used to prevent syncope and asks if this could be an option.

How should you respond?

A. Refer him for consideration of a pacemaker
B. Refer him for an implantable loop recorder to assess the likelihood of real-life event correlation with cardio inhibition
C. Suggest that if he continues to faint despite lifestyle changes then it will be considered
D. Reiterate and explain the findings of the tilt and the need to make conservative changes and to address his triggers
E. Repeat the tilt test to confirm the diagnosis

15. An 82-year-old man is referred to your afternoon clinic after recurrent episodes of transient loss of consciousness whilst at the breakfast table or washing up after having breakfast. His wife describes him as looking pale and vacant before slumping in his chair. He has fallen on two occasions but fortunately suffered no serious injury. He has a history of type 2 diabetes mellitus, peripheral neuropathy, hypertension, angina, and enlarged prostate. He takes all his medications an hour before breakfast whilst still in bed. His wife has a blood pressure machine which shows systolic BP readings of between 105 and 110 mmHg after these events. He has a normal resting 12-lead ECG and physical examination is unremarkable.

Which of the following actions would you undertake FIRST?

A. 24-hour ambulatory blood pressure monitor
B. Ambulatory ECG monitor (Holter)
C. Echocardiogram
D. Supine and standing blood pressure test
E. Insertion of an implantable loop recorder

16. A 48-year-old woman has presented to her local emergency department as well as other hospitals in her area multiple times over the last 6 months complaining of presyncope and syncopal episodes. These are associated with palpitations, shortness of breath, and rising anxiety. Each event's history is consistent with a clinical diagnosis of a tendency to reflex syncope with typical triggers of stress and dehydration. Echocardiogram and ambulatory ECG monitor (Holter) have been normal although an event has never been captured. You are asked to review her during her latest visit. She has attended with her family who are afraid to leave her on her own because of her symptoms. Her ECG is normal, and all her observations are within normal limits.

Which action would you take?

A. List for an implantable loop recorder to capture an event
B. Recommend referral to counselling and talking therapies
C. Discharge with further reassurance, the diagnosis is clear
D. Repeat the ambulatory monitor and echocardiogram
E. Request tilt test and specialist syncope review

17. A 25-year old athlete who was being screened privately for a security officer job was found to be bradycardic on his resting ECG and his GP arranged a 24-hour ambulatory ECG monitor (Holter). He was referred to your clinic as the monitor identified an abnormal finding at 4 am while the patient was asleep (Figure 4.2.4). He has no history of syncope or presyncope and is very fit and well, denying any medical health issues. His resting ECG shows sinus bradycardia with a heart rate of 52 bpm. His echocardiogram is normal. Physical examination is unremarkable.

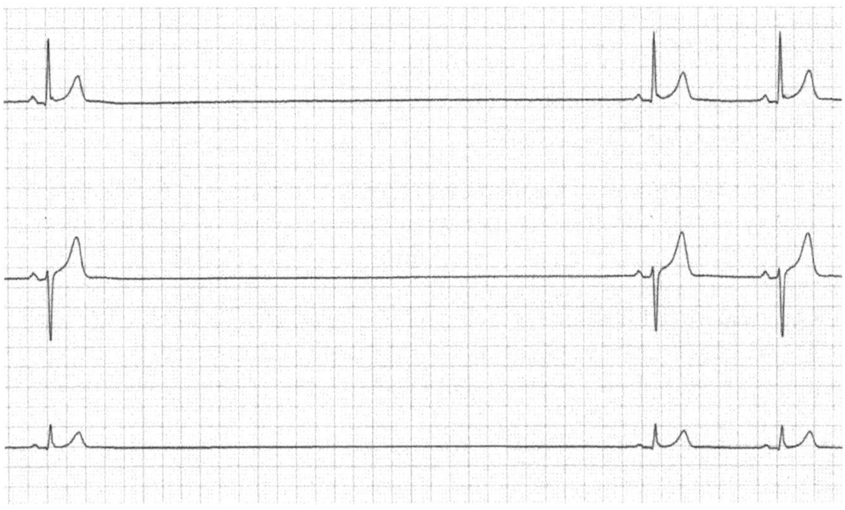

Figure 4.2.4

What would your next step in management be?

A. Pacemaker implant
B. Implantable loop recorder
C. Cardiac MRI
D. Admit for observation
E. Reassure and discharge

18. In your clinic you see a 33-year-old carpenter with a body mass index (BMI) of 36 kg/m^2, type 2 diabetes mellitus, and oesophageal reflux. He had an unheralded syncope whilst having dinner at a comedy club. He does not recall the exact events leading to it but remembers enjoying the show. He was described as jerking for few seconds with his eyes open. His recovery was quick and his ECG normal. He recalls a similar event a few years ago but that was never investigated.

Which examination is most likely to elicit the diagnosis?

A. Tilt table test
B. Echocardiogram
C. Ambulatory ECG monitor (Holter)
D. Implantable loop recorder
E. Exercise tolerance test

19. A 68-year-old man with a history of Parkinson's disease is referred to clinic by his GP after suffering two episodes of loss of consciousness whilst playing golf, both occurring after lunch in the clubhouse. These events were brief and not associated with any chest pain, shortness of breath, or palpitations. He felt a little tired before both. He has a normal 12-lead ECG and physical examination is unremarkable.

Which of the following would you NOT recommend as a first step?

A. Avoid alcohol and a large meal before golf
B. Maintaining good hydration
C. Grade 2 waist high compression stockings
D. Implantable loop recorder
E. Isometric counter pressure manoeuvres whilst playing

20. An 80-year-old man has a typical history of faints as a young adult with a clear prodrome of feeling sweaty and nauseous, particularly when having to stand in a warm environment. He was referred to clinic because of a recent syncopal episode whilst returning from walking his dog. He recalls only 1–2 seconds of feeling 'a strange giddiness' before finding himself on the floor with cuts and bruises on his arm as he landed on a rose bush which broke his fall. His ECG shows first degree atrio-ventricular block with a PR of 210 ms, left axis deviation and a narrow QRS complex. During tilt table test, he suffered a brief loss of consciousness following glyceryl tri-nitrate (GTN) provocation. He had significant prodromal warning identical to his faints as a young man. He demonstrated a mixed (VASIS 1) collapse pattern. His blood pressure was 75/35 mmHg and heart rate 49 bpm at tilt end.

Which of the following actions is correct?

A. The positive tilt test confirms a diagnosis of vasovagal syncope: conservative advice
B. His recognition of familiar symptoms on the test confirms the diagnosis of vasovagal syncope: conservative advice
C. He should be commenced on fludrocortisone in addition to conservative advice
D. He should be referred for consideration of a pacemaker
E. The test should be regarded as a false positive and an implantable loop recorder should be inserted

chapter 4.2

TRANSIENT LOSS OF CONSCIOUSNESS

ANSWERS

1. **C.** His history is suggestive of possible carotid sinus hypersensitivity, triggered by head turning or pressure on the neck. Whilst all listed investigations have a role in the work-up of varying syncope presentations, carotid sinus massage with tilt table test is most likely to have the highest diagnostic yield from the proposed investigations.

2. **E.** Having had a previous episode of cough syncope he is identified by DVLA as a high-risk group predisposed to cough syncope. Therefore, even if the acute respiratory infection was short lived, he is at a higher risk of cough syncope regardless. As his recent syncopal episodes did **not** occur within 24-hours of each other they are counted as multiple episodes in a 5-year period and so the guidance is not to drive for 12 months.

3. **C.** Her ECG shows manifest pre-excitation with presence of a delta wave and so an accessory pathway (AP) is the likely cause of her symptoms. Exercise tolerance tests can sometimes be useful as a test to deem an AP 'safe' by estimating the effective refractory period of the pathway with abrupt loss of pre-excitation during exercise. However, in the presence of syncope the risk of sudden cardiac death in this group is higher and an electrophysiological study combined with ablation would be the appropriate and safest way forward of all options presented.

4. **D.** The history and sequence of events as well as the signs of increased vagal activity (vomiting) in this case are diagnostic of vasovagal syncope. Her preceding illness, depending on the cause, can be a trigger or contributing factor (dehydration) to this presentation. Reassurance and reinforcement of conservative measures (increased salt intake, adequate hydration, compression stockings and counterpressure manoeuvres) would be the most appropriate action here.

5. **A.** Macrolides and tricyclic antidepressants are well recognized as QT prolonging drugs, and selective serotonin reuptake inhibitors such as citalopram can prolong the QTc. Indapamide has a prolonging effect on the QT by blocking potassium channels. Sumatriptan has no effect on the QT, although has been implicated in causing arrhythmias through a different mechanism.

6. **C.** An Implantable loop recorder is premature in this setting, whilst the rest of the investigations would all be reasonable and more likely to reach a rapid diagnosis here.

7. **D.** Syncope in pregnancy is common. In a patient who has a tendency to vasovagal syncope, as her childhood history would suggest, pregnancy will have an exacerbating effect. This is due to increased vagal tone by increased intra-abdominal pressure combined with reduced venous return due to inferior vena cava compression. Tilt-table testing is avoided during pregnancy. Neither an ambulatory monitor nor an implantable loop recorder would have a significant diagnostic yield in a patient with a normal echo and normal resting ECG.

8. **D.** The prodrome and history is consistent of a vasovagal syncope triggered by vasodilation from the hot shower. The patients' medical history of 'hypotension' should steer suspicion to

an autonomic cause. The patient's jerking movements are most likely due to an anoxic response to cerebral hypoperfusion at being kept upright after having suffered a vasovagal event. Anoxic seizures in this setting can sometimes have a more prolonged recovery which can confound the diagnosis. A tilt table test, if it reproduces typical symptoms, would be diagnostic.

9. E. The tilt table test here has provoked a typical vasodepressor (VASIS-3) response, i.e. characterized by a blood pressure drop with the heart rate not dropping more than 10% from peak at the time of syncope (as indicated here by the fifth interrupted vertical line). A pacemaker would not be able to prevent syncope in this setting. All the other choices would be viable, although conservative measures such as good hydration, increased salt intake, and counterpressure manoeuvres should ideally be tried first.

10. E. The patient is 39 years old with a presentation of syncope which has been replicated on tilt as vagal in origin. We know that there is no increased risk of mortality in the setting of prolonged vagal mediated pauses and any benefit derived from pacing would be aimed at preventing injury. He has adequate prodromal warning to take evasive action to avoid injury and has been given advice to help mitigate the onset of symptoms. In this age group, the risks of a pacemaker implant with the associated long- and short-term morbidity would need to be strongly considered. ISSUE 3 studied patients above 40 years old with implantable loop recorder guided pacing therapy. An implantable loop recorder would be helpful in correlating symptoms with real-life events and discern whether his symptoms are always accompanied by significant cardiac pauses, although the threshold for pacing would still be very high given his age.

11. D. His ECG demonstrates Brugada Type 1 pattern. Although there is a postural element in this patient's history, a spontaneous Brugada Type 1 pattern in context of an acute illness and with a background of multiple episodes of syncope in the past, male gender and family history of unexplained young death places him in a high-risk category for sudden cardiac death. An electrophysiology study with a VT stimulation test would help better risk stratify him and he should then be discussed at an electrophysiology multi-disciplinary team meeting to consider the need for an implantable cardioverter-defibrillator. Of note, one cannot assume from their history that the collapse was arrhythmic—the ECG showed sinus tachycardia with a Brugada pattern, and vasovagal syncope does exist with Brugada syndrome. The SCORE model can help risk assess patients with Brugada syndrome (Sieira et al. A score model to predict risk of events in patients with Brugada Syndrome. Eur Heart J. 2017 Jun 7;38(22):1756–1763. doi: 10.1093/eurheartj/ehx119).

12. B. This lady has recurrent, typical vasovagal syncope with a consistent prodrome. As a mnemonic, the conditions of the '3 Ps' (position, provocation, and prodrome) have been met and she can therefore continue to drive without notifying the DVLA.

13. A. During psychogenic pseudo syncope (PPS) patients will almost universally have their eyes closed avoiding direct gaze contact. This fact, along with the rest of the options in this question, are highly predictive of PPS.

14. D. This patient has a vasovagal tendency with a mixed cardioinhibitory and vasodepressor response to tilt. A pacemaker will not eliminate the vasodepressor response and the patient will still experience syncope despite having a device implanted. The lifetime risk of a device implant in a young patient is high (15–20%) and in this setting will offer minimal benefit. The patient needs to be counselled appropriately on lifestyle modifications with positive reinforcement.

15. D. His antihypertensives, antianginals, and prostate medication are very likely to have a synergistic compounding effect in reducing his blood pressure. As the patient takes his medication lying in bed the acute effect can be mitigated but is exacerbated as soon as he is in an upright position sitting at the table or standing up. Although syncope while sitting can be a red flag for conduction disease, in this context and with a normal surface ECG, drug-induced orthostatic hypotension is much more likely.

16. E. Although the clinical diagnosis may not be in doubt here the patient continues to be symptomatic and has sought help on repeated occasions. This may be through a lack of confidence in the diagnosis or inadequate education regarding the diagnosis and management. If these are not addressed, evidence suggests that such patients suffer significant morbidity with a detrimental socioeconomic impact. A specialist syncope unit will help reinforce the diagnosis, direct lifestyle changes, and empower the patient to deal with their condition effectively.

17. E. This is a young athletic patient with a baseline high vagal tone. He has not had any high-risk features in his presentation. Although the asymptomatic sinus pause seen (Figure 4.2.4) is longer than the guideline-suggested 6 seconds, the morbidity associated with pacing an asymptomatic young patient in this setting would be unacceptable as pacing would offer virtually no benefit in terms of either symptoms or mortality. The ISSUE 3 trial, which used implantable loop recorder directed pacing, only studied patients over 40 so there are no data in this young group of patients.

18. A. The history here is most suggestive of laughter-induced (situational) syncope, an extreme vagal response to laughter. The mechanism usually involves an exaggerated autonomic response to the Valsalva manoeuvre while laughing or coughing. One would expect a vasodepressor response to similar provocation with 'beat to beat' monitoring during a tilt test.

19. D. Parkinson's disease patients can suffer from autonomic dysfunction which can exacerbate post-prandial vagal effects and produce symptoms of syncope later in life. Conservative measures as laid out above are all appropriate, and a tilt table test would also help solidify diagnosis. The yield of an implantable loop recorder in this setting would be very low. It could be considered down the line if recurrent episodes of unheralded syncope take place despite adequate conservative measure implementation suggesting potential underlying conduction disease as a cause, but would not be appropriate as a first step.

20. E. Although this patient certainly suffers from vasovagal syncope, it is important to assess the presenting history. The tilt test indeed replicated his previous early adulthood faints, but his most recent syncopal episode was different in nature and not replicated. Therefore, whilst he may have a tendency to faint, the test should be viewed as a false positive. By age alone he is at a high-risk group for underlying conduction disease and his recent event should be investigated with an implantable loop recorder.

chapter 4.3 ATRIAL FIBRILLATION AND FLUTTER

QUESTIONS

1. A 60-year-old gentleman with a past medical history of hypertension is newly diagnosed with AF. It is recommended to:

A. Give him flecainide orally to chemically cardiovert him
B. Cardiovert him electrically in the next 48 hours
C. Assess for any significant bleeding risks and then anticoagulate with a non-vitamin K oral anticoagulant
D. Prescribe aspirin 75mg od for stroke prevention
E. Assess for the presence of asymptomatic coronary artery disease

2. You are asked to review a 78-year-old lady who has the following ECG (Figure 4.3.1):

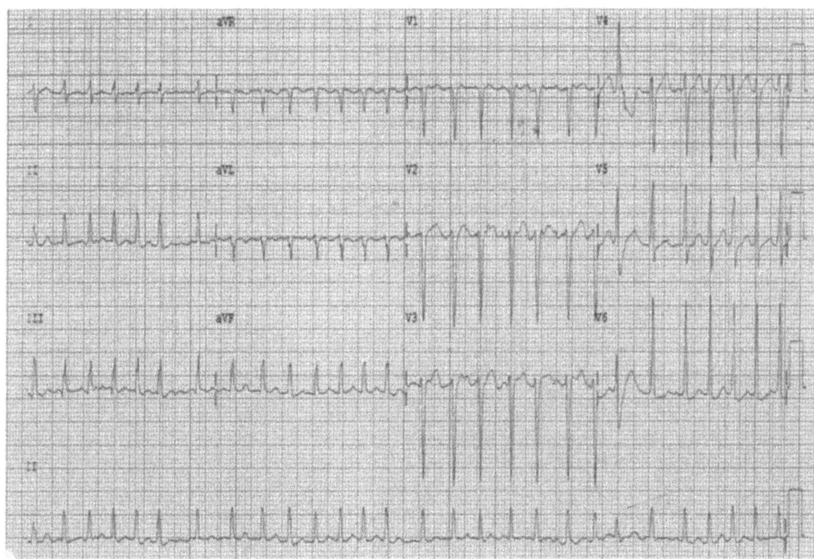

Figure 4.3.1

The appropriate strategy for rate control is:

A. Oral digoxin
B. Oral beta-blocker
C. IV amiodarone
D. Oral dihydropyridine calcium channel blocker
E. Pacemaker implantation and AV node ablation

3. **For a patient aged 75 with a history of hypertension and diabetes and an eGFR of 15 ml/min the most appropriate oral anticoagulant is:**

A. Dabigatran
B. Rivaroxaban
C. Apixaban
D. Edoxaban
E. Warfarin

4. **A 72-year-old man is due to undergo external DC cardioversion. He should:**

A. Discontinue any anti-arrhythmic medication
B. Have an echocardiogram to assess LV function
C. Not drive for 48 hours afterwards
D. Be on uninterrupted therapeutic anticoagulation for at least 3 weeks beforehand
E. Have a transoesophageal echocardiogram (TOE) performed if he is not anticoagulated and has been in AF for more than 12 hours

5. **A 68-year-old lady with a previous transient ischaemic attack (TIA) and hypertension is admitted with an acute coronary syndrome. She has a single stent inserted in her left anterior descending artery. Her echocardiogram pre-discharge shows a LVEF of 30%. In terms of anticoagulation, she:**

A. Should receive triple therapy for 6 months, then dual therapy for 6 months, then an oral anticoagulant alone
B. Should be given aspirin and a NOAC for 12 months, then aspirin alone
C. Can just take dual antiplatelet therapy for 1 year, then start an oral anticoagulant
D. May be started on clopidogrel and warfarin and after 1 year discontinue clopidogrel
E. Should be offered triple therapy for 1 week, followed by clopidogrel and a NOAC up to 12 months, then a NOAC only

6. Regarding the same patient (a 68-year-old lady with a previous TIA and hypertension, admitted with an acute coronary syndrome who has a single stent inserted in her left anterior descending artery and for whom an echocardiogram pre-discharge shows a LVEF of 30%), her approximate annual risk of a thrombo-embolic event is:

A. 4%
B. 6%
C. 8%
D. 10%
E. 15%

7. The following is true for catheter ablation:

A. The success rate for a single procedure for paroxysmal AF at one year without anti-arrhythmic drugs is 50–60%
B. There is randomized controlled evidence for mortality and morbidity benefit in patients with symptomatic AF
C. It is appropriate to consider this as first-line therapy in a young, symptomatic patient with paroxysmal AF and a structurally normal heart
D. The success rates for persistent AF are better than paroxysmal AF ablation
E. The risk of cardiac perforation and tamponade quoted in the literature is approximately 4%

8. A 48-year-old man with no previous medical history presents with palpitations for 6 hours. He is found to be in AF with a heart rate of 110 bpm and blood pressure 110/70 mmHg. There are no signs of heart failure clinically and his chest X-ray is normal. The optimum treatment is:

A. Treat with anticoagulation and beta blocker for 3 weeks, then DC cardioversion
B. TOE and urgent DC cardioversion
C. Intravenous flecainide
D. Intravenous amiodarone
E. Refer for catheter ablation

9. An 82-year-old man presents to the Emergency Department with shortness of breath and pre-syncope with the following ECG and rhythm strip (Figure 4.3.2):

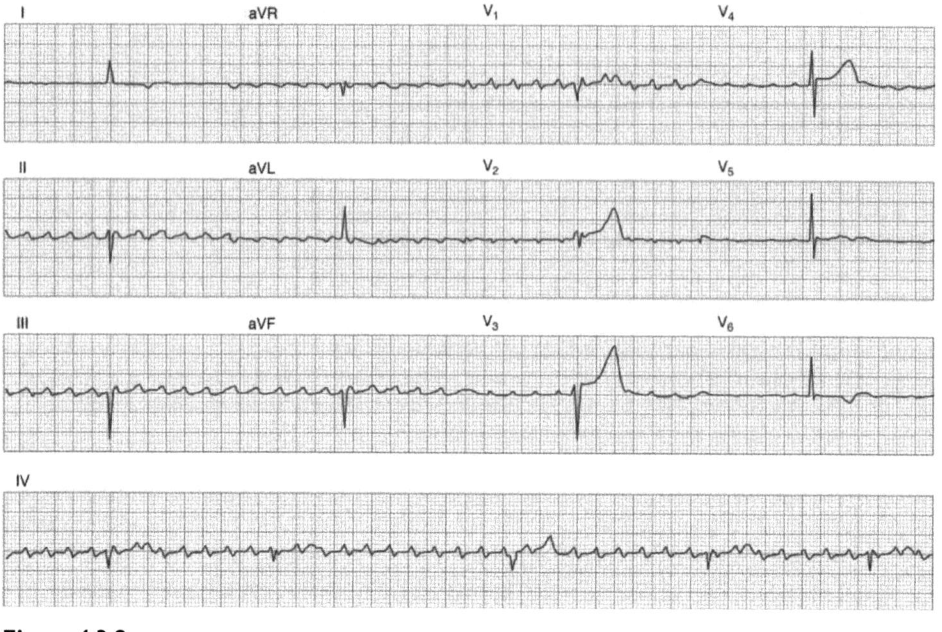

Figure 4.3.2

The most appropriate long-term treatment is:

A. Anticoagulation and rate control
B. DC cardioversion
C. Oral flecainide
D. Catheter ablation
E. Permanent pacemaker insertion

10. A 68-year-old gentleman underwent coronary artery bypass graft surgery (CABG) 4 days ago. He now has this ECG (Figure 4.3.3):

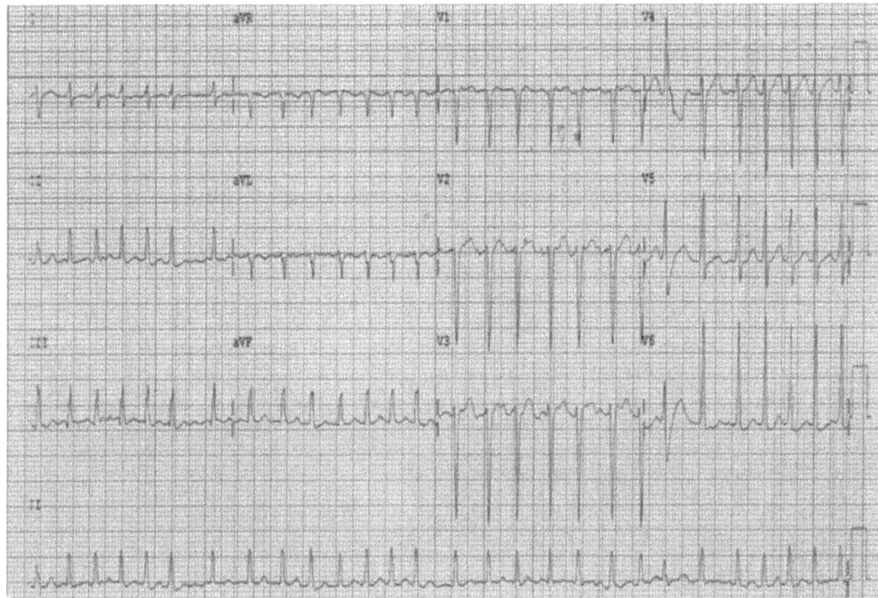

Figure 4.3.3

He is asymptomatic with a blood pressure of 120/80 mmHg and no clinical signs of heart failure. Pre-operatively, his LV function was normal. In terms of anticoagulation, he should:

A. Be given aspirin and clopidogrel for 3 months
B. Be treated with aspirin, and either warfarin or a NOAC pre-discharge
C. Be given aspirin plus venous thromboembolism (VTE) prophylaxis until discharge
D. Receive warfarin or a NOAC only
E. Be given aspirin and unfractionated IV heparin until discharge

11. This same patient (68-year-old gentleman 4 days post CABG with the above ECG (Figure 4.3.3) who is asymptomatic, has a blood pressure of 120/80 mmHg, no clinical signs of heart failure, and normal LV function pre-operatively) should be:

A. Urgently cardioverted electrically
B. Given IV flecainide to chemically cardiovert him
C. Given oral amiodarone
D. Given a beta-blocker or other rate-controlling drug
E. Given digoxin orally

12. A 42-year-old lady with a history of rheumatic heart disease and a mechanical mitral valve replacement (MVR) 10 years ago presents with palpitations. Her ECG is shown (Figure 4.3.4).

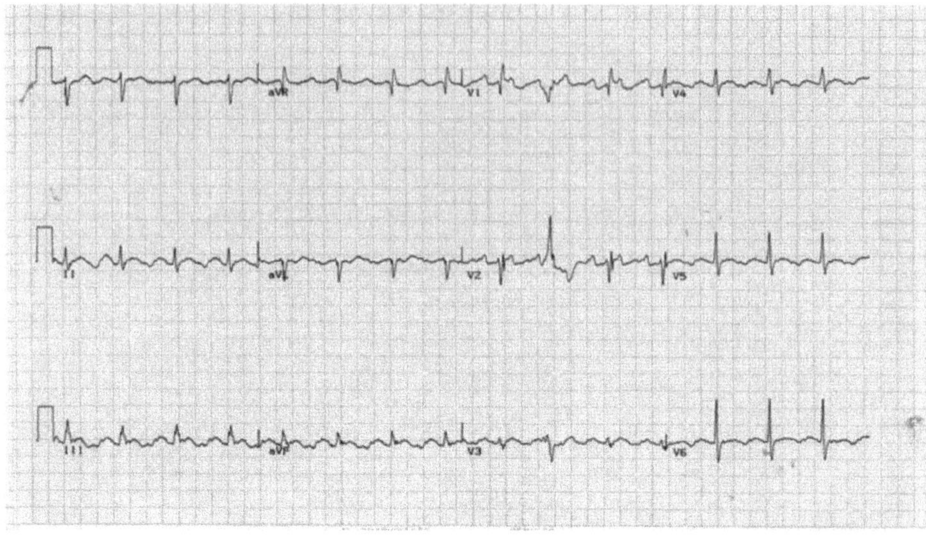

Figure 4.3.4

Her heart rate is 90 bpm, blood pressure 106/60 mmHg, there are no clinical signs of heart failure, and her echocardiogram shows the MVR is functioning well. The most appropriate treatment is:

A. Long-term rate control
B. Elective DC cardioversion
C. Amiodarone orally
D. Catheter ablation
E. Pacemaker implantation and AV node ablation

13. A 48-year-old man with no previous medical history presents to the Emergency Department with palpitations for 6 hours. He is found to be in typical atrial flutter with a heart rate of 150 bpm, blood pressure of 110/70 mmHg, there are no signs of heart failure clinically, and the chest X-ray is normal. This is his second presentation with atrial flutter in the last 12 months. The optimum treatment is:

A. Anticoagulation and beta-blocker for 3 weeks, then DC cardioversion
B. TOE and urgent DC cardioversion
C. Intravenous flecainide
D. Intravenous amiodarone
E. Refer for catheter ablation

14. Which of the following statements regarding atrial flutter is not true?

A. The risk of thromboembolic events is lower than AF
B. Catheter ablation may be considered as first line treatment
C. If the ventricular rate is greater than 150, a beta-blocker may be used for rate control
D. Anticoagulation prescription is indicated if the CHA_2DS_2-VASc score is ≥ 2
E. Typical flutter is a circuit in the right atrium

15. A 73-year-old lady with hypertension, diabetes, and AF is due to have elective total hip replacement. She takes apixaban 5 mg bd. Which of the following statements is true?

A. Her apixaban should be continued throughout the perioperative period
B. It is necessary to convert her to warfarin pre-operatively and continue this perioperatively
C. Her apixaban can be discontinued and appropriate venous thromboembolism (VTE) prophylaxis used until the apixaban can be restarted
D. Her risk of VTE perioperatively is lower than someone without AF
E. An ablation of the AF pre-operatively would lower stroke risk

16. A 65-year-old man with hypertension is incidentally diagnosed with AF. Which of the following is recommended in the 2020 ECS guidelines?

A. DC cardioversion should be performed urgently
B. There is no need for anticoagulation
C. He should be labelled as having persistent AF
D. A beta-blocker should be prescribed immediately
E. A transthoracic echocardiogram should be performed

17. In a patient with heart failure and AF, which of the following is true?

A. Catheter ablation offers no prognostic benefit
B. AF-induced cardiomyopathy should be considered
C. If cardiac resynchronization therapy is indicated, then AV node ablation must also be performed
D. If the AF is asymptomatic, there is no benefit from a rhythm-control approach
E. Mortality is the same as a patient with heart failure and no AF

chapter 4.3

ATRIAL FIBRILLATION AND FLUTTER

ANSWERS

1. C. As the exact onset of AF is not known it is not appropriate to cardiovert this gentleman either chemically or electrically until he has been anticoagulated for at least 3 weeks. If the exact onset of the AF was known and was less than 48 hours then one could consider cardioverting him without requiring a period of anticoagulation first. Aspirin is no longer recommended within the guidelines as stroke prevention for AF. If the patient's CHA_2DS_2-VASc score is ≥ 1 and bleeding risk has been assessed and addressed then anticoagulation is most commonly recommended using a non-vitamin K oral anticoagulant (NOAC), in preference to warfarin. Although underlying coronary artery disease can be associated with AF, in the absence of symptoms and risk factors in a gentleman of this age it would not be appropriate to investigate this. Some people will want to make sure there is no significant coronary artery disease prior to using class I antiarrhythmic drugs such as flecainide, but as that would not be considered as treatment for him at this stage there is no requirement to assess for coronary artery disease.

2. B. In this particular patient a rate control strategy is an appropriate initial strategy, with subsequent investigation and anticoagulation. Digoxin can be used for rate control but is not very effective at controlling rate with exertion. Therefore, given this lady's fast ventricular rates, it is unlikely this would control her rates sufficiently. Amiodarone is actually quite an effective rate-controlling drug but would not be used in this instance for that purpose given important potential side effects, and it also might potentially cardiovert her which should not be done without 3 weeks of formal anticoagulation. Pacemaker implantation and AV node ablation is a very effective form of rate control but normally medical therapy will be tried in the first instance before committing a patient to invasive procedures and their potential risks. The first-line choice for most patients in this scenario is an oral beta-blocker unless there is a clear contraindication. In that case a rate-limiting calcium channel blocker would be an option, possibly as a first-line choice, but not a non-rate limiting (dihydropyridine) calcium channel blocker.

3. E. None of the non-vitamin K oral anticoagulants are licensed for use in patients with this degree of renal impairment. Dabigatran, rivaroxaban, and edoxaban should not be used in patients with creatinine clearance < 30 ml/min, and apixaban should not be used in patients with creatinine clearance <15 ml/min or serum creatinine > 2.5 mg/dL (221 μmol/L).

4. D. Antiarrhythmic medication will often be continued before and after an external cardioversion to try and help maintain sinus rhythm. Most patients will have had an echocardiogram prior to cardioversion, predominantly to assess left atrial size which gives some indication of the likelihood of success, but also to assess ventricular and valve function. However, this is not absolutely mandatory. Generally patients are advised not to drive for 24 hours after the cardioversion. If patients have been in AF for more than 48 hours they should be therapeutically anticoagulated for at least 3 weeks before the cardioversion and for at least 4 weeks after the cardioversion. If the patient has been in AF for less than 48 hours (and there is no doubt about this) then the patient can have the cardioversion done without formal anticoagulation. A TOE can be performed if the patient has been in AF for more than 48 hours to specifically exclude left atrial appendage thrombus and allow an external cardioversion to be performed without 3 weeks of anticoagulation.

5. A. The most recent ESC guidelines regarding anticoagulation in the setting of AF and acute coronary syndromes with PCI are presented in Figure 4.3.A1. The default strategy for a patient with AF meeting criteria for anticoagulation who undergoes PCI as treatment for their ACS is up to 1 week of triple antithrombotic therapy, dual antithrombotic therapy using a NOAC at the recommended dose for stroke prevention and a single oral antiplatelet agent (preferably clopidogrel) for up to 12 months, followed by NOAC only. Other strategies may be considered depending on an individual's ischaemic and bleeding risk. Ticagrelor and prasugrel should not be avoided as part of triple antithrombotic therapy.

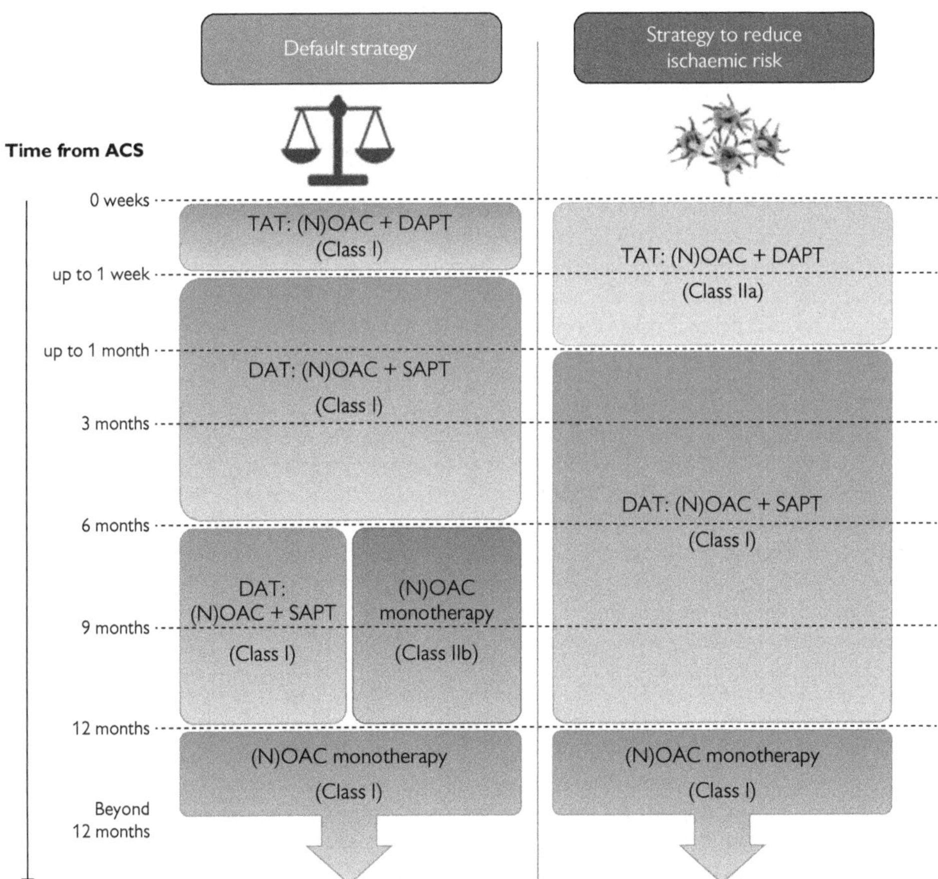

Figure 4.3.A1 Reproduced from Byrne RA, Rossello X, Coughlan JJ, et al; ESC Scientific Document Group. 2023 ESC Guidelines for the management of acute coronary syndromes. Eur Heart J. 2023 Oct 12;44(38):3720-3826. doi: 10.1093/eurheartj/ehad191. © European Society of Cardiology. With permission from Oxford University Press.. Acronyms – ACS = acute coronary syndrome, DAPT = dual antiplatelet therapy, DAT = dual antithrombotic therapy, (N)OAC = non-vitamin K antagonist oral anticoagulant, OAC = oral anticoagulation, SAPT = single antiplatelet therapy, TAT = triple antithrombotic therapy

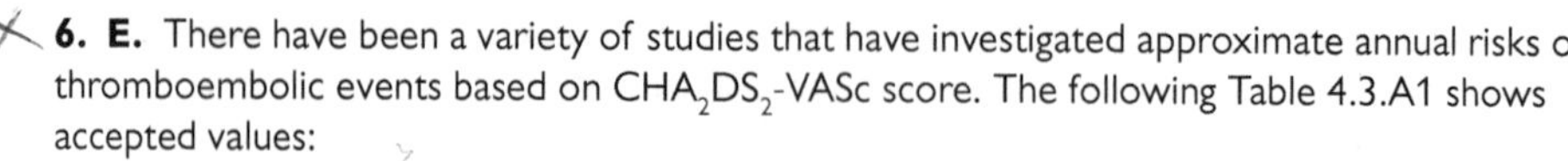

6. E. There have been a variety of studies that have investigated approximate annual risks of thromboembolic events based on CHA_2DS_2-VASc score. The following Table 4.3.A1 shows accepted values:

Table 4.3.A1

CHA_2DS_2-VASc	0	1	2	3	4	5	6	7	8	9
Adjusted stroke rate (%/year)	0.3	0.9	2.9	4.6	6.7	10.9	13.6	15.7	15.2	17.4

This patient has a score of 7 so the thromboembolic event risk is approximately 15%. It is worth noting that the risk with a score of 8 is slightly lower than that of 7. In reality it is agreed that the risk gradually increases so in fact it is probably slightly higher, but the data from studies that these numbers are based on provide these figures.

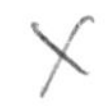

7. C. Current success rates for a single AF ablation procedure for paroxysmal AF without the use of any anti-arrhythmic medication range from 70–90% depending upon technique and literature source. All results are significantly better than 50–60%. In general, studies have all demonstrated better success rates with paroxysmal AF ablation then with persistent AF ablation. The one randomized control trial that has reported on mortality and morbidity in patients with AF undergoing ablation (CABANA) did not demonstrate a benefit with the pre-determined intention-to-treat analysis. This trial did demonstrate the safety of catheter ablation and in general the risk of cardiac perforation or tamponade is approximately 1–2%. The ESC guidelines suggest that AF ablation can be considered first-line therapy in a young, symptomatic patient with paroxysmal AF and a structurally normal heart.

8. C. As this patient seems to be able to give a fairly accurate time of onset of the symptoms and this is less than 48 hours it is unnecessary to anticoagulate, rate control, and then externally cardiovert. It is also unnecessary to perform a TOE even if external cardioversion is performed immediately. Catheter ablation would not be an appropriate initial strategy for this patient, even if his heart is structurally normal as he needs treatment for his current symptoms. Whilst intravenous amiodarone could be used there are some risks associated with this, particularly if given peripherally, and the time to cardiovert is significantly longer than with intravenous flecainide. In some countries other drugs, such as ibutilide and vernakalant, may be considered, but in many countries the first-line choice would be intravenous flecainide.

9. E. This patient has symptoms that could be related to the atrial arrhythmia itself and therefore rhythm control might improve his symptoms. However, external cardioversion is unlikely to be effective long term at this age. Catheter ablation in this age group also has a higher risk and potentially lower success rates. In the absence of an assessment of underlying coronary artery disease the use of flecainide would be relatively contraindicated. In this particular situation implantation of a permanent pacemaker is the most appropriate therapy as that is likely to improve symptoms with the lowest risk and longest-term success. He does need anticoagulation as well but rate control is clearly not needed as the patient is already bradycardic.

10. B. In this patient they need formal anticoagulation for the AF but also an antiplatelet agent for the recent bypass graft surgery. In the longer term they can be managed with formal anticoagulation alone. None of the other treatment strategies are appropriate.

11. D. It is appropriate to simply rate control this patient: the beta-blocker is more effective than digoxin and is first-line therapy. Many of these patients will spontaneously revert to sinus rhythm during follow-up without the need for any form of rhythm control therapy. If the patient were haemodynamically compromised then they would be urgently cardioverted electrically, or if it was felt that it was important to restore sinus rhythm then antiarrhythmic medication might be used, but neither of those is the case in this patient.

12. B. Even in a patient with mitral valve surgery atrial flutter (which this ECG shows) is most likely to be right atrial, unless left atrial ablation has been performed at surgery. Although the appearance is not typical it may be a clockwise right atrial flutter rather than the typical anticlockwise type. There is increasing use of catheter ablation early in the treatment of patients with right atrial flutter and therefore this may be considered, but given the possibility of a left atrial flutter it would be reasonable to perform an external cardioversion first. Whilst amiodarone could be used to chemically cardiovert the patient this may not be successful, potentially will take several weeks, and there is a small risk of significant side effects. Rate control is a strategy that may be appropriate, particularly if the patient is asymptomatic, but an initial attempt at rhythm control, especially in a lady of this age, would be preferred. Therefore long-term rate control is not a preferred treatment strategy. At her age pacemaker implantation and AV node ablation would not be considered appropriate either.

13. E. Where the ECG is suggestive of typical atrial flutter it is reasonable to consider catheter ablation as a first-line treatment given high success rates and low risk of complication. There is no need to anticoagulate prior to cardioversion as the onset of symptoms is less than 48 hours and management is therefore the same as AF. For the same reason he would not need a TOE if external DC cardioversion is performed. The use of antiarrhythmic drugs to chemically cardiovert flutter, as in AF, has limitations. Amiodarone may take a long time to chemically cardiovert even if administered intravenously. Flecainide has the potential risk of paradoxically accelerating the ventricular rate (because of its potential for slowing the cycle length of the atrial flutter and therefore increasing the possibility of 1:1 conduction to the ventricles).

14. A. Catheter ablation is increasingly considered as a first-line treatment for typical right atrial flutter. This is normally an anticlockwise circuit in the right atrium. Beta-blockers are typically the first-choice drug for rate control. Anticoagulation for patients with atrial flutter is performed along the same guidelines as for AF and the thromboembolic risk with atrial flutter is deemed to be the same as that for AF.

15. C. Management of anticoagulation for AF perioperatively depends upon the risk of thromboembolism whilst the anticoagulation is interrupted compared to the risk of haemorrhagic complication from the operation if anticoagulation is continued or started too soon. For most forms of surgery it is appropriate to discontinue non-vitamin K oral anticoagulants for the surgery itself. If the patient has a very high risk of thromboembolic events whilst off anticoagulation then heparin may be administered to bridge this. However, most of the time it is only necessary to use standard VTE prophylaxis. The risk of perioperative VTE is at least as high as someone without AF and ablation of AF has not been demonstrated to reduce stroke risk and therefore would not help perioperatively.

16. E. In the most recent guidelines rate control is still appropriate in the first instance. Anticoagulation is indicated and this type of AF is defined as 'first diagnosed' rather than persistent. It may be appropriate to prescribe a beta-blocker for rate control if ventricular rates are fast but this is not something that has to be done immediately. It is, however, deemed necessary to assess the substrate of AF including performing a transthoracic echocardiogram.

17. B. Many studies have demonstrated that patients with heart failure and AF have a higher mortality than those in sinus rhythm. There are a few studies, including CASTLE-AF, that have demonstrated ablation of AF in patients with heart failure confers prognostic benefit. A rhythm control strategy, including ablation, is particularly beneficial for patients in whom AF has potentially induced the cardiomyopathy, and this possibility should be considered. Because of the potential for improvement in LV function with a rhythm control strategy there may be prognostic benefit even in asymptomatic individuals. According to ESC guidelines, cardiac resynchronization therapy is indicated in patients with AF and the same criteria as those with sinus rhythm. However, to maximize benefit it is necessary to maximize biventricular pacing, and whilst this may be achieved with rate controlling therapy alone, sometimes AV node ablation is required.

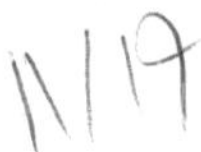

chapter 4.4

ARRHYTHMIAS AND IMPLANTABLE CARDIAC DEVICES

QUESTIONS

1. **A 56-year-old man attends the Emergency Department with a 9-hour history of chest pain. His admission ECG shows ST-segment elevation in the anterolateral leads and he is managed with primary PCI to the proximal LAD. There is no significant bystander disease. Post-PCI ECG shows sinus rhythm with a QRS duration of 98 ms. Transthoracic echo before discharge 2 days later shows severe LV systolic impairment with an LVEF of 24%. The RV is normal and there is no significant valve pathology.**

   Regarding his risk of sudden cardiac death, in addition to optimizing his medical heart failure therapy, what is the most appropriate next step?

   A. A dual chamber ICD should be implanted before discharge
   B. A CRT-D should be implanted before discharge
   C. He should be started on oral amiodarone before discharge
   D. A repeat echo should be undertaken after 6–12 weeks and decision made thereafter
   E. A repeat echo should be undertake after 4 months and decision made thereafter

2. **A 67-year-old woman attends the Emergency Department with a 5-day history of stuttering chest pain on exertion that has been constant for the last 12 hours and is still present. Her ECG shows ST-segment elevation in the anterolateral leads. She is managed with attempted PCI to the proximal left anterior descending (LAD) coronary artery but this fails for technical reasons. She is therefore not revascularized and the LAD remains occluded. By this time she is pain free and declines emergent coronary artery bypass grafting (CABG). Three days into her presentation she experiences an episode of sustained VT associated with dizziness and marked hypotension that resolves spontaneously after approximately four minutes. Resting ECG shows sinus rhythm with a normal PR interval and QRS duration 98 ms. Transthoracic echo shows severe LV systolic impairment. The RV is normal and there is no significant valve pathology. Cardiac MRI shows the LAD territory is infarcted and non-viable, with a calculated LVEF of 18%.**

   Regarding her risk of sudden cardiac death, in addition to optimizing her medical heart failure therapy, what is the most appropriate next step?

   A. A dual chamber ICD should be implanted before discharge
   B. A CRT-D should be implanted before discharge
   C. She should be started on oral amiodarone before discharge
   D. A repeat echo should be undertaken after 6 weeks and decision made thereafter
   E. A repeat echo should be undertaken after 4 months and decision made thereafter

3. **A 55-year-old woman with a diagnosis of dilated cardiomyopathy attends the cardiology clinic. She has been established on optimal medical heart failure therapy for the last 5 months, with a resting heart rate of 74 bpm in long-standing persistent atrial fibrillation. Her ECG shows LBBB with QRS duration 160 ms. Echo demonstrates severe biventricular systolic impairment. There is no significant valve pathology. Cardiac MRI confirms these findings with an LVEF of 18%. There is a small amount of subepicardial late gadolinium enhancement (LGE). She declines to undergo genetic testing. She is currently in NYHA class II, able to walk about 0.5 km on the flat.**

   Regarding device therapy, which of the following would be most appropriate to offer her?

   A. No device and advise continue medical therapy alone
   B. A single chamber ICD
   C. A CRT-P
   D. A CRT-D
   E. A subcutaneous ICD

4. An active 65-year-old woman presents with shortness of breath on exertion for 2 months, worse for the previous week with two episodes of pre-syncope in the last 24 hours. Her echocardiogram shows good biventricular systolic function with normal left atrial size. Her ECG shows newly diagnosed atrial fibrillation with complete heart block. An ECG from her GP surgery 6 months ago shows sinus rhythm.

What type of pacemaker should she be offered?

A. A single chamber pacemaker programmed VVIR
B. A single chamber pacemaker programmed AAIR
C. A dual chamber pacemaker programmed DDD-VVIR
D. A dual chamber pacemaker programmed DDDR
E. An exercise test should be undertaken to help decide

5. An 83-year-old man with a dual chamber pacemaker implanted for Mobitz II second-degree heart block 1 year ago presents to clinic with shortness of breath on exertion for the last 6 months, currently able to walk about 50 metres on the flat before stopping due to breathlessness. There is no associated chest pain. Echo shows new severe LV systolic impairment with LVEF 27%. The RV is normal and there is no valve pathology. ECG shows atrial sensing with RV pacing and device interrogation shows that his device is atrial pacing only 5% of the time but is RV pacing 45% of the time.

What would you advise to help him?

A. Optimse medical heart failure therapy and upgrade to CRT-P
B. Optimse medical heart failure therapy and upgrade to CRT-D
C. Optimse medical heart failure therapy and review his current device settings with a focus on AV interval and lower rate limit
D. Optimse medical heart failure therapy and obtain a coronary angiogram
E. Investigate for other causes of shortness of breath, such as anaemia or respiratory pathology

6. During a routine generator change, an 86-year-old man with no underlying rhythm and a single chamber RV pacemaker suddenly becomes asystolic when the generator is removed from the pocket. The RV lead is quickly disconnected from the generator and connected to PSA (pacing system analyser) leads. It begins pacing and all parameters are acceptable, similar to previous pacing checks.

What is the most likely explanation for this?

A. The RV lead has been damaged while dissecting into the pocket
B. The RV lead insulation has failed
C. The pacemaker was programmed to pace in unipolar mode
D. The pacemaker was programmed to pace in bipolar mode
E. The old generator was not functioning normally due to low battery life remaining

7. An 81-year-old woman with the below ECG (Figure 4.4.1) presents with two syncopal events. Both occurred while walking and with no warning. Recovery was rapid when she awoke on the floor. Her echocardiogram shows good biventricular systolic function.

What is the most appropriate device to offer her?

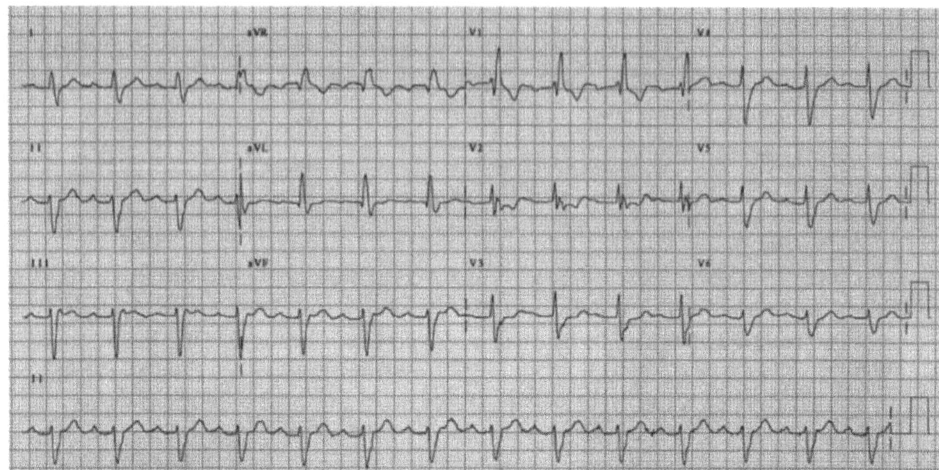

Figure 4.4.1 *https://www.stemlynsblog.org.*

A. Implantable loop recorder
B. Single chamber atrial pacemaker
C. Single chamber ventricular pacemaker
D. Dual chamber pacemaker
E. CRT-P

8. A 51-year-old man with type 2 diabetes, newly diagnosed familial hypercholesterolemia, and diffuse coronary artery disease presents with shortness of breath on exertion and a syncopal event. His ECG shows marked first-degree heart block (PR interval 320 ms) with intermittent Mobitz II second-degree heart block in the absence of any negatively chronotropic drugs. The QRS duration is 100 ms. His echocardiogram shows severe LV systolic impairment with normal RV function. A coronary angiogram from 2 months ago shows no targets for revascularization with no evidence of left main stem (LMS) disease. Perfusion cardiac MRI at that time showed no inducible ischemia.

How should he be managed?

A. Medical heart failure therapy should be optimized and he should be offered an updated echocardiogram after 3 months to decide
B. A dual chamber pacemaker should be offered
C. CRT-P should be offered
D. CRT-D should be offered
E. A dual chamber ICD should be offered

9. A frail 86-year-old patient with a CRT-P for non-ischaemic LV systolic impairment with LBBB presents with shortness of breath on exertion for the last 4 months. Her device interrogation shows new atrial fibrillation that corresponds to her symptom duration. The biventricular pacing percentage is 83%. Echocardiography shows moderate LV systolic impairment with severe left atrial dilatation. She is already taking oral anticoagulation.

What would you advise in order to help?

A. List for DC cardioversion
B. Start oral amiodarone
C. Increase her beta blocker dose
D. Start entresto
E. Review her device settings to try to reduce her biventricular pacing percentage 

10. A 70-year-old woman with a dual chamber pacemaker is seen in pacing clinic. Her original device was implanted 14 years ago and she underwent a generator change 2 years ago. The new generator has unexpectedly already reached ERI (elective replacement indicator). There is noise on the RV channel and RV lead pacing parameters are as follows:

- Threshold 1.6 V at 0.4 ms
- Impedance: 128 ohms

What is the most likely explanation for this?

A. RV lead insulation failure
B. RV lead fracture
C. RV lead displacement
D. Atrial lead insulation failure
E. Failure to adequately connect the leads to the generator at generator replacement

11. A 26-year-old woman presents to the Emergency Department with palpitations and the below ECG (Figure 4.4.2). She has no past medical history, looks well, has no chest pain, and blood pressure is 130/80 mmHg. This is her third episode of significant palpitations this year but all others have stopped spontaneously without her attending hospital.

What is the most appropriate long-term management to offer her?

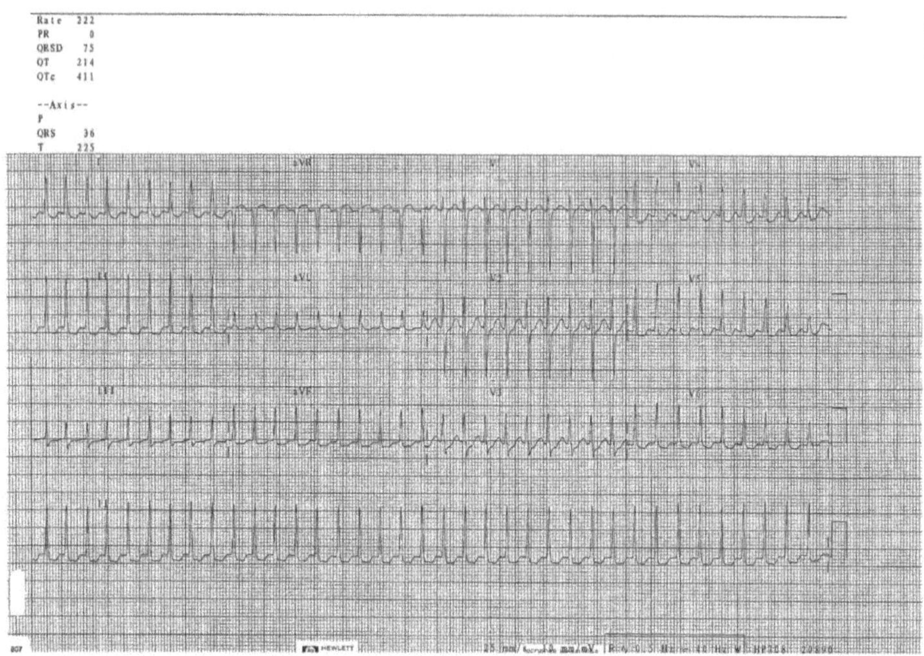

Figure 4.4.2

A. Pill-in-the-pocket verapamil
B. Regular verapamil
C. Pill-in-the-pocket beta blockers
D. Electrophysiology (EP) study and ablation
E. Follow-up in clinic to monitor symptom frequency and decide based on this

12. A 35-year-old patient presents to clinic. He has had an ECG undertaken as part of a health screening medical assessment (Figure 4.4.3) and is entirely asymptomatic.

How should he be managed?

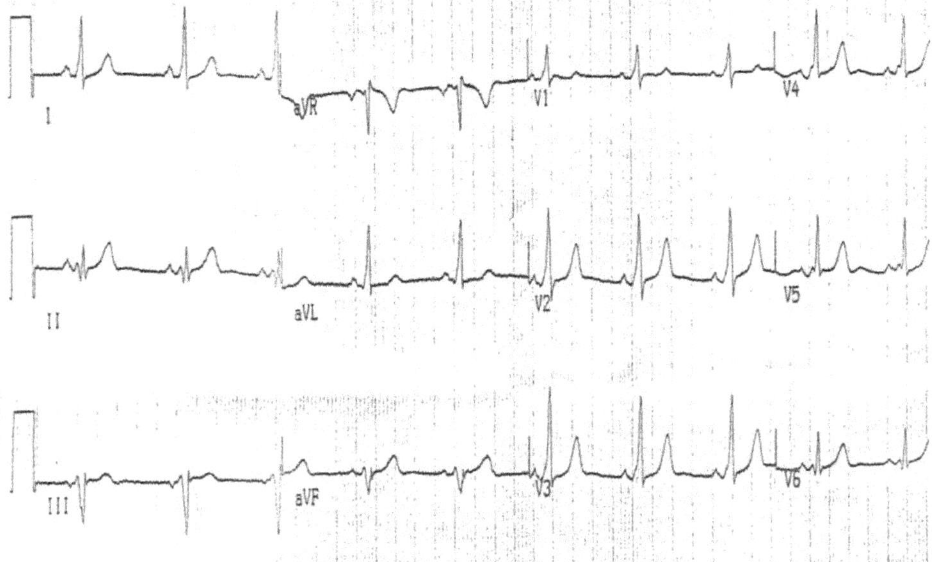

Figure 4.4.3

A. Reassurance and discharge
B. Treadmill test to assess for rapid antegrade conduction via an accessory pathway
C. Electrophysiology (EP) study to assess for rapid antegrade conduction via an accessory pathway
D. Pill-in-the-pocket flecainide for use in the event of future palpitations
E. Regular follow-up to monitor for the development of symptoms

13. The same 35-year-old patient did not want to have an electrophysiology (EP) study. He did undergo an echocardiogram that demonstrated a structurally normal heart, and a treadmill test that demonstrated the accessory pathway (AP) was still able to conduct antegradely at his maximum heart rate. He is now in the Emergency Department with palpitations and an ECG showing narrow complex tachycardia consistent with orthodromic AVRT. His blood pressure is 130/90 mmHg, he looks well, and has no chest pain. This is his second attendance in the last month. He is still unwilling to undergo EP study +/- ablation.

What medical therapy would you recommend?

A. IV adenosine acutely, verapamil thereafter
B. IV adenosine acutely, beta blockers thereafter
C. IV adenosine acutely, flecainide thereafter
D. Sedation and DC cardioversion, flecainide thereafter
E. Sedation and DC cardioversion, verapamil thereafter

14. A 40-year-old woman presents to Emergency Department with the below ECG (Figure 4.4.4). Her blood pressure is 86/50 mmHg. An echocardiogram undertaken by her GP 3 months prior to admission shows a structurally normal heart.

What management would you recommend?

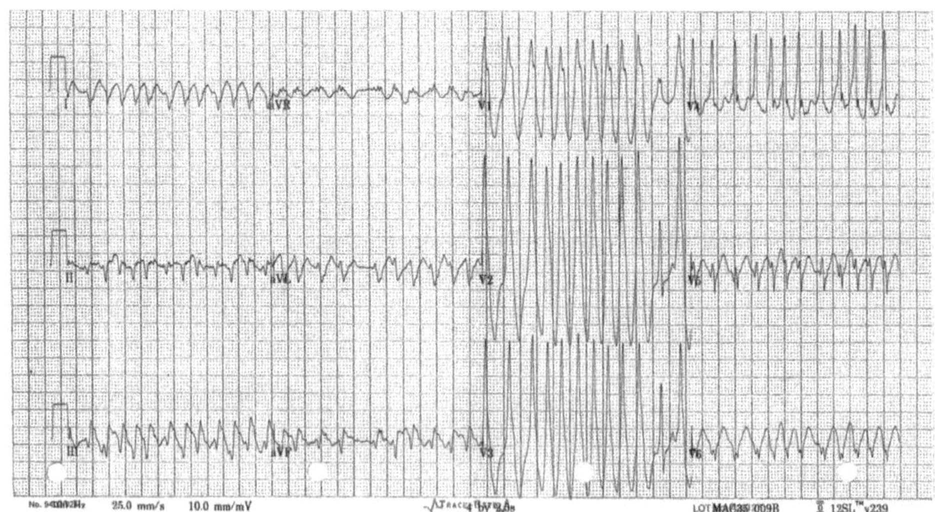

Figure 4.4.4

A. Sedation and DC cardioversion
B. IV flecainide
C. IV amiodarone
D. IV verapamil
E. IV adenosine

15. A 64-year-old man with a history of PCI to the right coronary artery (RCA) 7 years ago and moderate LV systolic impairment (EF 42%) presents to Emergency Department with intermittent chest pain. His admission ECG shows 2 mm ST depression in the inferior leads, with normal corrected QT interval. Troponin T is elevated at 660 ng/L. He has been pain free for 20 minutes, but during your assessment he becomes pre-syncopal with polymorphic VT seen on his cardiac monitor. This spontaneously cardioverts after about 1 minute, before he can be DC cardioverted.

How should he now be managed?

A. IV magnesium, admit to CCU
B. IV lignocaine, admit to CCU
C. Refer for primary PCI
D. IV amiodarone, admit to CCU
e. IV metoprolol, admit to CCU

16. A 19-year-old presents to the Cardiology Outpatient clinic following an ECG undertaken as part of a screening medical (Figure 4.4.5). She is entirely asymptomatic and has had an echocardiogram ahead of the appointment showing a structurally normal heart.

How would you manage her?

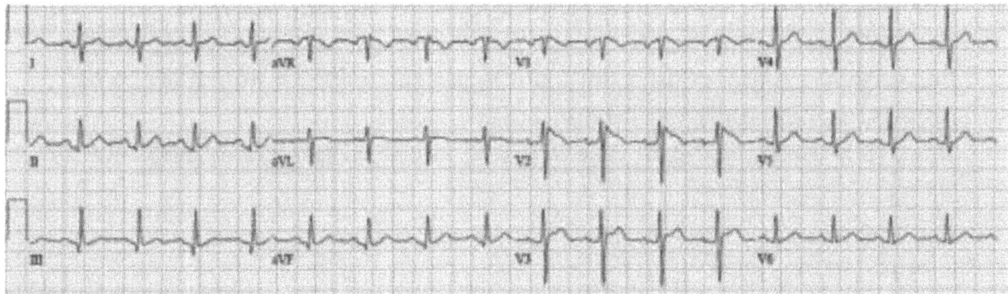

Figure 4.4.5 *https://www.heartrhythmcasereports.com/article/S2214-0271(20)30053-1/pdf*

A. Treadmill test to assess for arrhythmia on exertion
B. Advise her about the avoidance of fever, excess alcohol intake, large meals, and specific medications that could precipitate ventricular arrhythmias
C. Offer her an ajmaline challenge
D. Offer her a single chamber ICD
E. Advise her that family screening is not necessary

17. Which of these drugs increase the risk of ventricular arrhythmias in patients with Brugada Syndrome?

A. Flecainide
B. Amitriptyline
C. Lithium
D. Cocaine
E. All of the above

18. A 28-year-old man is referred to clinic with a history of recurrent syncope. He has no past medical history and takes no regular medications (prescribed or over the counter). His GP has performed an ECG showing a corrected QT interval of 486 ms. A repeat ECG in clinic shows a corrected QT interval of 498 ms.

Which of these statements is true?

A. This is not sufficient to diagnose long QT syndrome
B. Genetic testing will not be of use in this case
C. He should be commenced on beta-blockers and listed for an ICD
D. He should be commenced on beta-blockers and not listed for an ICD
E. He will have to remember which drugs he should avoid

19. A 29-year-old patient is referred to clinic following positive genetic testing. Her brother has been diagnosed with catecholaminergic polymorphic VT (CPVT), with a pathogenic variant identified in the *RyR2* gene. She has the sane variant. She is asymptomatic and has recently undergone a normal treadmill test with no evidence of bidirectional or polymorphic VT.

Which of the following statement is true regarding her management?

A. She should consider taking beta-blockers
B. She does not have CPVT, despite her genotype, as she does not have any inducible VT on exertion
C. She does not need to make any lifestyle changes
D. Flecainide is likely to increase her risk of ventricular arrhythmias
E. She should be offered an ICD

20. A 58-year-old man with a history of coronary artery bypass grafting (CABG) 15 years ago presents to the Emergency Department in cardiac arrest with a broad complex tachycardia. He is electrically cardioverted to sinus rhythm and makes a good recovery. In addition to a number of other interventions, he is advised to have a dual chamber ICD implanted. He works as a Heavy Goods Vehicle driver and therefore has both a group 1 and group 2 driving licence.

Based on UK DVLA guidelines, what would you advise him regarding the impact of an ICD on his ability to drive?

A. Both his group 1 and group 2 licences will be permanently revoked and he will not be able to drive again

B. His group 2 licence will be permanently revoked but he may be able to regain his group 1 licence and drive again after 1 month

C. His group 2 licence will be permanently revoked but he may be able to regain his group 1 licence and drive again after 6 months

D. Therapy from the ICD will not impact his ability to drive in future

E. Changes to anti-arrhythmic drugs will not impact his ability to drive in future

chapter

4.4

ARRHYTHMIAS AND IMPLANTABLE CARDIAC DEVICES

ANSWERS

1. D. With revascularization and optimal medical heart failure therapy, this patient's LV systolic function may significantly improve over time. According to ESC guidelines, implantation of an ICD for primary prevention of sudden cardiac death (SCD) <40 days after an ACS is a class III indication (contraindicated). A repeat TTE should be undertaken after 6–12 weeks and if the LVEF remains ≤35% implantation of a primary prevention ICD should be offered. In this case the QRS duration is narrow (<120 ms) and there is no pacing indication so a single chamber VR ICD would be appropriate. Oral amiodarone is not necessary.

2. A. This patient has severe LV systolic impairment that is unlikely to recover with time and medical heart failure therapy, after presenting with an ACS that has not been appropriately revascularized. She has also experienced a sustained ventricular arrhythmia >48 hours following an ACS presentation and ESC guidelines support ICD implantation <40 days after an ACS in this scenario. As her QRS duration is narrow (<120 ms) there is no indication for CRT. The normal PR interval and QRS duration suggest she is unlikely to require RV pacing, which could be detrimental in the setting of LV systolic impairment. A dual chamber DR ICD is therefore appropriate.

3. D. Although there is less evidence for the role of CRT in patients with AF than those in sinus rhythm, guidelines still support offering CRT based on the same indications. This patient has severe LV impairment despite >3 months of optimal medical therapy for HFrEF and a broad QRS in LBBB pattern. She should therefore be offered CRT. The choice of CRT-P vs CRT-D can be difficult in non-ischaemic LV systolic impairment, due to the (generally) lower risk of ventricular arrhythmias in this patient population. Taking account of the results of the large DANISH trial, which demonstrated that ICD therapy offered a mortality benefit in patients who are <68 years old who have non-ischaemic LV impairment, as well as the LGE suggestive of scar that could act as a substrate for ventricular arrhythmia on her CMR, it would be reasonable to recommend CRT-D in this case. Of course, taking patient preference into account is mandatory and MDT discussion before implant is advisable. Genetic testing is also playing an increasingly important role in risk stratifying patients with DCM, as some pathogenic variants (such as those in the LMNA gene) are associated with a higher risk of sudden cardiac death and ESC guidelines support a lower threshold for primary prevention ICD implant in these patients.

4. C. This patient has high-degree AV block which is an ESC class I indication for pacing both in the presence and absence of symptoms. She is currently in AF and therefore her atrium cannot be paced. However, this is a new diagnosis. It may be paroxysmal meaning she may require atrial sensing +/- pacing when in sinus rhythm (SR). Furthermore, she may decide to pursue rhythm control at a later date, again meaning that she would require atrial channel sensing +/- pacing. Therefore, a dual chamber pacemaker is most appropriate here, programmed to mode switch between DDD and VVI pacing based on her rhythm (DDD in SR, VVI in AF). As she is currently in AF, she will require VVI pacing with rate response to be programmed on to allow her continue at her previous activity level.

5. C. The first step in this case is to try to reduce his burden of RV pacing, which is likely to have contributed to his LV systolic impairment. Evidence suggests that patients whose device delivers RV pacing ≥40% of the time have a higher incidence of heart failure and mortality and ESC Pacing and CRT guidelines from 2021 state that upgrade from RV pacing to CRT can be considered in patients who require RV pacing >20% of the time. Device companies have each developed their own algorithms to try to reduce RV pacing. All are broadly based on increasing the AV delay in an attempt to allow intrinsic conduction from the atria to ventricles as much as possible. The lower rate limit should also be programmed to appropriate rate (e.g. 60bpm during the day and 50bpm at night). Medical heart failure therapy should be optimized in addition to this. If these steps fail, RV pacing burden cannot be reduced and the LV remains severely impaired then upgrade to CRT should be offered and is an ESC class I indication. Guidelines do not specify whether this should be CRT-P or CRT-D and this decision should be individualized in each patient that requires CRT upgrade. A coronary angiogram is not necessary at this stage as there is no history of angina.

6. C. Pacemakers that are programmed to pace in unipolar mode will stop pacing when the generator is removed from the pocket. This is because the generator is part of the unipolar circuit (acting as the anode) and the pacing circuit is broken by removing the generator from the body. This does not happen to pacemakers that are programmed in bipolar mode. This problem illustrates the importance of understanding pacing settings and patient factors such as the presence or absence of underlying rhythm before undertaking generator changes.

7. D. This patient has trifasicular block, which is evidence of advanced conduction system disease on her ECG: first-degree heart block, RBBB, and left axis deviation. Given her typical syncopal symptoms, it is likely she is experiencing transient episodes of complete heart block and an implantable loop recorder is not required to confirm this diagnosis in this setting. She should be offered a dual chamber pacemaker as her atrial channel will need to be sensed +/- paced and ventricular channel will need to be both sensed and paced. She has normal LV systolic function and therefore there is no indication for CRT.

8. D. This patient has a class 1 indication for pacing. This cannot be delayed and therefore answer A is not appropriate. He has marked first degree heart block and intermittent high grade AV block which means he is likely to experience a high burden of ventricular pacing. If RV pacing alone is offered, this is likely to worsen his already-impaired LV systolic function. This situation is therefore an ESC class I indication for de novo CRT implant, even though his intrinsic QRS is narrow. The presence of ischaemic heart disease with severe LV systolic impairment is also an indication for ICD therapy. Therefore, the most appropriate choice is CRT-D. Unlike in the majority of CRT implants, there would be no benefit in trying to maximize biventricular pacing as his intrinsic QRS complex is narrow.

9. C. This patient is likely to be short of breath because her heart rate in atrial fibrillation is faster than it was in sinus rhythm, which is reducing her biventricular pacing percentage as her device will be programmed not to pace her ventricles above a certain heart rate. The benefit of CRT is greatly reduced if the percentage of biventricular pacing is low and the minimum percentage that is usually targeted is 95%. Amiodarone may help to control her rate but has more significant side effects and should usually only be used on a long-term basis when other therapies have failed. Pursuing rhythm control with DC cardioversion is not likely to be appropriate given her frailty, left atrial dilatation, and the likelihood that AF will recur. An additional option here is AV node ablation, should an increase in rate control drugs fail to adequately slow her intrinsic AV node conduction and increase biventricular pacing percentage to the required level.

10. A. Rapid battery depletion with low RV lead impedance is suggestive of RV lead insulation failure. Energy is lost at the site of insulation failure causing the generator to lose battery reserve. It is likely that this patient will need a generator change and a new RV lead implanted.

11. D. This ECG is consistent with AV nodal re-entrant tachycardia (AVNRT). Offering an EP study with ablation as first-line therapy for patients with symptomatic recurrent episodes is an ESC class 1 indication. Either regular or pill-in-the-pocket therapy with calcium channel blockers or beta-blockers can be considered if ablation is not desirable or feasible.

12. C. An EP study and interrogation of the accessory pathway (AP) to assess for rapid antegrade conduction is a class IIa indication. This is because APs that can conduct rapidly can lead to sudden cardiac death in patient who develop AF, as the pathway conducts very rapidly from the fibrillating atria to the ventricles causing very rapid ventricular rates that lead to cardiac arrest. This is a class 1 indication in patients with high-risk occupations, such as professional drivers and athletes. Non-invasive assessment with treadmill testing is a class IIb indication and can be considered. However, it is not as reliable as invasive assessment.

13. C. IV adenosine is first line therapy for AVRT (both orthodromic and antidromic) and is likely to terminate the tachycardia. Electrical cardioversion should always be readily available due to the small risk of inducing AF that may be pre-excited and rapidly conducted. Sedation and cardioversion should be considered if this fails or in patients who are haemodynamically unstable. Options for ongoing medical therapy are limited in patients with manifest pre-excitation of their ECG, including only propafenone and flecainide. AV nodal blocking drugs such as verapamil and beta blockers should be avoided where possible in this patient population, due to risks associated with the development of pre-excited AF.

14. A. This ECG demonstrates pre-excited AF. This patient is haemodynamically unstable and should be promptly electrically cardioverted according the Advanced Life Support (ALS) guidelines. If she was haemodynamically stable IV flecainide would have been an option, as she is has a recent echocardiogram showing no evidence of structural heart disease. Amiodarone, verapamil, and adenosine block the AV node. This can increase conduction down the accessory pathway and increase ventricular rate, which can precipitate worsening haemodynamic status or cardiac arrest. They are all contraindicated in this situation (class III recommendation).

15. C. Unstable ventricular arrhythmia in the context of an ACS presentation is an indication for primary PCI. All of the other options are reasonable medical interventions to help with stabilization, but primary PCI is likely to be the definitive therapy.

16. B. This ECG demonstrates pre-excited AF patient has a resting ECG with spontaneous type 1 Brugada pattern. She should be given the lifestyle advice documented above in answer B. As she is asymptomatic she should not be offered an ICD—this would be indicated if she had a history of syncope (class IIa) or had spontaneous sustained VT (class 1). It would of course also be indicated as secondary prevention if she had survived an aborted cardiac arrest (class 1). An ajmaline challenge is not necessary as she already has type 1 pattern on her ECG. Family screening is required and should be offered as Brugada syndrome is inherited (autosomal dominant).

17. E. The list of drugs that should be avoided, as well as those that are safe, is freely available at brudagadrugs.org.

18. D. Two ECGs with a corrected QT interval >480ms is sufficient for a diagnosis of Long QT Syndrome (LQTS) to be made (ESC class I). Genetic testing will be helpful, in particular with family screening. The history of syncope is concerning for episodes of ventricular arrhythmia but the guidelines support offering beta-blockers as first-line therapy, with an ICD if patients experience recurrent syncope despite adequate beta blockade. Other treatment options include left cardiac sympathetic denervation and sodium channel blockers, such as flecainide or mexiletine in LQTS type 3. He does not need to remember all the drugs that are contraindicated—these are listed and freely available at crediblemeds.org.

19. A. ESC guidelines regarding CPVT all have a low level of evidence, graded as C. They advise that patients with a positive pathogenic genetic variant identified as part of family screening should consider taking beta-blockers, even in the presence of a normal exercise test (class IIa). She does have a diagnosis of CPVT, based on her genetics alone. Lifestyle changes including avoidance of competitive sports, strenuous exercise, and stressful environments are advised (class I). Flecainide is actually a useful anti-arrhythmic in CPVT, and can be added to beta-blocker therapy in patients who experience recurrent VT despite adequate beta blockade (class IIa). An ICD is usually only offered to patients who survive an aborted cardiac arrest (class I), or who experience recurrent syncope or documented VT despite beta blockade and flecainde (class IIa).

20. C. According to UK DVLA guidelines, this patient's group 2 licence will be revoked permanently and he will unfortunately need to find alternative employment. His group 1 licence will be restored after 6 months as long as he has not had any therapy from the device or changes to his anti-arrhythmic therapy. ICD therapy (anti-tachycardia pacing or shocks) has the following driving restrictions:

- ICD therapy that is not associated with incapacity
    - Must not drive for 6 months
- ICD therapy that is associated with incapacity
    - Due to inappropriate therapy, e.g. AF or programming issue: 1 month only if the cause is completely controlled to the satisfaction of the cardiologist
    - Due to appropriate therapy for VT/VF, with subsequent treatment to prevent recurrence (change of drugs, VT ablation): 6 months
- If neither of the above categories apply, must not drive for 2 years

This information is difficult for patients to retain and a recent study found that up to 30% of patients with ICDs do not follow driving restrictions. Clear oral and written communication is likely to be of benefit.

chapter

5

HEART FAILURE

chapter

5.1

HEART FAILURE SYNDROMES

QUESTIONS

1. **A 42-year-old woman presents with breathlessness on exertion that has been present for many years. She stopped smoking a year ago just before the birth of her second child. She says her ankles are swollen, but there is no pitting oedema. Blood pressure is 157/92 mmHg and heart rate 70 bpm (sinus rhythm). She is 173-cm tall and weighs 115 kg. Echocardiogram is challenging but shows normal left ventricular systolic function. NT-proBNP is 240 ng/L.**

   According to UK guidelines, what is the likely diagnosis and what would you do next?

   A. Heart failure with preserved ejection fraction: cardiac MRI
   B. No cardiac diagnosis: reassure, encourage exercise and weight loss
   C. Underlying ischaemic heart disease: coronary artery imaging
   D. Peripartum cardiomyopathy: cardiac MRI
   E. Paroxysmal arrhythmia: Holter

2. **A 74-year-old woman with type II diabetes is hospitalized for the first time with progressive dyspnoea and orthopnoea over three months. On examination an ejection systolic murmur with a quiet S2 is noted. The patient is comfortable at rest. Blood pressure is 142/68 mmHg and SpO_2 is 95% on room air. The chest X-ray reports bilateral pleural effusions. ECG shows sinus rhythm 85 bpm and voltage criteria for left ventricular hypertrophy. The patient is managed with IV diuretics and clinically improves. The haemoglobin level is normal. Transthoracic echocardiography shows severe LV systolic impairment and a heavily calcified trileaflet aortic valve with a valve area of $0.8cm^2$. Doppler (continuous wave) interrogation of the aortic valve is shown in Figure 5.1.1.**

   Which of the following would NOT be indicated in the further management?

   A. Continue diuretics to relieve congestion
   B. Perform invasive coronary angiography
   C. Dobutamine stress echocardiogram (DSE) to assess for LV contractile reserve
   D. Refer for surgical aortic valve replacement if acceptable surgical risk
   E. Antihypertensive medical therapy

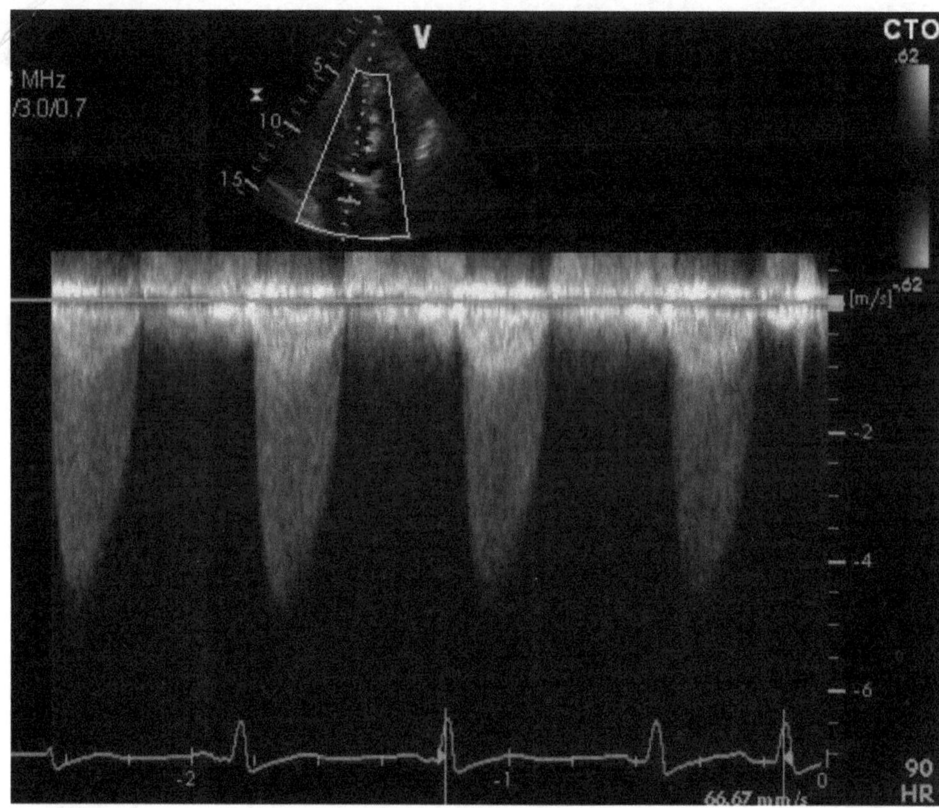

Figure 5.1.1

3. A 57-year-old woman presents reporting breathlessness with leg and abdominal swelling. She has had rheumatoid arthritis for 25 years (well controlled on infliximab), hypertension (treated with valsartan 160 mg once daily), and diabetes (treated with metformin and gliclazide). She has pitting oedema to mid-thigh, ascites, and her JVP is raised to her ear lobe. Pulse is 76 bpm in atrial fibrillation, blood pressure 116/74 mmHg, and NT-proBNP is 1450 ng/L.

What is the likely diagnosis?

A. Heart failure with preserved ejection fraction
B. Heart failure with reduced ejection fraction
C. Heart failure caused by atrial fibrillation
D. Constrictive pericarditis
E. Nephrotic syndrome

4. **An 80-year-old Caucasian man was admitted with progressive dyspnoea and peripheral oedema, and he was noted to be in atrial fibrillation with complete heart block. He had a history of median nerve decompression 8 years previously. Echocardiography showed septal thickness of 17 mm, severe LV systolic impairment, and a small pericardial effusion. NT-proBNP was 2100 ng/L. He underwent a successful pacemaker implant (CRT-P). Cardiac planar nuclear scintigraphy using a ^{99m}Tc-DPD labelled tracer is shown in Figure 5.1.2.**

   Which of the following is NOT correct regarding the underlying diagnosis?

   A. Serum/urine electrophoresis and free light chains should be measured
   B. It is a disease predominantly affecting older males
   C. Lumbar spinal canal stenosis and biceps tendon rupture are recognized clinical features
   D. Endomyocardial biopsy is the gold standard when other diagnostic tests are inconclusive
   E. The *V122I* mutation is the commonest mutation in those of Caucasian origin

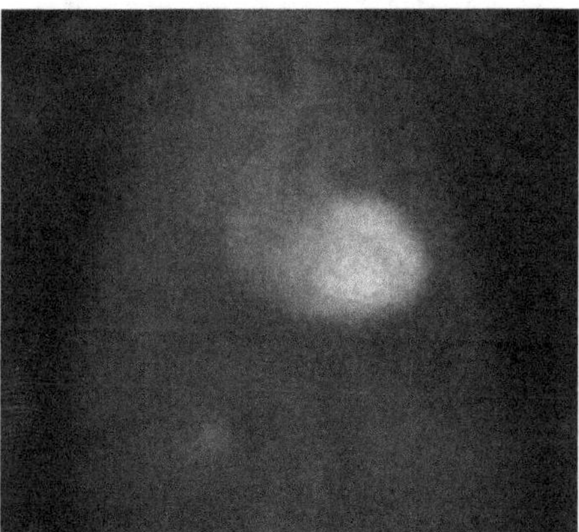

Figure 5.1.2

5. **A 26-year-old man presents with rapidly progressive breathlessness over the preceding 10 days, accompanied by some chest tightness. He has pitting oedema below his knees, a raised JVP, and a loud third heart sound. Blood pressure is 95/62 mmHg with a heart rate of 104 bpm. ECG shows sinus rhythm with left bundle branch block. Bedside echocardiogram shows a dilated heart with a visually estimated ejection fraction of approximately 10%.**

   What is the likely diagnosis?

   A. Giant cell myocarditis
   B. Acute myocardial infarction
   C. Dilated cardiomyopathy
   D. Lamin A/C cardiomyopathy
   E. Hyperthyroidism

6. A 48-year-old woman with type II diabetes had an anterior STEMI treated with primary PCI to the LAD 4 years previously. LV ejection fraction at the time was 35–40% and background medical therapy included aspirin, furosemide 40mg bd, carvedilol 6.25 mg bd, spironolactone 25mg od, ramipril 1.25mg bd, and a statin. The patient had stopped smoking following the MI and was compliant with medications. Home blood pressure readings were satisfactory (SBP <130 mmHg) and she was in stable NYHA functional class II. The patient presented with two abrupt episodes of florid pulmonary oedema at rest within a month and acutely required IV nitrate and CPAP therapy. ECG showed sinus rhythm with no new changes. Further investigation confirmed patent LAD stent and coronary arteries. Cardiac MRI reported mild mitral regurgitation, RVEF 65% and LVEF 33%, and late gadolinium enhancement (LGE) images are shown in Figure 5.1.3. CT imaging is provided in Figure 5.1.4, and after appropriate management there were no further episodes of pulmonary oedema.

Which of the following is the most likely cause of the pulmonary oedema?

A. Acute myocardial infarction
B. Acute takotsubo syndrome
C. Severe aortic valve stenosis
D. Renovascular disease
E. Phaeochromocytoma

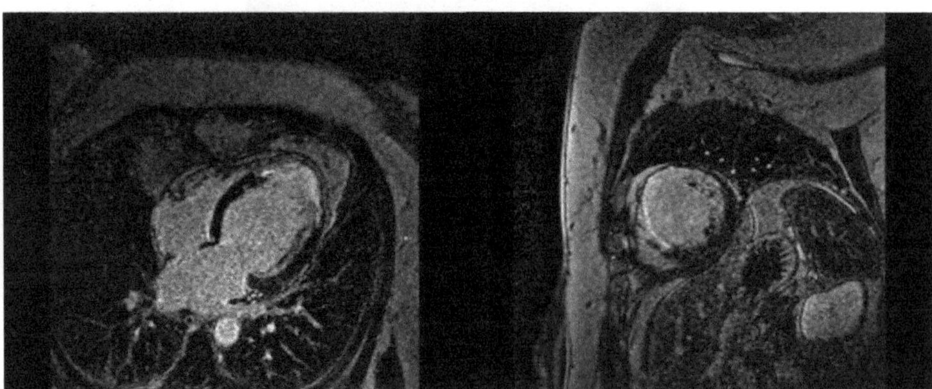

Figure 5.1.3 LGE imaging from cardiac MRI

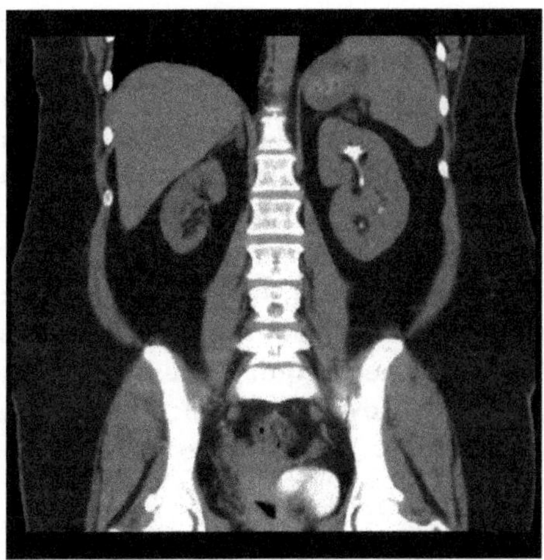

Figure 5.1.4 Coronal cut of CT imaging

7. A 60-year-old man with an established diagnosis of non-ischaemic dilated cardiomyopathy had undergone a CRT-D implant 10 years previously following initial presentation with monomorphic VT and complete heart block. He had a subsequent history of atrial flutter ablation and VT ablation on two occasions. There was a family history of sudden death and pacemaker implant in several relatives.

The patient had young children. After 8 years he had developed decompensated heart failure (NT-proBNP 4974). At clinical review, blood pressure is 92/57 mmHg, pulse 60 bpm and regular, and he experiences a significant symptomatic improvement after the addition of diuretics. ECG showed biventricular pacing with new, persistent AF. Echocardiography revealed a dilated LV (7 cm) with an ejection fraction of 25%, mild-moderate RV dysfunction, moderate mitral regurgitation (MR), and an estimated pulmonary arterial systolic pressure of 60 mmHg. NT-proBNP remained elevated (2132 ng/L). Long-term medical therapy consisted of ramipril 2.5mg bd, eplerenone 25mg od, furosemide 40mg bd, anticoagulation, carvedilol 12.5mg bd, and amiodarone 200mg od. DC cardioversion was unsuccessful. A cardiopulmonary exercise test (CPET) was performed: respiratory exchange ratio (RER) 1.19, peak VO_2 12.4ml/kg/m^2, and VE/VCO2 slope (minute ventilation/carbon dioxide production) was 52. Postural hypotension was an intermittent problem. Device interrogation revealed 99% bi-ventricular pacing and persistent AF with no sensed R wave.

Which of the following would you do next?

A. Offer sacubitril valsartan

B. Refer for genetic testing and transplant assessment

C. Refer for percutaneous mitral valve intervention (E.g. MitraClip)

D. Refer for AF ablation

E. Perform coronary angiography

8. A 55-year-old male is admitted with 3 months of progressive dyspnoea and peripheral oedema. The 12-lead ECG shows sinus rhythm at 100 bpm with no other abnormalities. Chest X-ray is unremarkable. NT-proBNP is 1780 ng/L. The JVP is elevated with prominent V waves. Pan-systolic and early diastolic murmurs are noted. A transthoracic echocardiogram shows a dilated right heart with diastolic septal flattening and mild RV systolic impairment. Figure 5.1.5 shows three images from the echocardiogram. A CT pulmonary angiogram reports no evidence of acute or chronic pulmonary embolic disease with normal lung appearances. On further enquiry, the patient reports intermittent abdominal pain and loose bowel motions.

What is your next step in management?

A. Refer for closure of an atrial septal defect (ASD)
B. Measure levels of serum chromogranin A and urinary 5-hydroxyindoleacetic acid
C. Right heart catheterization
D. Evaluate for cardiac sarcoidosis
E. Commence pulmonary vasodilator therapy

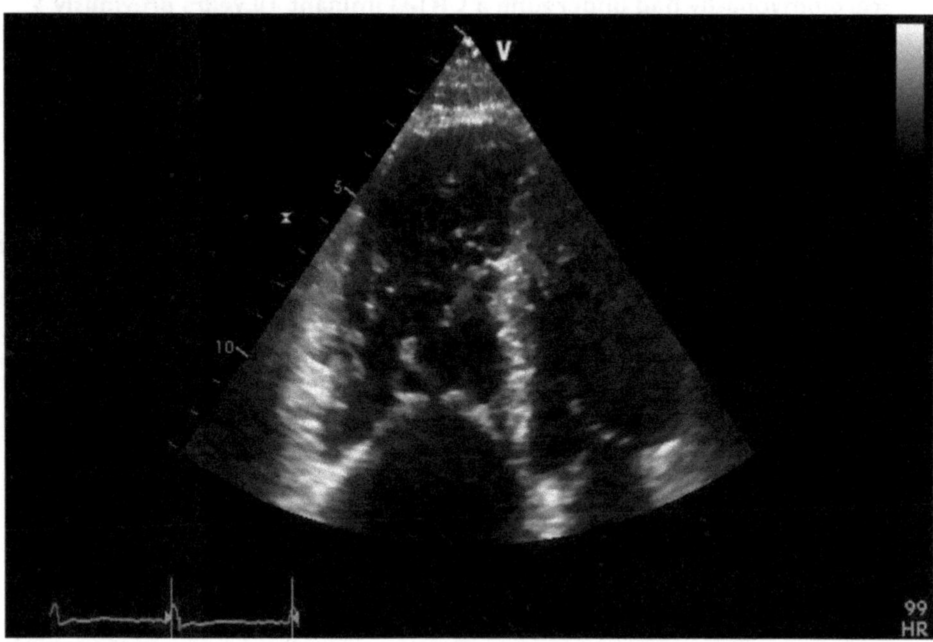

Figure 5.1.5

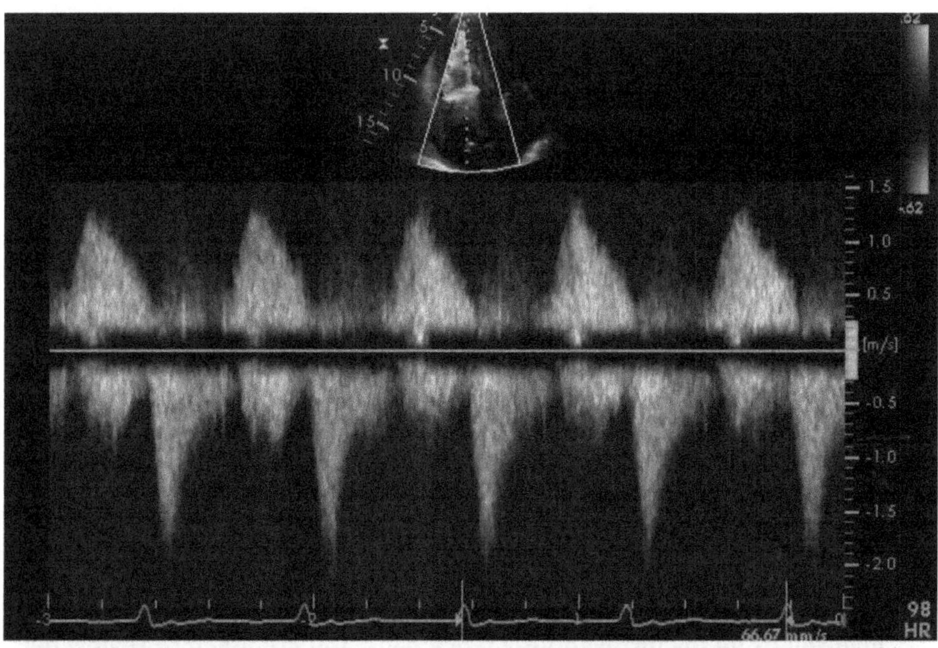

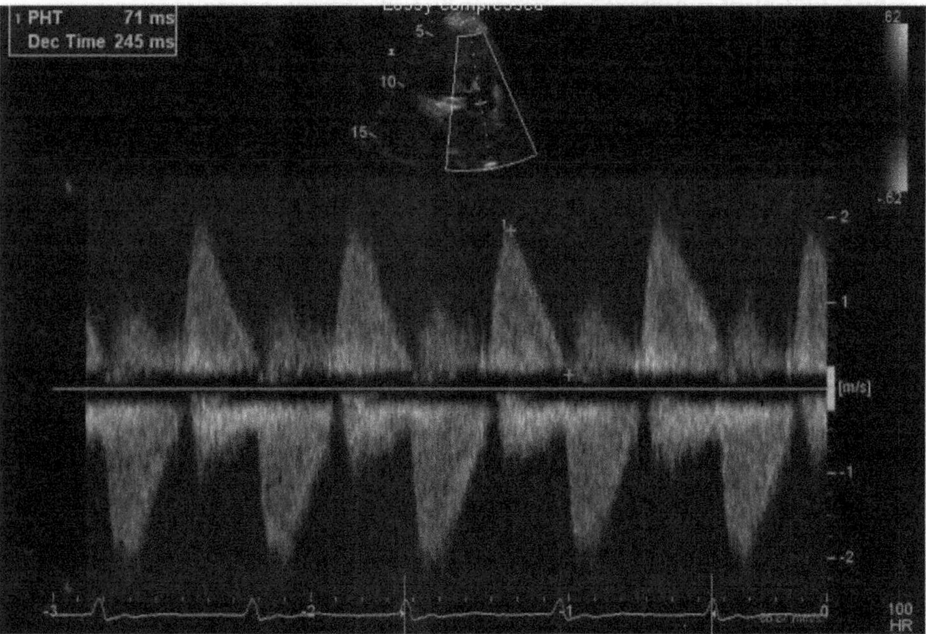

Figure 5.1.5 Continued

9. **A 62-year-old man with an anterior MI 2 years previously and a left ventricular ejection fraction of 32% still has NYHA class II symptoms despite treatment with enalapril 5 mg bd, dapagliflozin 10mg od, carvedilol 25 mg bd, eplerenone 25 mg bd, and bumetanide 1 mg od. He has an ICD in-situ. There are no signs of fluid retention, heart rate is 62 bpm (sinus rhythm), blood pressure 118/68 mmHg, and QRS duration is 119ms.**

   What is your next management step?

   A. Add digoxin for relief of symptoms
   B. Coronary angiography with a view to revascularization
   C. Switch enalapril to candesartan 16 mg od
   D. Switch enalapril to sacubitril/valsartan 49/51 mg bd
   E. Upgrade device to CRT-D

10. **A 52-year-old woman presents with gross fluid retention with a JVP raised above her ears and is found to have severe left ventricular systolic impairment (ejection fraction 28%). Heart rate is 100 bpm in sinus rhythm and blood pressure is 98/56 mmHg. Renal function is normal. She is treated with one dose of 80 mg furosemide intravenously, followed by 40 mg intravenously twice daily. You are asked to review her 48 hours after admission as she has lost no weight.**

    What is your next management step?

    A. Add an ACE inhibitor
    B. Transfer to the intensive care unit for ultrafiltration
    C. Add dobutamine 5 mcg/kg/min
    D. Convert to a furosemide infusion at a rate of 10 mg per hour
    E. Transfer to a referral centre for consideration of advanced heart failure therapies

11. **An 84-year-old man with chronic stable heart failure (NYHA class II symptoms) is reviewed in clinic. His heart rate is 84 bpm (sinus rhythm) and blood pressure 98/64 mmHg with no fluid retention clinically. He is taking bumetanide 1 mg alternate days, enalapril 5 mg bd, dapagliflozin 10mg od, carvedilol 6.25 mg bd and spironolactone 25 mg od.**

    What would your management plan be?

    A. Reassure all is well and review in 6 months
    B. Switch enalapril to sacubitril-valsartan
    C. Double carvedilol to 12.5 mg bd
    D. Add ivabradine 5 mg bd
    E. Add digoxin 250 mcg od

12. A 57-year old woman presented with exertional dyspnoea (NYHA II-III) and an NT-proBNP 1555 ng/L. ECG showed sinus rhythm and LBBB (QRS duration 150 ms). Echocardiography, CT coronary angiography, and cardiac MRI confirmed a diagnosis of non-ischaemic dilated cardiomyopathy (LVEDVi 110ml/m^2, LVEF 25%, good RV, and no scar). Cardiomyopathy genetics and biochemical panel were negative. The patient was optimized on enalapril 10mg bd, carvedilol 3.125mg bd, dapagliflozin 10mg od, ivabradine 5mg bd, bumetanide 1mg od, and spironolactone 25mg od. Due to the patient having a cough, enalapril was exchanged for sacubitril-valsartan 100mg bd. NT-proBNP fell to 473 ng/L within 3 months of diagnosis and was 50 ng/L g after 12 months. Eight months after diagnosis the ECG showed a QRS width of 100 ms. Repeat cardiac MRI 15 months later showed a non-dilated LV with LVEF 60% and no abnormal fibrosis/scar. The patient was in NYHA class I and at clinical review was euvolaemic.

The patient enquired about stopping medications. What would you advise?

A. Discontinue all cardiac medications
B. Discontinue the loop diuretic
C. Discontinue sacubitril-valsartan and carvedilol
D. Offer an ICD
E. Discontinue the spironolactone

13. You review a 68-year-old man who is asymptomatic despite an LV ejection fraction of 37% (due to underlying ischaemic heart disease). He is in AF with a rate of 90 bpm at rest and blood pressure is 136/82 mmHg. There are no signs of fluid retention. He is taking carvedilol 6.25 mg bd, sacubitril-valsartan 24/26 mg bd, eplerenone 25 mg od, dapagliflozin 10mg od, and bumetanide 1 mg once or twice a week.

What is your next management step?

A. Increase carvedilol to reduce heart rate below 70bpm
B. Increase sacubitril-valsartan to 49/51 mg bd
C. Discuss ICD implantation
D. Use ivabradine to reduce heart rate below 70 bpm
E. No change because clinically stable

14. A 68-year-old man with HFrEF is reviewed in the community heart failure clinic, 4 weeks after discharge from hospital with gross fluid retention. His medical therapy includes enalapril 5 mg bd, bumetanide 2 mg bd, bendroflumethaizide 5 mg od, and carvedilol 6.25 mg bd. Your nurse specialist colleague contacts you for advice. His blood pressure is 100/60 mmHg and heart rate 62 bpm. The patient's JVP is no longer visible and there has been a 20 kg reduction in body weight compared with that on admission. Renal biochemistry is: Na^+ 135 mmol/L, K^+ 5.6 mmol/L, urea 30.1 mmol/L, and creatinine 275 µmol/L (values prior to discharge were: K^+ 4.9 mmol/L, urea 12.1 mmol/L, and creatinine 150 µmol/L).

What would you advise?

A. Continue all medications and recheck renal biochemistry after 1 week
B. Add eplerenone to optimize HFrEF therapy and recheck biochemistry after 2 weeks
C. Stop enalapril indefinitely as renal artery stenosis is likely
D. Stop enalapril and loop diuretic and reassess with biochemistry in 1 week
E. Halve dose of enalapril and bumetanide, stop thiazide and recheck biochemistry after 1 week

15. A 67-year-old man presents with gross fluid retention due to severe left ventricular systolic impairment following a remote anterior MI. Heart rate is 110 bpm in atrial fibrillation and blood pressure is 98/56 mmHg. Creatinine is 264 µmol/L. He is treated with 80 mg furosemide intravenously once only, then a 10 mg per hour continuous infusion. You review him 24 hours after admission. His weight has decreased by 1 kg and creatinine has increased to 280 µmol/L.

What would you do next?

A. Increase furosemide to 20 mg per hour and add bendroflumethiazide 5 mg od
B. Stop furosemide and give 500 ml normal saline cautiously
C. Add dobutamine 5 mcg/kg/min
D. Add digoxin 250 mcg od
E. Transfer to intensive care for ultrafiltration

16. You review an 86-year-old man in clinic who has recovered from a recent episode of gross fluid retention secondary to anterior MI many years previously (LVEF 18%). He has NYHA class III symptoms. He is stable on carvedilol 6.25 mg bd, dapagliflozin 10mg od, enalapril 2.5 mg bd, and spironolactone 12.5 mg od. Blood pressure is 96/55 mmHg, heart rate 58 bpm (sinus), and creatinine 265 µmol/L. He has left bundle branch block (QRS 166 msec).

What would the most appropriate next management step be?

A. Up-titrate his ACE inhibitor
B. Switch to sacubitril-valsartan
C. Add digoxin
D. Implant a CRT-D
E. Implant a CRT-P

17. A 45-year-old woman with HFrEF (dilated cardiomyopathy) remains symptomatic (NYHA III) despite 6 months of optimal medical therapy (sacubitril-valsartan 100mg bd, spironolactone 50 mg od, carvedilol 6.25 mg bd, dapagliflozin 10 mg od, and furosemide 40 mg od). There is no history of syncope. The ECG shows sinus rhythm at 60 bpm, PR interval 250 ms, and LBBB (QRS duration 160 ms). A chest X-ray done 1 year previously is shown in Figure 5.1.6. Cardiac MRI shows a dilated left ventricle, LV ejection fraction of 25%, and patchy mid-wall myocardial fibrosis affecting the basal septum. An extra-cardiac biopsy is performed.

What should be your next management step?

A. Oral steroids
B. CRT-D implant
C. ICD implant
D. CRT-P implant
E. Refer for heart transplant assessment

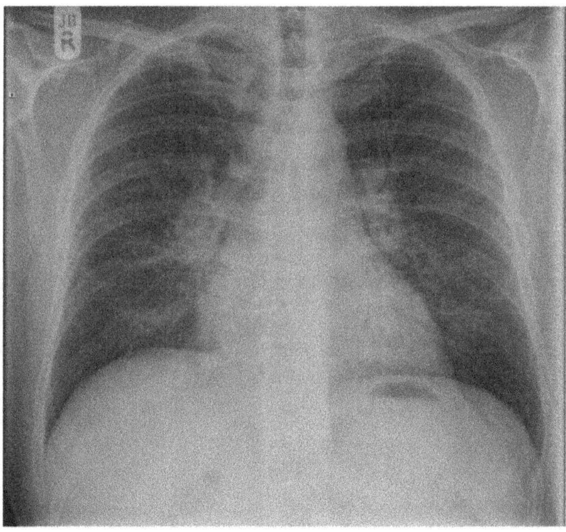

Figure 5.1.6

18. A 70-year-old woman presents with an episode of syncope. A 12-lead ECG captures intermittent episodes of second- and third-degree atrioventricular block. When in sinus rhythm, she has a PR interval of 300 ms, left axis deviation, and QRS width of 120 ms. She is not taking any negative chronotropic medications and there are no reversible causes for the AV block. Cardiac MRI reports an LVEF of 40% with no abnormal scar or fibrosis. NT-proBNP was 600 ng/L.

What type of pacemaker system would you advise?

A. AAI pacemaker
B. VVI pacemaker
C. Dual chamber pacemaker
D. CRT-P
E. CRT-D

19. A 58-year old woman with ischaemic cardiomyopathy (HFrEF) has persistent symptoms despite best tolerated doses of bisoprolol, enalapril, dapagliflozin, eplerenone, and bumetanide. QRS duration was 120 ms and an ICD had been previously implanted. At cardiopulmonary exercise testing (CPET) performance was significantly reduced. Resting haemodynamics at right heart catheterization were: mean RA pressure 11 mmHg, PA pressure 90/42 mmHg (mean 52 mmHg), PA wedge pressure (PAWP) 31 mmHg, and cardiac output (CO) 3 L/min.

Which one of the following aspects of advanced heart failure management is incorrect?

A. The transpulmonary gradient (TPG) and pulmonary vascular resistance (PVR) permit listing for orthotopic heart transplantation
B. Sildenafil therapy is not a proven treatment for pulmonary hypertension X
C. Insertion of a left ventricular assist device (LVAD) could offer a bridge to candidacy for cardiac transplant X
D. Loop diuretic dose can be increased X
E. Aortic valve regurgitation is a recognized complication of a continuous flow LVAD X

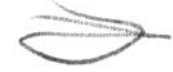

20. You are reviewing an 82-year-old lady with an established diagnosis of HFrEF. Medications include ramipril 1.25mg bd, dapagliflozin 10mg od, furosemide 40mg od, and bisoprolol 1.25mg od. Spironolactone was withdrawn due to symptomatic hypotension. The resting heart rate is 62 bpm (sinus rhythm), blood pressure is 88/60 mmHg, and there is no clinical congestion. Co-morbidities include COPD, CKD (eGFR 40), type II diabetes, and anaemia (Hb 95 g/dl, microcytosis, and transferrin saturation 10%). She is less independent than 1 year ago and recently has had a carer visiting once a day. There is evidence of mild frailty but no incontinence. The serum albumin is 28 g/L (reference range 32–38 g/L). On further enquiry you learn of poor sleep, low mood, and constipation.

What should you consider in your consultation?

A. Medications review to limit unnecessary poly-pharmacy
B. Consider intravenous iron for symptomatic benefit and the merits of GI investigation
C. Refer for a comprehensive geriatric assessment (CGA)
D. Refer to your local palliative care service
E. All of the above

21. A 75-year-old man with HFrEF (LVEF 30%) has had three admissions with decompensated heart failure within the past 18 months. After the second admission his therapy was optimized to include sacubitril-valsartan 100 mg bd, eplerenone 25 mg od, carvedilol 25 mg bd, and bumetanide 2 mg bd. He clinically appears euvolaemic. Blood pressure is 130/60 mmHg and pulse 60 bpm in sinus rhythm. You are satisfied that he is compliant with medication.

What would you consider next to reduce both HF hospitalization and mortality further?

A. Vericiguat
B. Dapagliflozin
C. Digoxin
D. Implant a pulmonary artery (PA) pressure monitoring device
E. All of the above

chapter 5.1

HEART FAILURE SYNDROMES

ANSWERS

1. **B.** This is a difficult area in that NICE and ESC guidelines differ. NICE suggests that an NT-proBNP < 400 ng/L excludes heart failure, whereas the ESC suggests a cut-off of 125 ng/L. However, this woman has a BMI of over 38 gk/m^2 and normal left ventricular function, therefore weight loss is the most appropriate intervention. Ischaemic heart disease presenting as long-standing breathlessness is uncommon, whilst peripartum cardiomyopathy presents within 6 months after delivery.

2. **C.** This case illustrates new onset decompensated heart failure associated with high gradient (peak Doppler velocity >4m/s) aortic valve stenosis. LV systolic function can be normal or reduced in high gradient aortic valve stenosis. The mismatch is related to ventricular–arterial uncoupling (high systemic afterload) but could also indicate another co-existing cause for LVSD, e.g. ischaemia, dual valve pathology or cardiac amyloidosis. DSE is indicated when there is low gradient aortic stenosis and reduced LVEF. Systemic hypertension should be managed to reduce LV afterload but with caution and both ACE inhibitors and angiotensin receptor blockers are not absolutely contraindicated. Coronary angiography is required to assess coronary anatomy to define the procedural risks and extent of intervention needed.

3. **D.** Hypertension and diabetes do predispose to heart failure (both with normal and reduced left ventricular ejection fraction), but with such gross fluid retention, constriction is more likely, related to her long-standing rheumatoid arthritis. Her NT-proBNP is relatively low for someone with AF and such severe fluid retention, and is also often relatively low in patients with constriction.

4. **E.** The previous history of carpal tunnel surgery, new onset heart failure, AF, and LVH in an elderly male strongly suggest a diagnosis of ATTR cardiac amyloidosis. The image shows grade III cardiac uptake and confirms the diagnosis. Typical features include lumbar spinal stenosis, peripheral neuropathy, and postural hypotension. More than 90% of patients are older men. Both wild type and variant (hereditary) forms are recognized. At least 80 different mutations in transthyretin (TTR) have been reported and common variants with cardiac involvement include T60A (mostly Caucasians) and V122I (4% of Afro-Caribbean carry the variant). Nuclear scintigraphy (99mTc labelled with the phosphate tracers DPD, PYP, or HMDP) and SPECT imaging are used semi-quantitively to assess cardiac uptake. AL cardiac amyloidosis can give a positive result (grade I/II) and so must be excluded for the bone tracer scintigraphy to be a valid diagnostic test. Genetic testing and extra-cardiac or cardiac biopsy are required if there is a mixed phenotype.

5. **A.** Giant cell myocarditis typically presents with rapidly progressive heart failure with a very short illness. Myocardial infarction is very unlikely in a young man particularly without a history of chest pain. Dilated cardiomyopathy typically has an insidious presentation over a far longer period of time. Lamin A/C cardiomyopathy typically presents later in life and should be suspected in cases of heart failure with arrhythmias and evidence of conduction system disease. Hyperthyroidism can present with heart failure, but other features of hyperthyroidism would be expected.

6. D. Cardiac MRI LGE images demonstrate transmural infarction consistent with previous antero-apical MI. The CT abdomen shows a shrunken right kidney and in the context of flash pulmonary oedema (FPO) strongly suggests severe renal artery stenosis (RAS). RAS (usually bilateral) is a recognized cause of FPO. In one series of stable patients with heart failure with reduced ejection fraction (HFrEF), 30% of patients had significant unilateral RAS and 7% had bilateral RAS. The mechanism of FPO involves an acute hypertensive crisis with rapid elevation in LV end diastolic pressure and consequently high hydrostatic pulmonary venous pressure (exceeding colloid oncotic pressure and lymphatic drainage capacity) resulting in alveolar oedema. In this case the management implied was a renal artery stent. Causes of FPO include severe (and usually acute) mitral valve disease (endocarditis, papillary muscle rupture, etc.), critical aortic valve stenosis, critical coronary ischaemia, large territory acute myocardial infarction phaeochromocytoma, renovascular disease (Pickering syndrome), and Takotsubo cardiomyopathy.

7. B. A history of AV block, atrial arrhythmias, a family history of sudden cardiac death (SCD) and pacemaker strongly suggests a genetic cause for his cardiomyopathy, and specifically a lamin mutation. Given the high risk of SCD with this mutation and adverse family history, cascade screening is advised. The patient also met criteria for advanced heart failure (defined as: NYHA III, persistently elevated NT-proBNP, pulmonary hypertension/RV dysfunction on optimal medical therapy with adverse prognostic CPET variables). Such patients should be referred in a timely manner to a transplant centre for further assessment. AF ablation is unlikely to be successful in this patient given the unsuccessful DC cardioversion on amiodarone. Furthermore, the patient has no intrinsic AV node conduction (no sensed R wave) due to the laminopathy partly explaining the 99% bi-ventricular pacing capture (and effectively behaving as if there has been an AV node ablation). Sacubitril-valsartan should be considered but due to symptomatic hypotension is unlikely to be tolerated. MitraClip with moderate MR and severe LVSD is unlikely to alter the disease trajectory significantly and probably better suited for selected patients with relatively smaller left ventricular volumes and severe functional MR.

8. B. The constellation of abdominal pain, diarrhoea, right heart failure, and a volum- loaded right heart suggest carcinoid syndrome. Other typical symptoms include facial flushing and wheeze. The tricuspid and pulmonary valve leaflets were thickened, retracted, and had a complete failure of coaptation. The resulting echo Doppler tracings demonstrate severe tricuspid regurgitation (forward peak velocity of >1 m/s and a dense triangular or 'dagger'-shaped spectral Doppler typical of torrential tricuspid regurgitation with rapid equalization of RA/RV pressures and thus underestimating the pulmonary arterial systolic pressure) and severe pulmonary regurgitation (steep PR slope with pressure half time <100 ms) indicating dual valve pathology caused by carcinoid heart disease. The patient had a GI neuroendocrine tumour with multiple liver metastases. Serum chromogranin A levels and 24-hour urine 5HIAA levels should be checked to confirm the diagnosis and management typically consists of medical therapy for right-heart failure (loop/thiazide diuretic and spironolactone), a long-acting somatostatin analogue, and/or valve surgery if considered a surgical candidate.

9. D. Sacubitril valsartan is indicated for symptomatic patients with LVEF <35% on a stable dose of ACEi/ARB. It will improve prognosis and is likely to improve symptoms. Digoxin might help symptoms, but would not affect prognosis. In the absence of chest pain, there is very little evidence to support revascularization. There is no evidence to support use of ARBs in preference to ACEi. According to ESC guidelines, CRT is not indicated when QRS <130 ms (and <120 ms in UK NICE guidelines).

10. D. The commonest cause for 'failure' to respond to diuretics is a failure to deliver adequate doses of diuretic. An ACE inhibitor would reduce the blood pressure further, though there is some evidence it may enhance diuretic effects. Ultrafiltration should be considered as a final resort, and there is no indication for positive inotropic agents as yet. Advanced therapy might be necessary eventually but is not the next management step.

11. D. The temptation to leave well alone is understandable, but wrong when further optimization is possible in a patient who remains symptomatic (NYHA class II in this case). The heart rate of 84 bpm is too high. His blood pressure is low, suggesting an increase in carvedilol (or switching to sacubitril-valsartan) is unlikely to be tolerated. Ivabradine will reduce heart rate without reducing blood pressure and the SHIFT trial suggests such a move will reduce the combined end-point of hospitalization for worsening heart failure or cardiovascular death. Interestingly, digoxin might reduce heart rate, but it's unlikely that there will ever be a repeat of the DIG trial with modern background medication and is not currently recommended in this clinical scenario.

12. B. This patient with idiopathic dilated cardiomyopathy (DCM) and HFrEF had gone into remission with complete recovery of LV function on medical therapy associated with a normal NT-proBNP and resolution of the LBBB. Available data (including the TRED-HF randomized trial) suggest that patients with DCM in remission should continue neurohormonal modulating therapy given the high risk of relapse. Thus, in the context of euvolaemia the patient may be advised to discontinue diuretic therapy, but all other cardiac medications should be continued long-term. There was no indication for an ICD, but such patients should be monitored long-term to ensure no there is no relapse.

13. B. The aim should be to up-titrate patients to target (or maximally tolerated) doses of all clinically indicated medications. Ivabradine is not indicated if the patient is in AF. An ICD is not indicated unless LVEF <35%. The role of beta-blockers in patients in AF (and the heart rate to target) remains unclear, and a target rate below 70 is too low in AF. Thus, sacubitril-valsartan therapy should be up-titrated to the maximum tolerated dose.

14. E. It is most likely that the high dose loop and thiazide diuretics have led to over-diuresis. If there is a 30–50% increase in serum creatinine (or values 265–310 µmol/L) and/or K+ >5.5, ESC and UK guidelines advise a reduction in ACEi dose and rechecking of renal function after 1 week. Concomitant medication should also be reviewed. Diuretic dose should be optimized to maintain euvolemia with the lowest achievable dose. Additional simple measures to consider include assessment of volume status, renal tract ultrasound (to exclude obstruction), and urine culture to exclude a urinary tract infection. If the rise in serum creatinine is >50% (or reaches >310 µmol/L, whichever is the lower) then the ACEi/ARB/ARNI/MRA should be stopped with regular monitoring of renal biochemistry until values have reduced or plateaued.

15. A. The commonest cause for 'failure' to respond to diuretic therapy is failure to deliver adequate doses. A common, but wrong, approach to deteriorating renal function in patients with fluid retention in heart failure is to stop (or decrease) diuretic, and even to give IV saline. This is entirely the wrong approach—clinically the patient has fluid overload. The solution is usually more diuretic—an important finding from the CARRESS trial was that even very high doses of diuretic (up to 30 mg per her of furosemide plus metolazone) in patients recruited because of worsening renal function was associated with both diuresis and improvement in renal function. Positive inotropic agents should only be used as a last resort, as, indeed, should ultrafiltration.

16. E. His renal dysfunction and hypotension preclude both ACEi up-titration and a switch to sacubitril-valsartan. Digoxin is not a good choice given his heart rate, rhythm and renal function, and device therapy would be precede digoxin in a stepwise escalation of therapy. He has LBBB with a broad QRS and remains in sinus rhythm so CRT is a good option. In view of his age and severe renal dysfunction, he is unlikely to be a candidate for a defibrillator.

17. B. The patient remains symptomatic on optimal medical therapy (OMT) with LVEF<35% and an ECG demonstrating LBBB with a QRS of >150 ms. This is an ESC class IA indication for CRT-D. The chest X-ray shows bilateral hilar lymphadenopathy and cardiac MRI highlights mid-wall myocardial septal scar suggesting cardiac sarcoidosis. No randomized trials have been performed to test the efficacy of steroid therapy in cardiac sarcoidosis but observational data suggest a role for steroids in early disease. Cardiac sarcoidosis can manifest with atrioventricular block, ventricular arrythmia, sudden death, and heart failure (affecting both ventricles). Such patients were not representative of the cohort in the DANISH trial (Køber et al., NEJM 2016) which demonstrated no overall mortality benefit (the primary end point with a median follow up 5.6 years) for an ICD (with or without CRT) in patients with non-ischaemic DCM. Heart transplant referral may be required at a later stage after escalation of heart failure therapy.

Køber L, Thune JJ, Nielsen JC, Haarbo J, Videbæk L, Korup E, Jensen G, Hildebrandt P, Steffensen FH, Bruun NE, Eiskjær H, Brandes A, Thøgersen AM, Gustafsson F, Egstrup K, Videbæk R, Hassager C, Svendsen JH, Høfsten DE, Torp-Pedersen C, Pehrson S; DANISH Investigators. Defibrillator Implantation in Patients with Nonischemic Systolic Heart Failure. N Engl J Med. 2016 Sep 29;375(13):1221–30. doi: 10.1056/NEJMoa1608029. Epub 2016 Aug 27. PMID: 27571011.

18. D. The patient has a clear indication for pacing and is likely to have a high pacing requirement. In patients with reduced LVEF, ESC recommends a biventricular pacemaker system is considered if a high degree of pacing is expected. This is based on the BLOCK HF trial (Curtis et al., NEJM 2013) which showed reduction in the primary endpoint of death, heart failure hospitalization, and increase in LV end systolic volume with biventricular pacing compared to conventional RV apical pacing in patients with impaired but not severely reduced LV systolic function. In the presence of high degree AV block, AAI pacing is clearly inappropriate. There is no indication for the addition of a defibrillator at this stage.

Curtis AB, Worley SJ, Adamson PB, Chung ES, Niazi I, Sherfesee L, Shinn T, Sutton MS; Biventricular versus Right Ventricular Pacing in Heart Failure Patients with Atrioventricular Block (BLOCK HF) Trial Investigators. Biventricular pacing for atrioventricular block and systolic dysfunction. N Engl J Med. 2013 Apr 25;368(17):1585–93. doi: 10.1056/NEJMoa1210356. PMID: 23614585.

19. A. If pulmonary artery (PA) systolic pressure is >60 mmHg and there is also an elevated transpulmonary gradient (TPG >15 mmHg) and/or pulmonary vascular resistance (PVR >5 WU) then this significantly increases the risk of right ventricular failure in the donor heart. In this patient the TPG (calculated as mean PA pressure − PA wedge pressure) is 21 mmHg and PVR (calculated as TPG ÷ CO) is 7 Wood units (or 560 dyne s cm^{-5}) are both significantly elevated and prohibit proceeding directly to heart transplantation. Medical therapy (increasing diuretic dose, addition of ARNI, inotropes, and vasodilators, etc.) and/or LVAD implant can help to reduce PAWP, augment cardiac output, and reduce PA pressure to reduce TPG and PVR and allow a patient to becoming eligible for heart transplantation. Complications of long-term intra-pericardial LVADs include bleeding (GI/cerebral), infection (device and driveline), thromboembolism (LVAD pump, stroke), right-heart failure, and aortic valve regurgitation. The latter can be due to worsening of pre-existing aortic valve disease and/or develop following implant and is related to infrequent opening of the valve during mechanical unloading of the LV. Sildenafil is licensed for group 1 pulmonary arterial hypertension (not group 2 with elevated PAWP).

20. E. This is not an uncommon scenario and is likely to be encountered more frequently. Elderly patients with heart failure frequently have significant co-morbidities which impact on well-being and prognosis. Microcytic anaemia and altered bowel habit could indicate poor dietary intake and/or intestinal malignancy. Several features in this case highlight that palliative care input would be beneficial. The CGA involves assessing an individual's physical, functional, mobility/balance, psychological, and socioeconomical requirements to develop personalized interventions and has been shown to improve patient outcomes. Honest and open discussions with patients and their family or carers is important to define goals and expectations of care. This helps to ensure patients are offered the best available services to both improve quality of life and plan end of life care.

21. B. Dapagliflozin significantly reduces both all-cause mortality and hospitalization (DAPA-HF trial; McMurray et al., NEJM 2019). Empagliflozin (EMPEROR-reduced trial; Anker et al., NEJM 2020) also met its primary endpoint. Vericiguat (VICTORIA trial; Armstorng et al., NEJM 2020) showed a significant reduction in recurrent hospitalization within 1 year in a high-risk population on excellent background medical therapy. Both digoxin (Digitalis Investigation Group, NEJM 1997) and an implantable PA monitor (CHAMPION study; Abraham et al., Lancet 2016) have shown significant reductions in HF hospitalization but not mortality. Larger randomized trials of implantable PA pressure monitoring are ongoing.

Abraham WT, Stevenson LW, Bourge RC, Lindenfeld JA, Bauman JG, Adamson PB; CHAMPION Trial Study Group. Sustained efficacy of pulmonary artery pressure to guide adjustment of chronic heart failure therapy: complete follow-up results from the CHAMPION randomised trial. Lancet. 2016 Jan 30;387(10017):453–61. doi: 10.1016/S0140-6736(15)00723-0. Epub 2015 Nov 9. PMID: 26560249.

Armstrong PW, Pieske B, Anstrom KJ, Ezekowitz J, Hernandez AF, Butler J, Lam CSP, Ponikowski P, Voors AA, Jia G, McNulty SE, Patel MJ, Roessig L, Koglin J, O'Connor CM; VICTORIA Study Group. Vericiguat in Patients with Heart Failure and Reduced Ejection Fraction. N Engl J Med. 2020 May 14;382(20):1883–93. doi: 10.1056/NEJMoa1915928. Epub 2020 Mar 28. PMID: 32222134.

Packer M, Anker SD, Butler J, Filippatos G, Pocock SJ, Carson P, Januzzi J, Verma S, Tsutsui H, Brueckmann M, Jamal W, Kimura K, Schnee J, Zeller C, Cotton D, Bocchi E, Böhm M, Choi DJ, Chopra V, Chuquiure E, Giannetti N, Janssens S, Zhang J, Gonzalez Juanatey JR, Kaul S, Brunner-La Rocca HP, Merkely B, Nicholls SJ, Perrone S, Pina I, Ponikowski P, Sattar N, Senni M, Seronde MF, Spinar J, Squire I, Taddei S, Wanner C, Zannad F; EMPEROR-Reduced Trial Investigators. Cardiovascular and Renal Outcomes with Empagliflozin in Heart Failure. N Engl J Med. 2020 Oct 8;383(15):1413-1424. doi: 10.1056/NEJMoa2022190. Epub 2020 Aug 28. PMID: 32865377.

Digitalis Investigation Group. The effect of digoxin on mortality and morbidity in patients with heart failure. N Engl J Med. 1997 Feb 20;336(8):525–33. doi: 10.1056/NEJM199702203360801. PMID: 9036306.

McMurray JJV, Solomon SD, Inzucchi SE, Køber L, Kosiborod MN, Martinez FA, Ponikowski P, Sabatine MS, Anand IS, Bělohlávek J, Böhm M, Chiang CE, Chopra VK, de Boer RA, Desai AS, Diez M, Drozdz J, Dukát A, Ge J, Howlett JG, Katova T, Kitakaze M, Ljungman CEA, Merkely B, Nicolau JC, O'Meara E, Petrie MC, Vinh PN, Schou M, Tereshchenko S, Verma S, Held C, DeMets DL, Docherty KF, Jhund PS, Bengtsson O, Sjöstrand M, Langkilde AM; DAPA-HF Trial Committees and Investigators. Dapagliflozin in Patients with Heart Failure and Reduced Ejection Fraction. N Engl J Med. 2019 Nov 21;381(21):1995–2008. doi: 10.1056/NEJMoa1911303. Epub 2019 Sep 19. PMID: 31535829.

15/21

chapter 5.2

CARDIOMYOPATHIES

QUESTIONS

1. A 45-year-old female patient is referred to the inherited cardiomyopathy clinic (ICC) for family screening. The patient's father had no known cardiac disease but had a cardiac arrest and post mortem has suggested a diagnosis of hypertrophic cardiomyopathy. Genetics panel result from the father has been inconclusive. She is entirely asymptomatic and plays sport regularly with no symptoms. She has two children aged 9 and 16 who are well. Other family members are well but do not live locally.

You would recommend:

A. Annual review in clinic to check symptoms
B. Genetic screening of the patient
C. Transthoracic echocardiogram and ECG and review annually in clinic
D. Transthoracic echocardiogram and ECG and if normal discharge from clinic
E. Transthoracic echocardiogram and ECG and if normal review every 2–5 years in clinic

2. A 22-year-old female patient presents to the A&E department after a seizure while walking. She has had a previous seizure at rest but did not seek medical attention. She is not aware of any relevant family history. Her ECG shows T-wave inversion in the anterolateral leads. Transthoracic echo reveals severe asymmetric hypertrophy of the basal to mid anterior septum (IVSd 31 mm) with evidence of SAM, and resting LVOT gradient of 40 mmHg. Cardiac MRI shows extensive replacement fibrosis in the hypertrophied region.

The best initial approach is:

A. Annual surveillance in cardiology clinic and neurology review for possible epilepsy
B. Genetic testing of patient for pathogenic mutations of HCM then treat depending on the mutation
C. Beta-blocker, genetic testing, and family screening of first-degree family members with ECG and echo then annual surveillance in clinic
D. Beta-blocker, Holter monitor, exercise test, genetic screening, and family screening of first-degree family members then treat according to results
E. Implant a cardioverter defibrillator (ICD) and annual review in clinic

3. **A 55-year-old male patient with a previous diagnosis of hypertrophic cardiomyopathy is referred to your clinic after moving into the local area. He has not been seen by a cardiologist for some years. He is well in himself and denies any specific symptoms though admits to a sedentary lifestyle. He is slightly overweight. He has an ejection systolic murmur, but observations, ECG, and clinical examination are otherwise normal.**

   You recommend:

   A. Lifestyle changes—encourage more physical activity to assess for exertional symptoms.
   B. Transthoracic echocardiogram and review annually in clinic
   C. Treadmill exercise test, transthoracic echocardiogram, and review every 2 years in clinic
   D. Treadmill exercise test, transthoracic echocardiogram, Holter monitor, and review annually in clinic
   E. Cardiac MRI only, to assess for fibrosis.

4. **A 28-year-old Afro-Caribbean man is referred after a routine ECG done by his GP shows voltage criteria for LV hypertrophy with T-wave inversion in the lateral leads. His transthoracic echocardiogram shows moderate concentric LVH of 14 mm and borderline dilatation of the left ventricle with LVEDD 6.0 cm but no other abnormalities. CMR shows no evidence of replacement fibrosis. He is physically very active and trains 5–6 times a week in the gym and reports no symptoms. He has no family history of note. He takes no regular medication and denies recreational drug use. Examination is normal, including blood pressure of 126/85 mmHg and HR 61 bpm.**

   You initially recommend:

   A. Genetic screening panel for HCM
   B. Period of detraining for 12 weeks then repeat echocardiogram
   C. Ambulatory BP monitor to check for hypertension
   D. Family screening of first-degree relatives for LVH
   E. Reassure and discharge without further investigations but advise reduction in level of exercise

5. You are asked to review a 30-year-old patient on the cardiology ward. She presented with aborted sudden cardiac death. Her echocardiogram and CMR show asymmetrical LVH with SAM and LVOT turbulence. She has an ICD in situ and is on appropriate medication and is ready for discharge. She has three children aged 4, 6, and 8 years and five siblings aged between 25 and 40 years. She has some questions regarding the chance of her other family members being affected. Her genetics screen results are awaited.

Regarding genetic screening:

A. In cases of HCM, only 20% patients are found to have an identifiable mutation in sarcomeric genes

B. All family members (adult and children) should have an echo and ECG and if a gene is identified in the index case then they should be offered genetic screening

C. All adult first-degree relative should be offered genetic screening to look for a pathogenic mutation if an abnormal gene is identified in the index case.

D. Most commonly HCM is inherited in an autosomal recessive mode

E. Her imaging findings confirm the diagnosis and there is no role for genetic screening

6. A 42-year-old patient with known apical HCM is referred to the A&E department with palpitations. On arrival he appears anxious but is haemodynamically stable with no signs of heart failure. His ECG shows atrial fibrillation with a ventricular rate of 124 bpm. Aside from the HCM he has no other past medical history.

You recommend:

A. Rate control with a beta-blocker and monitor until rate controlled then discharge and continue usual cardiology follow up

B. Rate control with a beta-blocker and monitor until rate controlled, anticoagulate regardless of CHADS VASc score.

C. Review echocardiogram and if left atrium is enlarged then proceed to DCCV immediately to avoid decompensation.

D. Admit to CCU and request inpatient AF ablation procedure

E. Rate control with a beta-blocker then discharge with Holter monitor to check for HR variability and AF burden.

7. A 50-year-old woman with a history of type 2 diabetes mellitus and hypertension presents to hospital with a 6-week history of progressive exertional dyspnoea and peripheral oedema. On arrival she has signs of congestive cardiac failure, with rapidly conducted atrial fibrillation with a LBBB pattern and a troponin of 200 ng/L. She has an angiogram which shows no obstructive CAD. She is rate controlled and given diuretics with good effect. Her transthoracic echocardiogram reveals severe systolic impairment with an LVEF of 24% and dilated LV volumes. ECG shows QRS duration 120 ms.

Prior to discharge, you recommend:

A. Rate control with beta-blocker and digoxin, ACEi, MRA, repeat echo in 6–8 weeks. Anticoagulate with warfarin or DOAC
B. Genetic testing for DCM
C. Anticoagulate with warfarin or DOAC and add amiodarone
D. Inpatient atrial fibrillation ablation
E. AV node ablation and CRT pacemaker as outpatient

8. A 36-year-old female presents with signs and symptoms of congestive heart failure on a background of recent coryzal illness. Her observations are stable. Her echocardiogram shows severe LVSD with an LVEF 34% and global hypokinesia with dilated LV volumes. Her CMR shows a rim of epicardial late gadolinium enhancement in the basal lateral wall. Coronary angiography was normal. ECG shows sinus rhythm with a narrow QRS. She takes no recreational or prescription drugs and drinks minimal alcohol. Her aunt died suddenly aged 40 years, but she has no details of this.

You recommend:

A. Primary prevention implantable cardioverter defibrillator (ICD)
B. Genetic screening for DCM and screening of all relatives with echo and ECG
C. Viral serology, TSH, ferritin, autoimmune screen, and cardiac biopsy
D. CRT pacemaker
E. Beta-blocker, ACEi, MRA, Holter monitor, genetic screening, and screening of first-degree relatives

9. A 42-year-old man presents with presyncope. His ECG on arrival to hospital shows sinus rhythm with a broad LBBB (QRS 145 ms). His echocardiogram shows severe biventricular failure with an LVEF 25% and dilated atrial and ventricular volumes. His observations are normal including his BP. He admits to drinking alcohol heavily but denies recreational drug use and is a non-smoker. He has no known family history of cardiac disease or sudden cardiac death. Stress perfusion cardiac MRI does not show any evidence of inducible ischaemia.

You recommend:

A. Lifestyle advice regarding alcohol abstinence and repeat echo in 6–8 weeks
B. Lifestyle advice regarding alcohol abstinence, repeat echo in 6–8 weeks, and review indication for CRT after echo in 6–8 weeks
C. Lifestyle advice regarding alcohol abstinence, start beta-blocker, ACEi, and MRA, inpatient implantable cardioverter defibrillator (ICD)
D. Lifestyle advice regarding alcohol abstinence, start beta-blocker, ACEi, and MRA, review indication for CRT after echo in 6–8 weeks.
E. Lifestyle advice regarding alcohol abstinence, start beta-blocker, ACEi, and MRA, invasive coronary angiogram

10. A man is referred for family screening to the cardiology clinic. He has a strong family history of dilated cardiomyopathy with his maternal grandmother, male cousin, and three aunts being known to have had the condition with three having had aborted sudden cardiac death, and a genetic mutation has been identified. He takes ramipril 2.5 mg OD for BP, otherwise has no past medical history, takes no other medications, and does not drink alcohol. He has a normal exercise capacity. Examination and observations are normal. ECG is normal. His echocardiogram shows normal LVEF and ventricular volumes with no valvular abnormalities.

You recommend:

A. Chase genetic screening of relatives and perform genetic screening of patient – if pathogenic mutation not present, discharge
B. Review in clinic and repeat echocardiogram, ECG and Holter monitor every 3–5 years
C. Increase ramipril to 5mg OD and add beta blocker and MRA as tolerated
D. Holter monitor recording and consider implantable cardioverter defibrillator (ICD)
E. Reassure and discharge

11. A woman is admitted 6 weeks after delivery of her first baby with decompensated heart failure. She has a high BNP and is clinically overloaded. Her echocardiogram shows a dilated LV with LVEF of 30%. There is severe functional MR. Her ECG shows SR with a broad QRS duration. She continues to deteriorate with impaired renal function and hepatic congestion despite aggressive medical therapy.

You recommend:

A. Referral to transplant centre for consideration of mechanical circulatory support or heart transplantation.
B. Inpatient CRT-D.
C. Continue with diuretics and consider renal replacement therapy
D. Palliative care input
E. Surgical review with view to mitral valve repair or replacement

12. A 75-year-old patient is seen in the community HF clinic. He has a known diagnosis of dilated cardiomyopathy with LVEF 40%, diet-controlled DM and hypertension. He currently takes bisoprolol 2.5 mg od, ramipril 2.5 mg bd and amlodipine 10 mg od. He describes increasing exertional shortness of breath and worsening peripheral oedema. His ECG shows SR with a borderline LBBB (QRS 128 ms). His HR is 80 bpm, BP 130/85.

You recommend:

A. Refer for outpatient CRT devicE.
B. Switch bisoprolol to ivabradine and review in 4 weeks.
C. Add spironolactone and review in 4 weeks.
D. Stop amlodipine and up titrate beta blocker and ACEi.
E. Switch ramipril to sacubitril valsartan.

13. A 74-year-old female patient with a history of rheumatoid arthritis and mild renal impairment presents with progressive malaise, weight loss, and signs of decompensated heart failure. Echo reveals moderate mitral regurgitation, mild aortic regurgitation, and concentric left ventricular impairment with poor long axis function, biatrial dilatation, and a small global pericardial effusion. ECG shows rate controlled atrial fibrillation and normal QRS duration. Bloods reveal worsening of renal function. Amyloidosis is suspected.

Regarding amyloidosis:

A. AL amyloid is caused by deposition of immunoglobulin light chains produced by plasma cells and is associated with myeloma
B. Senile systemic amyloidosis has a worse prognosis than acquired forms of amyloidosis
C. Digoxin is the first-line treatment of atrial fibrillation in amyloidosis
D. Prognosis for AL amyloid is better than senile amyloidosis
E. Treatment options for the different subtypes of amyloidosis are similar

14. A 39-year-old man presents with syncope while playing football. He has a past medical history of pulmonary sarcoidosis and previous MI with stent to LAD. ECG on arrival to hospital shows 2:1 heart block with a narrow QRS. Coronary angiography shows a patent stent with no obstructive CAD. Echocardiogram shows a dilated LV with moderate impairment of LV function (LVEF 45%). Cardiac MRI shows patchy LGE and cardiac sarcoidosis is suspected.

You recommend:

A. Increased steroid therapy and annual follow up
B. Increased steroid therapy and implant CRT-D
C. Dual chamber pacemaker
D. Electrophysiological (EP) study
E. Telemetry, increase steroid therapy, consider ICD

15. Regarding Anderson-Fabry disease:

A. Inherited in an autosomal recessive mode
B. Treatment is supportive
C. Aortic root dilatation is seen in approximately a third of patients
D. Coronary artery disease should always be excluded with angiography
E. Valvular regurgitation is uncommon

16. A 46-year-old man presents with out-of hospital VF arrest. His brother died suddenly a few months ago at the age of 32 and he was awaiting clinic review for family screening. He had previously been asymptomatic and was cycling to work. He takes no medication. His CMR shows features of ARVC: which of the following constitute a major criterion for ARVC?

A. Family history of premature sudden death
B. Regional RV hypokinesia
C. Inverted T-waves in V2 and V3, in presence of RBBB
D. Inverted T waves in right precordial leads (V1, V2 and V3) or beyond in individuals with complete pubertal development (in the absence of complete RBBB)
E. LBBB type tachycardia on ECG/ Holter/ during exercise testing

17. A 32-year-old patient presents with pre-syncope whilst out running. She is a keen runner and has never had similar symptoms. Her family history is unclear as she was adopted. Her ECG shows sinus rhythm with a narrow QRS and T-wave inversion in V2 and V3 and she has short runs on broad complex tachycardia on telemetry. Observations and examination are normal. Echo shows severe segmental RV dilatation with impaired RV function and a non-dilated LV with mild impairment. She is unable to have a CMR due to claustrophobia.

You recommend:

A. Myocardial biopsy
B. Increase exercise intensity
C. Beta blocker and implantable cardioverter defibrillator (ICD)
D. Negatively chronotropic calcium channel blocker
E. Beta blocker / ACEi / MRA

18. Regarding LV hypertrabeculation/non-compaction cardiomyopathy:

A. The myocardium normally becomes compacted at weeks 12–15 in utero
B. Usually an autosomal recessive mode of inheritance
C. Over 10 genes have been linked to left ventricular non-compaction (LVNC)
D. Thromboembolism is rare
E. ECG typically shows a low voltage QRS

19. A 42-year-old man presents with left arm weakness and is found to have evidence of an embolic stroke on CT head. He undergoes transthoracic echocardiography which reveals a dilated left ventricle with globally impaired function (LVEF 25%) and a large LV thrombus. CMR shows a thinned LV wall with hypertrabeculation; ratio of non-compacted to compacted is >2 in end-systole. His ECG shows SR with a narrow QRS. His bloods show a raised BNP but are otherwise within normal limits. He has a history of mild hypertension but no significant family history. He responds well to initial therapy and is started on anticoagulation.

You recommend:

A. Cardiac catheterization
B. Beta-blocker, ACEI/ARB, MRA
C. Beta-blocker, ACEI/ARB, MRA, primary prevention ICD
D. Beta-blocker, ACEI/ARB, MRA, Holter monitor, and consideration of ICD
E. Transoesophageal echo and bubble contrast echo

20. A 75-year-old lady with mild Alzheimer's is admitted after developing chest pain after locking herself in the bathroom. Her ECG is normal on admission, but her troponin is raised; she is admitted for angiography. This shows unobstructed coronary arteries. Her echocardiogram shows apical ballooning and moderate impairment of the LV. She is diagnosed with Tsakotsubo cardiomyopathy.

Regarding Tsakotsubo cardiomyopathy

A. Inpatient hospital mortality is 10–20%

B. Recurrence rates of up to 22% have been reported

C. Thromboembolism is a common consequence

D. Most patients have long term reduced ejection fraction on echo

E. Repeat cardiac imaging should be performed annually

chapter

5.2

CARDIOMYOPATHIES

ANSWERS

1. E. The 2023/24 ESC Guidelines on Hypertrophic Cardiomyopathy recommend genetic and clinical testing of adult relatives of a patient with hypertrophic cardiomyopathy. Genetic screening should be performed in the index case and if a pathogenic mutation is identified should be cascaded to all first-degree adult relatives. When no definite genetic mutation is identified in the proband or genetic testing is not performed, clinical evaluation with ECG and echocardiography should be considered in first-degree adult relatives and repeated every 2–5 years (or 6–12 monthly if non-diagnostic abnormalities are present).

2. D. Patients with syncope should undergo 12-lead ECG, standard upright exercise test, and 48-hour ambulatory ECG monitoring and, if a bradyarrhythmia is identified, it should be treated in accordance with current ESC Guidelines on cardiac pacing. Exercise stress echocardiography should be considered, particularly in patients with exertional or postural syncope, to detect provocable LVOT. As unexplained non-vasovagal syncope is a risk factor for sudden cardiac death, particularly when it occurs in young patients in close temporal proximity to their first evaluation, treatment with a prophylactic implantable cardioverter defibrillator (ICD) may be appropriate in individuals with other features indicative of high sudden death risk; however, in this case, this would follow after the appropriate investigations.

3. D. A clinical evaluation, including 12-lead ECG and TTE, is recommended every 12–24 months in clinically stable patients. Forty-eight-hour ambulatory ECG is recommended every 12–24 months in clinically stable patients, every 6–12 months in patients in sinus rhythm with left atrial dimension 45 mm, and whenever patients complain of new palpitations. CMR may be considered every 5 years in clinically stable patients, or every 2–3 years in patients with progressive disease. Symptom-limited exercise testing should be considered every 2–3 years in clinically stable patients, or every year in patients with progressive symptoms.

4. B. There are a number of clinical features that can help distinguish between hypertrophic cardiomyopathy and athletic heart, and this is an important distinction to make. In the absence of a validated 'gold standard', the diagnosis of HCM in an athlete requires integration of a number of different parameters of varying sensitivity and specificity. These include demographics, ECG, and structural, functional, and genetic factors. No response to detraining for 12 weeks in this situation would then require further assessment.

5. C. In the majority of cases, HCM is inherited as an autosomal dominant genetic trait with a 50% risk of transmission to offspring. Some cases are explained by de novo mutations, but apparently sporadic cases can arise because of incomplete penetrance in a parent and, less commonly, autosomal recessive inheritance. In patients fulfilling HCM diagnostic criteria, sequencing of sarcomere protein genes identifies a disease-causing mutation in up to 60% of cases. When a definite causative genetic mutation is identified in a patient, his or her relatives should first be genetically tested, and then clinically evaluated if they are found to carry the same mutation. The children of patients with a definite disease-causing mutation should be considered for predictive genetic testing—following pre-test family counselling—when they are aged 10 or more years. In first-degree child relatives aged 10 or more years, in whom the genetic status is unknown, clinical assessment with ECG and echocardiography should be considered every 1–2 years between 10 and 20 years of age, and every 2–5 years thereafter.

6. B. In haemodynamically stable patients, oral beta-blockers or non-dihydropyridine calcium channel antagonists are recommended to slow the ventricular response to AF. Use DC cardioversion if haemodynamically unstable. Given the high incidence of stroke in patients with HCM and paroxysmal, persistent, or permanent AF, it is recommended that all patients with AF should receive anticoagulation. In general, lifelong therapy with oral anticoagulants is recommended, even when sinus rhythm is restored.

7. A. AF is the most common arrhythmia in HF irrespective of concomitant LVEF: it increases the risk of thromboembolic complications (particularly stroke) and may impair cardiac function, leading to worsening symptoms of HF. Incident HF precipitated by AF is associated with a more benign prognosis, but new-onset AF in a patient with established HF is associated with a worse outcome, probably because it is both a marker of a sicker patient and because it impairs cardiac function. Initial treatment is with beta blockade. If there is evidence of marked congestion, then digoxin is preferred initially. If there is haemodynamic instability, then IV digoxin or amiodarone can be administered. Emergency electrical cardioversion is recommended for patients with haemodynamic collapse. DCM is idiopathic in 50% of cases, about one-third of which are hereditary. Genetic testing could be discussed at follow up.

8. E. Epicardial LGE suggests a non-ischaemic cardiomyopathy but is non-specific. No indication for a CRT device currently as narrow QRS. Holter monitor to look for NSVT as part of risk stratification and then consider ICD. DCM is idiopathic in 50% of cases, about one-third of which are hereditary. There are already more than 50 genes identified that are associated with DCM. Many genes are related to the cytoskeleton. The most frequent ones are titin, lamin, and desmin. Genetic screening may be appropriate and if positive could be offered to first-degree relatives. If genetic screening is negative, then screening of first-degree relatives with ECG, echo, and clinical review may be appropriate.

9. D. The association between alcohol intake and the risk of developing de novo HF is U-shaped, with the lowest risk with modest alcohol consumption (up to 7 drinks/week). Greater alcohol intake may trigger the development of toxic cardiomyopathy, and when present, complete abstention from alcohol is recommended. CRT is recommended for symptomatic patients with HF in sinus rhythm with a QRS duration of 130–149 msec and LBBB QRS morphology and with LVEF ≤35% despite optimal medical therapy in order to improve symptoms and reduce morbidity and mortality.

10. A. If there is a pathogenic mutation is found in affected cases in the family, then this can be looked for and if not present, the patient reassured and discharged. Otherwise the patient needs regular review and risk stratification.

11. A. To manage patients with AHF or cardiogenic shock (INTERMACS level 1), short-term mechanical support systems, including percutaneous cardiac support devices, extracorporeal life support (ECLS), and extracorporeal membrane oxygenation (ECMO), may be used to support patients with left or biventricular failure until cardiac and other organ function has recovered.

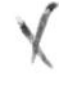

12. D. His QRS is too narrow to consider CRT. Although his heart rate is >70 bpm, the beta-blocker should be increased first before considering ivabradine. Spironolactone could be initiated although his EF is >35% so there is less strong evidence for this. Amlodipine may well be contributing to his ankle swelling and so should be stopped and his ACEi and BB up titrated. No indication for sacubitril valsartan as EF is >35%.

13. A. Acquired amyloid (AL) is deposition of fibril proteins from immunoglobulin light chains produced by plasma cells. It is associated with myeloma or monoclonal gammopathies. Secondary amyloid (AA) is associated with chronic inflammatory conditions such as rheumatoid arthritis, ankylosing spondylitis, and familial Mediterranean fever. The amyloid fibrils consist of protein A. Senile amyloidosis carries a better prognosis than AL amyloid. Digoxin should be used with caution as higher risk of toxicity in amyloidosis, beta-blockers should also be used cautiously due to the risk of AV block. Nephrotic syndrome and renal failure are common at presentation.

14. E. Immunosuppression with steroids and implantation of a device is indicated. Look for evidence of NSVT and consider ICD (CRT not indicated as narrow QRS duration).

15. C. Anderson Fabry disease is a genetic condition inherited in an X-linked fashion. It affects men more commonly than women: women can be affected but typically present with a milder form of disease and at a later age. The genetic mutation affects the function of alpha-galactosidase given as the treatment. Diagnosis is usually made by measurement of enzyme activity but genetic testing is available. Aortic root dilatation is seen in a third of patients. Microvascular disease and premature coronary atherosclerosis can occur. Valvular regurgitation is common but usually mild.

16. D. The diagnostic criteria for Arrhythmogenic Cardiomyopathy has evolved. According to the 2020 International Criteria for the Diagnosis of ARVC, only D is a major criteria. The other answers listed are minor criteria for diagnosis.

17. C. The pattern of clinical and imaging findings suggests ARVC with one major criterion (severe segmental RV dilatation) and two minor criteria (T-wave inversion in leads V2 and V3; no RBBB; LBBB type tachycardia on ECG). Activity levels should be restricted from endurance and competitive sports. Standard heart failure therapy if symptoms. Medical treatment is with amiodarone, beta blockers, or propafenone. ICD is indicated if high risk of sudden cardiac death. High risk markers include:

- syncope due to documented arrhythmia,
- severity of the electrical manifestations of the disease
- presence of non-sustained ventricular tachycardia, a high ventricular ectopic frequency, and a positive EP study
- severity of structural heart disease

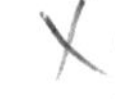

18. C. More than 10 genes have been linked to LVNC. These include mutations in the Tafazzin gene, alpha-dystrobrevin, and several sarcomeric proteins. Inheritance is usually autosomal dominant.

19. D. The hypertrabeculation suggest a diagnosis of LV hypertrabeculation/non-compaction cardiomyopathy. Coronary artery disease is unlikely to be the cause but could be investigated non-invasively. Standard heart failure therapy is recommended. ICD implantation is recommended for patients with sustained VT, recurrent unexplained syncope, or LV ejection fraction <35% on optimal medical therapy with non-sustained VT on Holter monitor

20. B. In-hospital mortality is around 2–5% mainly due to refractory cardiogenic shock or ventricular fibrillation. Recurrence rates up to 22% have been reported over 5-year follow-up. Thromboembolism occurs in around 4%. Most patients recover fully with no long-term symptoms.

chapter

5.3

PERICARDIAL DISEASE

QUESTIONS

1. **Which of the following statements is false regarding the presenting signs and symptoms of acute pericarditis?**

   A. Chest pain is present in 85–90% of cases
   B. Pericardial effusion is seen in 60% of cases
   C. Electrocardiographic changes are observed in 60% of cases
   D. A pericardial friction rub is heard in >67% of cases
   E. Elevated troponin generally indicates myocarditis/myocardial involvement

2. **Which of the following is true regarding the triage and risk stratification of patients with acute pericarditis?**

   A. Minor predictors of poor outcome include immunosuppression, oral anticoagulant use, and myopericarditis
   B. It is mandatory to search for the aetiology in all cases of acute pericarditis
   C. Major predictors of poor outcome include fever >38°C, pericardial effusion >10mm, and subacute onset
   D. Clinical presentation with no specific aetiology suspected (likely idiopathic or viral) warrants hospital admission and aetiology search
   E. Clinical presentation with only one predictor of poor outcome may be managed on an outpatient basis

3. **Which of the following is true regarding the management of acute pericarditis?**

   A. Colchicine is recommended as an alternative to aspirin or NSAIDS and is associated with lower recurrence rates
   B. Physical activity should be restricted to sedentary activity alone for 3 months after the initial onset of symptoms in all patients diagnosed with acute pericarditis
   C. Corticosteroids are considered second-line therapy, due to the risk of favouring chronic evolution of the disease and promoting dependence
   D. Asprin, ibuprofen, and colchicine must all be administered in tapering dose regimens in order to prevent recurrence
   E. CRP is not a useful marker of response to treatment

4. Regarding prognosis in acute pericarditis:

A. Constrictive pericarditis develops in <5% of patients with idiopathic pericarditis

B. Constrictive pericarditis develops in 20–30% of patients with tuberculous or purulent pericarditis

C. Constrictive pericarditis develops in 5–10% of patients with malignant or immune-mediated pericarditis

D. Colchicine reduces the recurrence rate of acute pericarditis by 20–25%

E. 2–3% of patients with idiopathic acute pericarditis who are not treated with colchicine will develop recurrent or incessant disease

5. Regarding recurrent pericarditis:

A. Viral aetiology is identified in around 40% of cases when pericardial fluid and tissue is analysed

B. In contrast with a first episode of pericarditis, corticosteroids are considered first line therapy for recurrent pericarditis

C. Third-line corticosteroid sparing agents include intravenous immunoglobulin, anakinra, and azathioprine

D. Colchicine should be administered for 3 months

E. Influenza vaccination should be considered in all patients with recent recurrent pericarditis, in order to prevent further recurrence

6. In pericarditis with myocardial involvement:

A. Definite confirmation of myocardial involvement cannot be made in the absence of biopsy even when advanced imaging techniques (CMR, PET) are available

B. Predominant myocarditis with suspected pericardial involvement should be termed 'myopericarditis'

C. Focal or diffuse impairment of left ventricular systolic function is a feature of myopericarditis

D. Coronary angiography is recommended to rule out acute coronary syndromes in all cases

E. Strenuous physical activity may be resumed when symptoms have resolved and CRP has normalized in non-athletes, or after 3 months have passed since initial symptom onset in athletes

7. Regarding the aetiology of pericardial effusions:

A. Approximately 90% are idiopathic in developed countries

B. 1–2% are iatrogenic in developed countries

C 40–50% are due to connective tissue diseases in developed countries

D. Tuberculosis is the cause in 15–25% of cases in developing countries

E 10–25% are malignant in developed countries

8. The following symptoms may all result as a direct mechanical consequence of a large pericardial effusion except:

- **A.** Orthopnoea
- **B.** Dysphagia
- **C.** Hoarse voice
- **D.** Hiccups
- **E** Unilateral upper limb weakness

9. Which of the following statements is true regarding pericardial effusions?

- **A.** CT or CMR should be performed in all moderate or large pericardial effusions
- **B.** Large effusions without inflammatory signs or tamponade are usually associated with an idiopathic aetiology
- **C.** Aspirin, NSAIDS, and colchicine are generally effective in reducing the size of most pericardial effusions
- **D.** Pericardiocentesis should be considered for effusions >10 mm in depth which are chronic (>3 months old), due to a 30–35% risk of progression to tamponade
- **E.** Idiopathic pericardial effusions with multiple recurrences have a high rate of progression to constrictive pericarditis

10. Regarding cardiac tamponade:

- **A.** Pulsus paradoxus is defined as an inspiratory decrease in systolic arterial pressure >10mmHg with the breath held at end inspiration
- **B.** Pulsus paradoxus is a consequence of interventricular septal shift
- **C.** Intrapericardial pressure-volume curves demonstrate a rapid initial rise in pressure with small volumes of fluid accumulation, followed by a plateau phase
- **D.** Electrical alternans represents alternating QRS amplitude according to the phase of respiration
- **E.** A normal cardiac silhouette on chest X-ray rules out the possibility of tamponade

11. Echocardiographic markers of early cardiac tamponade include all of the following except:

- **A.** Early diastolic right atrial collapse
- **B.** Early diastolic right ventricular collapse
- **C.** >25–30% increase in tricuspid inflow velocity during inspiration
- **D.** Inspiratory decrease in pulmonary vein diastolic forward flow
- **E.** Dilated IVC with reduced inspiratory collapsibility

12. Regarding the triage of cardiac tamponade:

A. Presentation with orthopnoea is a stronger indicator of the need for urgent pericardiocentesis than pulsus paradoxus

B. Malignant disease, tuberculosis, and systemic autoimmune disease are aetiological indicators of the need for urgent pericardiocentesis

C. On echocardiographic imaging, a 'swinging' heart is a stronger indicator of the need for urgent pericardiocentesis than left ventricular collapse

D. If the total risk score is <6, pericardiocentesis can be safely delayed and re-assessed by echocardiography after 5–7 days

E. Pericardial effusion associated with Type A aortic dissection warrants urgent surgical management if the risk score is ≥6

13. Regarding the clinical presentation of constrictive pericarditis:

A. The classical presentation is with signs and symptoms of biventricular heart failure

B. When occurring as a consequence of inflammatory pericarditis, the delay from inflammation to diagnosis of constrictive pericarditis is usually >10 years

C. Kussmaul sign may be present in the absence of a haemodynamically significant pericardial effusion

D. Fatigue, peripheral oedema, dyspnoea, pleural effusions, and ascites are suggestive of concomitant myocardial dysfunction

E. The presence of a pericardial knock is indicative of a concomitant pericardial effusion

14. In the differentiation between constrictive pericarditis and restrictive cardiomyopathy:

A. Low ECG voltages are more suggestive of constriction

B. The absence of pericardial calcification on echocardiography or CT effectively rules out constrictive pericarditis

C. Echocardiographic colour M-mode flow propogation velocity (Vp) <45 cm/s is more in keeping with restrictive cardiomyopathy

D. Significant variation in mitral and tricuspid inflow velocities is non-specific and does not assist in the differentiation between constriction and restriction

E. Tissue Doppler E′ velocity <8 cm/s is more in keeping with constrictive pericarditis

15. Regarding cardiac catheterization for suspected pericardial constriction:

A. Confirmatory left and right heart catheterization is indicated in all suspected cases if pericardectomy is being considered

B. A 'square-root' sign may be present due to a late diastolic dip and plateau in LV and RV pressures

C. RVEDP is usually greater than LVEDP

D. RVEDP > 1/3 RV systolic pressure is more in keeping with restrictive cardiomyopathy

E. a systolic area index >1.1 is suggestive of constriction

16. In the treatment of constrictive pericarditis:

- **A.** Anti-inflammatory therapy alone may be an effective treatment
- **B.** Pericardectomy is always indicated for pericardial constriction secondary to radiotherapy
- **C.** Pericardectomy is the only effective treatment
- **D.** Pericardiocentesis alone cannot be an effective treatment
- **E.** ACE-inhibitors are prognostically beneficial in chronic constriction

17. Effusive-constrictive pericarditis:

- **A.** Is characterized by the failure of right atrial pressure to fall by >30%, or to less than 10 mmHg, after pericardiocentesis
- **B.** Is usually caused by tuberculosis in developing and developed countries
- **C.** Requires cardiac catheterization for definitive diagnosis
- **D.** Definitive diagnosis may be established by multimodality imaging (echo, CT, CMR)
- **E.** Is usually secondary to cardiac surgery or radiotherapy in developed countries

18. Markers of poorer outcome after surgical pericardectomy include all of the following except:

- **A.** Child–Pugh score >7
- **B.** Prior ionizing mediastinal radiation
- **C.** Extensive pericardial calcification
- **D.** Low serum sodium
- **E.** Cardiac index <1.2 $l/m^2/min$

19. Regarding multimodality imaging in pericardial diseases:

- **A.** Echocardiography and CMR are of equivalent utility in assessing cardiac systolic function, diastolic function, and ventricular interdependence
- **B.** CT and CMR are of equivalent utility in assessing pericardial thickness and calcification
- **C.** Echocardiography and CT are of equivalent utility in assessing cardiac morphology (including tissue characterization)
- **D.** CT and CMR are of equivalent utility in assessing pericardial inflammation
- **E.** Echocardiography and CMR are of equivalent utility in characterizing pericardial masses

20. Regarding pericardial syndromes during pregnancy and breastfeeding:

- **A.** Hydropericardium occurs in up to 4% of pregnant females
- **B.** Aspirin or NSAIDs are the treatments of choice for acute pericarditis occurring after 20 weeks of pregnancy
- **C.** Aspirin is the treatment of choice for acute pericarditis occurring during the first 20 weeks of pregnancy
- **D.** Colchicine can be safely used as an adjunct to aspirin or NSAIDs throughout pregnancy
- **E.** Aspirin is the drug of choice for acute pericarditis during breastfeeding

21. When performing pericardiocentesis:

A. The risk of significant complications is in the order of 5–10%
B. For echo-guided pericardiocentesis, the ideal entry site is from the sub-xiphoid approach
C. The internal mammary artery lies 1–2 cm lateral to the left parasternal border
D. When performing angiography-guided pericardiocentesis, the LAO cranial view generally provides the best visualization of the puncturing needle and its relation to the diaphragm and pericardium
E. The procedure should never be performed 'blindly' (i.e. without either echocardiographic or angiographic guidance)

22. Regarding interventional and surgical techniques for pericardial diseases:

A. Autoreactive and lymphocytic pericardial effusions may be treated with intrapericardial cisplatin or thiotepa
B. Balloon pericardiotomy should be considered for recurrent malignant pericardial effusions
C. Uraemic pericardial effusions may be treated with intrapericardial triamcinolone
D. A pericardial window creates a passage from the pericardial space into the peritoneum
E. Complete pericardectomy involves removal of the visceral pericardium only, leaving the parietal pericardium in situ

23. Regarding post-cardiac injury syndromes (PCIS):

A. It may occur in the absence of acute inflammation
B. High-dose corticosteroid at the time of cardiac surgery is effective in preventing PCIS
C. Early post-infarct pericarditis is often an indication of subacute ventricular rupture
D. Late post-infarct pericarditis (Dressler's syndrome) typically occurs 28 days post-MI
E. Around 3% of patients experiencing PCIS after cardiac surgery will go on to develop constrictive pericarditis

24. Which of the following statements is true regarding diseases of the pericardium?

A. Chylopericardium, also known as cholesterol pericarditis, occurs as a sequela of tuberculous pericarditis, rheumatoid pericarditis, and trauma
B. The use of anticoagulants is an established precipitant of tamponade in patients with acute pericarditis
C. Pericardial cysts usually communicate freely with the pericardial fluid
D. Up to 30% of patients with hyperthyroidism may have a pericardial effusion
E. Left atrial early diastolic collapse is a useful indicator of tamponade in patients with pulmonary hypertension

25. When considering the aetiology of pericarditis and pericardial effusions:

A. Viral serology is indicated in the investigation of suspected viral pericarditis

B. Analysis of tumour markers from pericardial fluid has a high diagnostic yield in suspected malignant effusions

C. Pericardial fluid unstimulated interferon-gamma (uIFN-γ) assay has superior accuracy for the diagnosis of tuberculous pericarditis than pericardial fluid adenosine deaminase (ADA) assay

D. TRAPS mutations should be sought in pericarditis suspected to be secondary to Still's disease

E. Pericardial fluid should be tested for ANA, ENA, and ANCA if an effusion is suspected to be secondary to autoimmune disease

chapter

5.3

PERICARDIAL DISEASE

ANSWERS

1. D. Chest pain, typically sharp/pleuritic and exacerbated by lying flat is reported by the majority of patients with acute pericarditis. A pericardial friction rub is a squeaky or rasping noise typically heard best with the diaphragm of the stethoscope over the left sternal border. Rubs are heard in less than 33% of cases. They are often transient in nature and can be accentuated by manoeuvres such as lying the patient flat. Typical ECG changes are observed in 60% of cases and include widespread concave ST-segment elevation and PR segment depression (Stage 1), PR-segment normalization with progressive T-wave flattening and inversion (Stage 2), and generalized T-wave inversion (stage 3) progressing to ECG normalization (stage 4). A pericardial effusion, usually small in size, is seen in 60% of cases. Biomarkers of myocardial injury generally indicate some degree of concomitant myocarditis.

2. A. It is not mandatory to search for aetiology in all cases, particularly in countries with low tuberculosis prevalence, since the clinical course of most cases of pericarditis is benign and aetiology search has a low yield. Obvious non-viral, non-idiopathic aetiology is associated with worse clinical outcomes. Major predictors of adverse outcome include fever >38°C, subacute onset, pericardial effusion > 20 mm, cardiac tamponade, and lack of response to aspirin or NSAIDs after 1 week of therapy. Minor predictors of poor outcome are myopericarditis, immunosuppression, trauma, and oral anticoagulant therapy. In cases where there is a likely non-viral aetiology or where there are any predictors of poor outcome, the patient should be hospitalized and aetiology search undertaken. Where the aetiology is likely viral/idiopathic, a trial of empiric aspirin or NSAIDs is warranted. Hospitalization is only warranted in these cases when there is a lack of response to initial therapy.

3. C. Physical activity should be restricted to sedentary only (in non-athletes) until symptoms have resolved and CRP has normalized, with no specific recommendation for timescale. For athletes, CRP, ECG, and the echocardiogram should have normalized, and 3 months should have elapsed since the onset of symptoms before competitive sports may be resumed. Colchicine has been shown in large studies to improve the rate of response to standard therapy (aspirin and/or NSAIDs) and prevent recurrences when administered in conjunction with first-line therapy. Tapering should be considered for aspirin and NSAIDs, although this is not mandatory for colchicine. Corticosteroids are considered second-line agents due to the risk of promoting chronic pericarditis and dependence. Other drug therapies should be targeted to specifically identified aetiological factors if present. Serial CRP monitoring is a useful marker of response to therapy.

4. B. Constrictive pericarditis develops in <1% of patients with acute idiopathic pericarditis, 2–5% of patients with immune-mediated or neoplastic aetiology, and 20–30% of patients with tuberculous or purulent aetiology. From 15% to 30% of patients with acute idiopathic pericarditis who are not treated with colchicine develop recurrent (return of symptom after at least a 4–6 week symptom-free period) or incessant pericarditis (persistent symptoms >4—6 weeks without any obvious remission). Colchicine reduces the recurrence rate by approximately half. Around 50%

of patients with acute pericarditis not treated with colchicine will develop recurrent pericarditis, particularly if treated with corticosteroids.

5. C. Recurrent pericarditis is defined by a return of symptoms after at least a 4–6-week symptom-free period. Diagnosis is established using the same criteria as for acute pericarditis. In developed countries, the aetiology is usually not identified although it is presumed to be immune-mediated in most cases. Nonetheless, virology studies of pericardial fluid and tissue have identified viral pathogens in 20% of cases. First-line therapy remains aspirin or NSAIDs with colchicine. As for a first episode of acute pericarditis, corticosteroids are considered second-line agents for patients experiencing an inadequate response to first-line therapy. Careful tapering of steroid dosing is required over the course of several months, with close attention to the recurrence of symptoms or increasing inflammatory markers. Colchicine should be continued for 6 months in recurrent pericarditis. Azathioprine, IVIG, and anakinra (a recombinant IL-1B antagonist) may be used as third-line agents in steroid-dependent recurrent pericarditis once an infective aetiology has been excluded. Pericardiectomy may be considered as a last resort.

6. A. Cases with definite criteria for acute pericarditis and concomitant elevation of serum biomarkers of myocardial injury but no significant left ventricular systolic dysfunction are termed 'myopericarditis', which accounts for the majority of combined acute myocardial and pericardial syndromes. In contrast, where there is predominant myocardial involvement with significant acute LV impairment and evidence of pericardial involvement, the term 'perimyocarditis' is applicable. Significant new LV systolic impairment is not a feature of myopericarditis. Definite confirmation of myocardial involvement can only be made on biopsy. Nonetheless, CMR is a Class 1 recommendation to support the diagnosis of myocardial involvement in view of the fact that biopsy may not be practicable in all centres and is associated with a risk of procedural complications. Coronary angiography is also a Class 1 recommendation but its use should be tailored according to the clinical presentation and patient risk factors for coronary disease, and is not mandated in all cases. Avoidance of strenuous physical activity is recommended for 6 months for all patients with myocarditis (athletes and non-athletes).

7. E. In the last 20 years, five major series have been published on the characteristics of moderate and large pericardial effusions. In developed countries, up to 50% are idiopathic, 10–25% malignant, 15–25% iatrogenic, and 5–15% due to connective tissue diseases. In developing countries, >60% of cases are secondary to tuberculosis.

8. E. Classical symptoms of a pericardial effusion include exertional dyspnoea and orthopnoea, due to impaired cardiac filling as a consequence of increased intrapericardial pressure. Other non-specific symptoms include chest pain, fullness, cough, weakness, fatigue, anorexia, and palpitations. Fever may be present if there is an infectious or immune-mediated aetiology. Rarer presenting symptoms include nausea due to diaphragmatic compression, dysphagia due to oesophageal compression, hoarse voice (recurrent laryngeal nerve compression), and hiccups (phrenic nerve compression). Limb weakness is not a recognized mechanical consequence of pericardial effusion.

9. B. The mainstay of investigations for pericardial effusion is transthoracic echocardiography which should be performed in all suspected cases. Chest X-ray and assessment of inflammatory markers is also recommended in all cases. Cardiac CT or CMR are recommended in cases where there is suspicion of a loculated effusion, pericardial thickening or mass, or associated chest wall abnormalities. In cases where inflammatory markers are elevated, treatment should be as for acute pericarditis, with empiric administration of anti-inflammatory drugs. Aspirin, NSAIDs, colchicine, and corticosteroids are generally not effective in reducing the size of non-inflammatory effusions. Large effusions without signs of inflammation or tamponade are usually associated with an idiopathic aetiology, whilst tamponade without inflammation is often associated with neoplasia. Pericardiocentesis should be considered in effusions >20 mm in depth which persist >3 months, due to a 30–35% of progression to tamponade. Idiopathic effusions rarely progress to constrictive pericarditis even with multiple episodes of recurrence.

10. B. Pulsus paradoxus is a key diagnostic finding in tamponade and is defined as an inspiratory decrease in systolic blood pressure >10 mmHg during normal breathing, and is a consequence of exaggerated ventricular interdependence. When the overall volume of the cardiac chambers becomes fixed due to pericardial fluid accumulation, an increase in the size of one ventricle must occur at the expense of a reciprocal decrease in the size of the other ventricle. Hence during inspiration, increased venous return to the right heart results in increased RV dimensions, interventricular septal shift towards the left, and a decrease in left ventricular size and consequent fall in systolic blood pressure. Intrapericardial pressure initially increases slowly whilst the pericardium is able to accommodate increased fluid volume, until a plateau is reached whereby minimal additional fluid leads to rapid increases in pressure. Electrical alternans is the electrocardiographic phenomenon of alternating low and normal QRS amplitudes which reflects the 'swinging' motion of the heart within a large pericardial effusion. A normal cardiac silhouette does not exclude tamponade, since a small but rapidly accumulating effusion, for example after iatrogenic coronary artery perforation, may lead to dramatic increase in intrapericardial pressure. In contrast, a large effusion may accumulate over weeks or months without the development of tamponade due to accommodatory changes in pericardial compliance.

11. A. Right ventricular pressure is around 0–8mmHg in diastole, at which point the RV will collapse if intrapericardial pressure is elevated. Right atrial pressure is lowest (near 0 mmHg) during late diastole and early systole and will therefore be most prone to collapse at this stage of the cardiac cycle. When the overall volume of the cardiac chambers becomes fixed due to pericardial fluid accumulation, an increase in the size of one ventricle must occur at the expense of a reciprocal decrease in the size of the other ventricle—the phenomenon of ventricular interdependence. During inspiration, increased venous return to the right heart results in increased RV dimensions, interventricular septal shift towards the left, and a decrease in left ventricular size and consequent reduction in mitral inflow velocity with a concomitant increase in tricuspid inflow velocity. The opposite effects on mitral and tricuspid inflow are observed during expiration. Respiratory variation in mitral and/or tricuspid inflow velocities >25–30% is a marker of tamponade in the presence of a pericardial effusion. A concomitant inspiratory decrease in pulmonic vein diastolic forward flow into the left heart is also observed. Impaired diastolic right ventricular filling results in dilatation of the IVC with reduced inspiratory collapsibility.

12. A. The ESC Working Group on myocardial and pericardial diseases has proposed a triage system to determine the urgency of pericardiocentesis in cardiac tamponade. A combined score is derived from aetiological factors, clinical presentation, and imaging findings. Amongst aetiological factors, the highest risk is attributed to malignant and tuberculous effusions (2 points each), whilst systemic autoimmune diseases are considered to pose the lowest risk (-1 point). Orthopnoea without rales on auscultation is considered the single highest risk clinical presentation (3 points). Circumferential effusion >2 cm in diastole is the most highly scoring imaging finding (3 points), whilst left ventricular collapse scores 2 points. A combined score ≥6 warrants urgent pericardiocentesis. A combined score <6 allows for pericardiocentesis to be delayed for 12–48 hours. Urgent surgical management is warranted regardless of risk score in cases of Type A aortic dissection, ventricular free wall rupture after myocardial infarction, severe recent chest trauma, and in iatrogenic cases where bleeding cannot be controlled percutaneously.

13. C. Constrictive pericarditis is characterized by impaired diastolic filling of both ventricles due to a stiff, non-compliant pericardium and presents primarily with signs and symptoms of right-heart failure. When occurring as a result of an inflammatory pericarditis, the delay from initial inflammation to chronic constriction is highly variable and may even evolve directly from subacute or chronic inflammation. Classical presenting signs and symptoms are fatigue, peripheral oedema, dyspnoea, pleural effusions, and ascites resulting from impaired right ventricular diastolic filling rather than intrinsic myocardial dysfunction. A pericardial knock may be heard due to rapid ventricular filling which is abruptly halted by the non-compliant pericardium and is unrelated to the presence or absence of pericardial effusion. Kussmaul sign, a paradoxical rise in jugular venous pressure on inspiration, may be present due to increased ventricular interdependence. Kussmaul sign is not specific for constriction and is not dependent on the presence of effusion.

14. C. Restrictive cardiomyopathy is a common differential diagnosis of constrictive pericarditis. Kussmaul sign may be observed in both, whilst a pericardial knock is suggestive of constriction. Low ECG voltages and atrial fibrillation are common in both, whilst a pseudo-infarction pattern is more frequently observed in restrictive cardiomyopathy. Biatrial dilatation is characteristic of both conditions. Pericardial thickening and calcification (CXR, echo, CT, CMR) would point towards constriction, although neither is necessary for constrictive physiology to develop. Ventricular interdependence in constriction results in significant respiratory variation in mitral inflow (>25%) tricuspid inflow (>40%), and pulmonary vein D-wave velocity (>20%), none of which are characteristic in restrictive cardiomyopathy. Intrinsic myocardial disease in restrictive cardiomyopathy often results in left ventricular hypertrophy with reduced cavity size, impaired LV long axis, and impaired diastolic function (tissue Doppler E′ velocity <8 cm/s, E/A ratio >2, short deceleration time, colour M-mode flow propogation velocity <45 cm/s). CMR may be additionally useful for characterizing myocardial tissue abnormalities in restrictive cardiomyopathy, which should not be a feature of pure constriction.

15. E. Cardiac catheterization is indicated when non-invasive methods do not provide a definitive diagnosis of pericardial constriction. The square root sign is manifest as an early diastolic dip and subsequent plateau in the RV and LV pressure tracings, due to rapid early diastolic filling followed by impaired filling due to pericardial constraint. In normal physiology and in restrictive cardiomyopathy, RVEDP is usually lower than LVEDP. In constriction, increased RVEDP results in equalization of LVEDP and RVEDP (or <5 mmHg difference). The ratio of the right ventricular to left ventricular systolic pressure-time area during inspiration versus expiration (systolic area index) has been described as an index of increased ventricular interdependence: a value >1.1 is in keeping with constriction. In restrictive cardiomyopathy, there may be marked RV systolic hypertension (>50 mmHg) with RVEDP <1/3 RV systolic pressure. Conversely in uncomplicated constriction, RVEDP is usually elevated and RV systolic pressure is generally <50 mmHg (RVEDP >1/3 RV systolic pressure).

16. A. It is recognized that transient pericardial constriction may occur following acute pericarditis, probably due to ongoing pericardial inflammation. This form of constrictive pericarditis usually resolves within a few weeks with administration of anti-inflammatory therapy. CT or CMR may be helpful in demonstrating an inflamed pericardium. Hence in a patient with clinical evidence of pericardial constriction but no signs of chronicity (such as cachexia, pericardial calcification, or hepatic dysfunction), an empirical trial of anti-inflammatory therapy may be given. C is therefore incorrect. Pericardiocentesis alone may be an effective treatment for effusive–constrictive pericarditis, which may be seen in particular with tuberculous pericardial effusions. Pericardiocentesis combined with medical therapy for the primary aetiology (e.g. anti-tuberculous drugs) may therefore avoid the need for pericardectomy. Standard heart failure therapies are not indicated in pure constrictive pericarditis where intrinsic myocardial function is generally preserved. Pericardectomy is the mainstay of treatment for chronic constriction. However, it is associated with significant mortality and morbidity even in expert centres, and patients with advanced disease or multiple comorbidities should be considered for palliative/symptomatic treatment rather than surgery. Prior ionizing radiation is associated with a poor outcome because it induces myocardial as well as pericardial disease, and patients that have undergone prior mediastinal radiotherapy have a higher risk of death after radical pericardectomy. Careful patient selection in such cases is therefore of great importance.

17. D. Effusive–constrictive pericarditis is characterized by a constrictive pericardium with superimposed effusion, which, due to the high intrapericardial pressure, combine to give signs suggestive of tamponade. During pericardiocentesis, the failure of right atrial pressure to fall by >50%, or to less than 10 mmHg, is suggestive of ongoing pericardial constriction. This can be assessed by invasive haemodynamic monitoring during pericardiocentesis, or by non-invasive multimodality imaging. In developed countries, the most common aetiology is tuberculosis, whilst in developed countries most reported cases are idiopathic. Other reported aetiologies include radiotherapy, malignancy, chemotherapy, and post-cardiothoracic surgery.

18. C. Markers of poor outcome after surgical pericardectomy include cachexia, atrial fibrillation, low cardiac output (<1.2 $l/m^2/min$), hypoalbuminaemia due to protein-losing enteropathy, and/or impaired hepatic function secondary to congestion (Child–Pugh score >7), pulmonary hypertension, severe renal impairment, prior ionizing mediastinal radiation, low serum sodium, and older age. The extent of pre-operative pericardial calcification has no impact on survival after pericardectomy. Overall operative mortality for pericardectomy is 6–12% hence the procedure should only be performed in expert centres.

19. C. Echocardiography and CMR are both of excellent utility in assessing ventricular systolic function, septal motion, and ventricular interaction (free-breathing CMR cine imaging), and respiratory changes (phase-contrast CMR imaging of cardiac flow patterns). CT and CMR both demonstrate excellent utility in quantifying pericardial thickness, although CMR is poor at assessing pericardial calcification. Echocardiography and CT are equivalent in their ability to quantify cardiac morphology and tissue characteristics, although CMR is undoubtedly superior for this indication. CMR is also superior in the assessment of acute inflammation. Due to its unique ability to characterize tissue composition using T1 and T2 weighted imaging, including gadolinium enhanced techniques, CMR is also the technique of choice for the characterization of pericardial masses.

20. C. A benign, mild, asymptomatic pericardial effusion (hydropericardium) may develop in up to 40% of pregnant females. Clinical examination and the ECG are generally normal. High dose aspirin is the treatment of choice for acute pericarditis during the first 20 weeks of pregnancy, due to extensive knowledge of its safe use in early pregnancy in patients with antiphospholipid syndrome and pre-eclampsia. After 20 weeks, all NSAIDs other than low-dose aspirin (<100 mg/day) are contraindicated due to their ability to constrict the ductus arteriousus and impair foetal renal function. Colchicine is considered contraindicated throughout pregnancy and breastfeeding. NSAIDS, paracetamol, and steroids may all be used during breastfeeding, although aspirin is preferably avoided due to the risk of Reye's syndrome.

21. A. When performing percutaneous pericardiocentesis, the ideal entry site is at the point on the surface of the body where the effusion is closest to the transducer, the depth of effusion is greatest, and the risk of puncturing vessels or organs is the least. Commonly used access approaches include left parasternal, apical, and sub-xiphoid. The internal mammary artery runs 3–5 cm lateral to the left parasternal border and should be avoided. Angiography-guided pericardiocentesis is best performed using the lateral angiographic view, which generally provides the best visualization of the puncturing needle and its relation to the diaphragm and pericardium. The risk of significant complications during pericardiocentesis, such as arrhythmias, coronary artery or cardiac chamber puncture, haemothorax, pneumothorax, pneumopericardium, and hepatic injury, is in the order of 5–10%. Due to this relatively high risk of serious complications, pericardiocentesis should be performed under echocardiographic or angiographic guidance if at all possible, by experienced operators and with full laboratory staff assistance (physiologist, radiographer). However, the necessity to perform the procedure 'blindly' may arise when immediately life-threatening haemodynamic compromise occurs in a ward-based setting.

22. C. Neoplastic pericardial effusions may be treated with intrapericardial cisplatin or thiotepa in combination with systemic antineoplastic therapy. Autoreactive, lymphocytic, and uraemic pericardial effusions may respond to therapy with intrapericardial triamcinolone (300 mg/m^2). Balloon pericardiotomy creates a transient pericardio-(pleural)-abdominal window for drainage, although this should be avoided in neoplastic and purulent effusions due to the risk of disease spread. A pericardial window creates a passage from the pericardial space into the pleural space, and is often used to palliate recurrent pericardial effusions in patients who are either unfit for major surgical intervention or who have a limited life expectancy. Complete pericardiectomy involves removal of as much as possible of both the visceral (epicardial) and parietal pericardium.

23. E. Post-cardiac injury syndromes (PCIS) are a group of inflammatory pericardial conditions including post-MI pericarditis, post-pericardiotomy syndrome, and post-traumatic pericarditis. There is generally a latent period of a few weeks after the original cardiac insult and the PCIS are usually responsive to systemic anti-inflammatory therapy, implying a likely autoimmune aetiology. According to proposed diagnostic criteria, ≥2 of the following should be present; unexplained fever, pleuritic or pericarditic chest pain, pleural or pericardial rubs, pericardial effusion, or pleural effusion with elevated CRP. Perioperative colchicine has been shown to reduce the incidence of PCIS after cardiac surgery, although no benefit has been demonstrated from the prophylactic administration of systemic corticosteroids. Around 3% of patients developing PCIS after cardiac surgery will develop constrictive pericarditis, although other complication rates are low (recurrence 4%, tamponade 2%). Early post-MI pericarditis is usually self-limiting and responds to supportive treatment and anti-inflammatory therapy. Late post-MI pericarditis (Dressler's syndrome) typically occurs 1–2 weeks after an acute MI. It is associated with larger myocardial infarctions and has become rare (<1%) with the advent of primary percutaneous intervention.

24. E. Chylopericardium is a pericardial effusion composed of milky lymphatic fluid. This rare disorder may be primary or may be a consequence of damage to the thoracic duct by trauma, surgery, radiotherapy, subclavian vein thrombosis, tuberculosis, or malignancy. Cholesterol pericarditis is a separate entity in which clear, cholesterol-rich fluid accumulates within the pericardium, often as a sequela of tuberculous, rheumatoid, or traumatic pericarditis. Despite the widespread perception that the use of anticoagulants in patients with pericarditis will lead to haemorrhagic effusions or tamponade, studies of patients with acute pericarditis have failed to provide evidence for this. In patients with pulmonary hypertension, classical indicators of tamponade such as right atrial and right ventricular collapse may be masked due to high baseline right-sided pressures. In such cases, left atrial pressure may be lower than right atrial pressure and LA collapse may therefore be a more sensitive indicator of incipient tamponade. Pericardial cysts are rare cardiac masses with an incidence of 1:100,000 patients. They are often located in one of the cardiophrenic angles. They are often asymptomatic and require no treatment, although they can present with chest pain, dyspnoea, or palpitations. CMR has excellent utility in charcterizing the cystic nature of these structures, which do not communicate with the pericardial fluid. Up to 30%

of patients with hypothyroidism may have a pericardial effusion. These may be large in size but rarely cause tamponade.

25. C. Due to a poor diagnostic yield, routine viral serology is no longer recommended in the investigation of suspected viral pericarditis, with the exception of that occurring in the context of possible HIV or hepatitis C. Genome-wide search of pericardial fluid and/or tissue for specific infectious agents is now preferred to serology for most viruses if a definite diagnosis of viral pericarditis is needed. The diagnostic yield of tumour markers in pericardial fluid is controversial: several markers may be useful; however, none have demonstrated accuracy in distinguishing malignant from benign effusions. A definite diagnosis of tuberculous pericarditis requires isolation of tubercle bacilli from the pericardial fluid or tissue. However, a 'probable' diagnosis can be made in the presence of TB elsewhere in the body in combination with a lymphocytic pericardial exudate with elevated unstimulated interferon-gamma (uIFN-γ) or adenosine deamine (ADA) assay from the fluid. uIFN-γ has demonstrated superior accuracy for the diagnosis of tuberculous pericarditis compared to pericardial fluid ADA assay. FMF (familial Mediterranean fever) and TRAPS (tumour necrosis factor receptor-associated periodic fever) mutations should be sought in patients with pericarditis suspected to be associated with auto-inflammatory conditions presenting with periodic fevers. An elevated serum ferritin should be sought if an underlying diagnosis of Still's disease is suspected. Serum rather than pericardial fluid should also be tested for ANA, ENA, and ANCA if autoimmune pathology is suspected.

chapter 5.4

CARDIO-ONCOLOGY AND CARDIAC TUMOURS

QUESTIONS

1. A 67 year-old woman with a previous history of anthracycline exposure is referred by her GP for a cardiology review as she is complaining of exertional dyspnoea and tiredness. You elicit from the history that her cancer treatment was completed more than 10 years ago and she has only recently developed these symptoms. Which of the following statements regarding anthracycline-mediated cardiotoxicity is false?

A. Can present as acute, subacute, and chronic cardiotoxicities

B. If cardiac complications detected early cardiac outcomes better

C. Liposomal formulations may decrease risk

D. Administration of dexrazoxane may decrease risk of cardiotoxity

E. A cumulative dose of < 400 mg/m^2 of idarubicin is considered safe

2. A 67 year-old male is diagnosed with lung cancer. Radiotherapy is planned and in light of his past medical history of hypertension, diabetes, and myocardial infarction he is referred to cardiology for a pre-treatment assessment.

Which of the following is not a risk factor for radiation-induced heart disease (RIHD)?

A. The heart being in the radiotherapy field

B. Lower radiation fraction per dose

C. High cumulative total radiation dose

D. Concomitant radiotherapy with anthracyclines

E. Pre-existing cardiac disease

3. **A 38 year-old female presents to her GP with a decrease in exercise capacity and palpitations. She underwent mantle radiotherapy for lymphoma in childhood. She was told that she was cured and would not require regular follow-up.**

   Which of the following statement regarding RIHD is incorrect?

   A. Up to 20% of patients develop delayed chronic pericarditis within 2 years following irradiation
   B. Constrictive pericarditis following RIHD appears to be dose-dependent and related to the presence of pericardial effusion in the acute phase
   C. Valve stenosis is more common than valve regurgitation
   D. Coronary ostia and proximal coronary artery segments are involved
   E. Calcification of the ascending aorta and arch (porcelain aorta) may be a chronic complication

4. **An adult survivor of childhood cancer is followed up in the late effects clinic. These visits usually include a comprehensive physical screen for cardiac, metabolic, neurovascular, and psychological issues.**

   Which of the following is not recommended in the follow up of patients with chest radiation exposure?

   A. Yearly targeted clinical history and physical examination
   B. Yearly lipid profile and screen for cardiovascular risk factors
   C. Screening echocardiography after 1 year in high-risk patients
   D. Screening echocardiography after 10 years in low-risk patients
   E. Functional imaging after 5 to 10 years in high-risk patients

5. **A 42 year-old man on chemotherapy presents in the Emergency Department with atrial fibrillation.**

   Which of the following statements is not true about chemotherapeutics and arrhythmias?

   A. Ibrutinib is more commonly associated with supraventricular tachycardia
   B. Anthracyclines are associated commonly with atrial fibrillation
   C. Cyclophosphamide is more commonly associated with sinus tachycardia
   D. Arsenic trioxide typically results in a prolonged QTc
   E. 5-fluorouracil typically is associated with a sinus bradycadia

6. A 53 year-old patient with melanoma was treated with the immune check point inhibitor nivolumab. He presented in cardiovascular extremis to the Emergency Department of his local hospital having been found collapsed in the street.

Which of the following is unlikely to be a reason for his presentation?

A. Atrioventricular block
B. Myocarditis
C. Pericarditis
D. Acute aortic regurgitation
E. Acute plaque rupture

7. A 59 year-old female with hypertension is diagnosed with multiple myeloma. She is initially treated with dexamethasone, melphalan, thalidomide, and bortezomib. Due to refractory disease she was commenced on carfilzomib. Her baseline echocardiogram was normal. Three months later she is found to be in New York Heart Association 3 stage heart failure. Echocardiography confirms severe left ventricular systolic dysfunction (LVSD) and she is treated with candesartan, carvedilol, eplerenone, and ivabradine. Three months later 3D LV ejection fraction is 50% and global longitudinal strain (GLS) is −17%. The oncologists wish to restart carfilzomib.

Which of the following should not be considered in this context?

A. Adapt intravenous hydration normally given with carfilzomib
B. Serial echocardiography
C. Serial biomarker monitoring
D. Have a high threshold for diuresis to prevent tumour lysis syndrome
E. Rule out pulmonary hypertension, pulmonary embolism, chest sepsis, acute respiratory distress syndrome, and interstitial lung disease in case of further dyspnoea

8. A 35 year-old male with no past medical history was admitted with bowel obstruction. Following an emergency hemicolectomy, he was started on capecitabine and oxaliplatin for colon adnenocarcinoma. Two days later he was admitted to hospital with dyspnoea and chest pain. Cardiac magnetic resonance imaging showed severe global myocardial dysfunction with no evidence of myocardial oedema. Coronary angiography showed unobstructed coronary arteries. One day later he developed dysphasia which improved with conservative management as per Neurology advice. Serial echocardiography showed a resolution of cardiac function.

What is the unifying diagnosis?

A. Capecitabine-associated coronary spasm followed by stroke (complication of coronary angiography) X
B. Takutsubo syndrome and carotid artery dissection
• C. Capecitabine-associated coronary spasm and myocardial dysfunction, and toxic leukoencephalopathy
D. Oxaliplatin-related LVSD and stroke, complicating coronary angiography
E. Oxaliplatin-related embolic event affecting both the heart and brain

9. A 48 year-old woman recently started on trastuzumab develops heart failure. What advice would be incorrect to give to the patient?

• A. The trastuzumab is likely to be the cause as cardiotoxicity typically manifests at start of therapy X
B. Trastuzumab-cardiotoxicity is usually reversible X
C. Can recur after re-challenge even if LV systolic function has normalized X
D. Increased incidence if concomitant use of anthracyclines X
E. Traditional cardiovascular risk factors do not increase risk of cardiotoxicity X

10. A 64-year-old male receives axicabtagene ciloleucel, a chimeric antigen receptor (CAR) T cell product, for management of relapsed/refractory diffuse large B cell lymphoma (DLBCL). Four days later, he develops fevers (39.3 °C), a tachycardia (150 bpm), and hypoxia (oxygen saturations of 90% on room air). Later that evening, he becomes hypotensive (90/60 mmHg). An electrocardiogram (ECG) demonstrates atrial flutter with 2:1 AV conduction and a ventricular rate of 150 bpm. A chest radiograph demonstrates radiographic features of pulmonary oedema.

He is subsequently transferred to the ICU where he is supported with non-invasive ventilation and inotropes. Which of the following is the cardiovascular complication most commonly associated with CAR T cell therapy?

A. Profound hypotension requiring vasopressor and inotropic support
B. Left ventricular systolic dysfunction
C. Decompensated cardiac failure requiring intravenous diuretic agents
D. New-onset arrhythmias including supraventricular tachycardia and atrial fibrillation or atrial flutter
E. Asytolic cardiac arrest

11. Which of the following statements is true regarding cardiac tumours?

A. Cardiac rhabdomyosarcoma is the most common primary cardiac tumour in adults.
B. Compared to metastatic cardiac tumours, primary cardiac tumours are more common.
C. Primary malignant cardiac masses are most commonly found in the right atrium and pericardium.
D. The majority of primary cardiac tumours are malignant.

12. Which of the following malignancies rarely metastasize to the heart?

A. Breast cancer
B. Lung cancer
C. Melanoma
D. Prostate cancer

13. Which of the following syndromes are associated with cardiac myxomas?

A. Carney complex
B. Gorlin syndrome
C. Li-Fraumeni syndrome
D. Tuberous sclerosis

14. Which of the following tumours is normally found on the downstream side of valves?

A. Myxoma
B. Papillary fibroelastoma
C. Angiosarcoma
D. Lipoma

15. Surgical resection of which of the following tumours is recommended in asymptomatic patients?

A. Lipoma
B. Fibroma
C. Rhabdomyoma
D. Myxoma

chapter 5.4

CARDIO-ONCOLOGY AND CARDIAC TUMOURS

ANSWERS

1. E. The risk of anthracycline cardiotoxity increases with increased cumulative exposure to anthracyclines. The incidence of heart failure rises to >5% when the cumulative dose exceeds 400 mg/m^2 of doxorubicin. This is equivalent to 150 mg/m^2 of idarubicin, 800 mg/m^2 of daunorubicin, and 900 mg/m^2 of epirubicin. Anthracycline toxicity while commonly a subacute or chronic presentation can sometimes present as acute heart failure. The earlier changes in cardiac function are detected, and treatment instituted, the better the cardiac outcomes. Measures to decrease cardiotoxicity include liposomal formulations and the administration of dexrazoxane.

2. B. Lower radiation fraction per dose (<2Gy/day) and a low total cumulative dose (<30Gy) are associated with decreased incidence of RIHD. Measures are usually taken during radiotherapy planning and administration to reduce the exposure of the heart to the radiotherapy beam. Close sequential or concurrent treatment of some cancers (e.g. breast cancer) with anthracyclines and radiotherapy increase the risk of subsequent cardiotoxicity. Pre-existing cardiac disease is a risk factor for poorer cardiac outcomes.

3. C. Valvular regurgitation is commoner than stenosis. Twenty years after radiation involving the heart, incidence of mild aortic regurgitation (AR) is up to 45%, ≥ moderate AR 15%, and aortic stenosis up to 15%. Mild mitral regurgitation is seen in up to 48%. Stenotic lesions are commoner in the aortic valve and 6% of patients have clinically significant valve disease at 20 years. Adult survivors of childhood cancers are routinely followed up in late effects clinics. Their visits include interval echocardiography if they received radiotherapy to a field involving the heart and/or cardiotoxic chemotherapy.

4. C. Screening echocardiography is recommended 5 years after radiotherapy to detect evidence of valvular heart disease, pericardial complications, regional wall motion abnormalities, and systolic and diastolic dysfunction. Yearly physical examinations and history taking is recommended to detect early signs of radiotherapy-induced premature valve or coronary disease. Metabolic complications are common in childhood cancer survivors and lipid screens are recommended yearly.
Depending upon risk (level of radiation dose to heart, concomitant anthracyclines etc.) screening echocardiography may take place regularly.

5. A. Ibrutinib is more commonly associated with atrial fibrillation than supraventricular tachycardia. Anticoagulation in these patients is challenging due to often abnormal full blood counts and coagulation related to the underlying cancer and/or cancer treatment. The other arrhythmias are commonly associated with their respective cancer treatments.

6. D. While check point inhibitor toxicity can include acute myocardial infarction and regional wall motion abnormalities, significant secondary valve lesions are uncommon. While coronary vasculitis can rarely be seen, acute aortic regurgitation is not commonly seen as a complication of check point blockade. Management of acute cardiotoxicity is with a combination of high dose steroids, mycophenolate mofetil, immunoglobulin therapy, and occasionally exchange transfusion and abatacept. While acute cardiotoxicity is rare, morbidity and mortality are high.

7. D. In patients with a history of carfilzomib-associated LVSD, one of the commonest causes for dyspnoea on reintroduction of carfilzomib is a deterioration of LV systolic function and development of pulmonary oedema. While tumour lysis syndrome and renal dysfunction can be associated with diuretic use in this context, the mortality and morbidity risk is higher from acute LVSD and as such there should be a low threshold for diuresis.

8. C. Capecitabine can cause coronary spasm and myocardial infarction in unobstructed coronary arteries. Rarely this can lead to a transient global stunning of myocardial function, which usually recovers on removal of the insult (capecitabine) and initiation of heart failure therapy. Very rarely capecitabine can lead to diffuse subcortical and callosal white matter changes consistent with toxic leucoencephalopathy. Symptoms normally resolve with conservative management and removal of exposure to the precipitating agent.

9. E. Trastuzumab cardiotoxity typically manifests at the time of therapy. While LV systolic function can normalize with suspension of therapy and initiation of standard heart failure medications, LVSD can occur again with re-exposure to trastuzumab. Such patients should be followed closely (with scanning and biomarker monitoring more frequently than the standard 3-monthly intervals), ideally in a cardio-oncology service. There is an increased risk in those with pre-existing cardiovascular risk factors.

10. A. The most commonly associated cardiovascular complication of CAR T cell therapy is profound hypotension requiring inotropic and vasopressor support, which has a reported incidence of between 4 to 33% of patients receiving CAR T cell therapy. Decompensated cardiac failure resulting in pulmonary oedema and fluid overload requiring intravenous diuretic agents occurs in 4–6%, whilst left ventricular systolic dysfunction occurs in 2–10%. The incidence of new-onset arrhythmias, including supraventricular tachycardia, atrial fibrillation, or atrial flutter, in a retrospective analysis of 137 patients was 4%.

11. C. Secondary cardiac tumours are 22 to 132 times more common than primary tumours. Atrial myxomas are the most common primary cardiac tumour in adults. 90% of primary cardiac tumours are benign.

12. D. It is very uncommon for prostate cancer to metastasize to the heart.

13. A. Carney complex and its subsets (LAMB and NAME syndromes) are autosomal dominant conditions comprising cardiac myxomas, skin hyperpigmentation, and endocrine abnormalities. Gorlin syndrome is associated with cardiac fibroma whilst Li-Fraumeni is associated with increased general cardiovascular risk rather than cardiac tumours. Tuberous sclerosis is associated with rhabdomyomas.

14. B. Papillary fibroelastomas are usually found on the downstream side of valves. They are best visualized on echocardiography and can present with embolic complications.

15. D. Complete resection of myxomas is recommended to prevent embolic complications. The others are usually treated conservatively unless significantly symptomatic.

chapter 6

ACUTE CARDIOVASCULAR CARE

chapter

6.1

ACUTE CARDIOVASCULAR CARE

QUESTIONS

1. **A 65-year-old man attends the emergency department with a 2-day history of increased shortness of breath and fever. He describes a cough productive of green sputum. He has a history of hypertension, hypercholesterolaemia, and had a myocardial infarction 3 years previously. He has been breathing 80% oxygen via facemask for the past 1 hour. A set of vital signs are recorded.**

   Which of the following measurements would make you consider that this patient is critically unwell?

   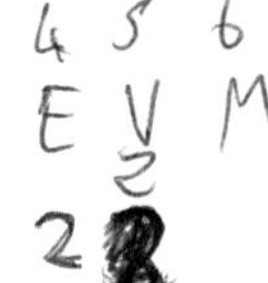

   A. Heart rate 98 bpm
   B. Blood pressure 115/58 mmHg
   C. Respiratory rate 32 bpm
   D. GCS 14
   E. Temperature 36.7°C

2. **You are called to the coronary care unit to review a deteriorating patient. When you arrive you check to see if they are responding by performing a sternal rub, to which they open their eyes and reach for your hand. You ask them their name and they make incoherent sounds which you are unable to decipher.**

   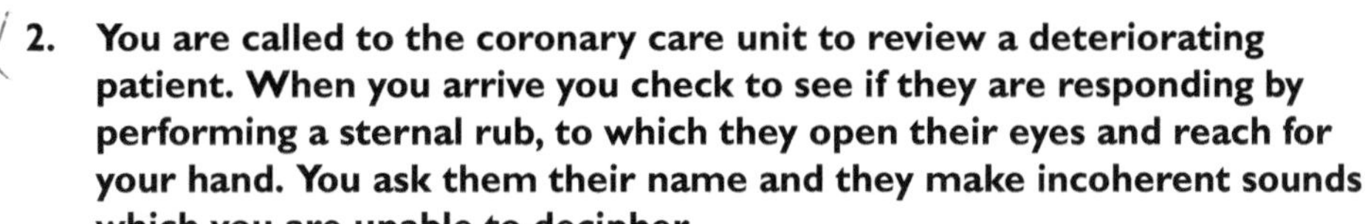

   What is this patient's Glasgow Coma Scale score?

   A. 6
   B. 7
   C. 8
   D. 9
   E. 10

3. **A patient is admitted after a prolonged out of hospital cardiopulmonary arrest. There has been a successful return of circulation but his temperature is 36 ˚C and you are asked how his temperature should be managed.**

   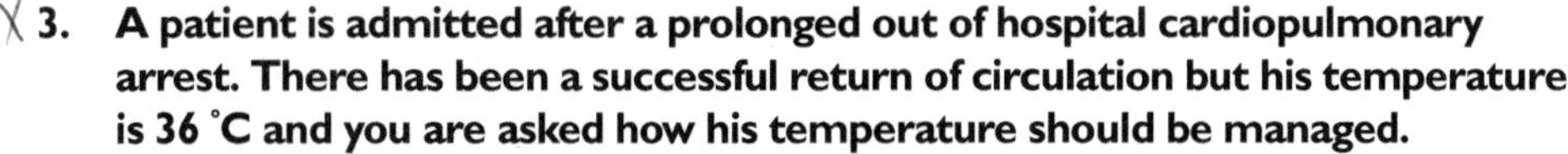

   Which of the following are the current guidelines in relation to this?

   A. Aim for a temperature of <36 °C for a minimum of 24 hours
   B. Cool to 32–36°C for a minimum of 72 hours
   C. Reduce the temperature to below 3°C for a minimum of 24 hours
   D. Only treat temperatures greater than 38°C
   E. Temperature management is not important in the post cardiac arrest period

4. A patient is admitted to the cardiac intensive care unit following a coronary artery bypass graft procedure, with three grafts performed. The temperature dropped to 33.4°C intra-operatively. The patient's temperature is currently reading 35.3°C.

Which of the following is not a commonly recognized complication of hypothermia?

A. Coagulopathy
B. Pain
C. Hyperkalaemia
D. Myocardial infarction
E. Impaired wound healing

5. You are called to review a patient on the ward who was admitted with an acute exacerbation of chronic obstructive pulmonary disease. They are maintaining their SaO_2 at 94%, but their respiratory rate has been rising over the past number of hours and is currently 32 bpm. An ABG has been performed and the parameters are as follows: pH 7.29, pO2 9.8kPa, pCO_2 8.7kPa. The patient's GCS is 15; however, they are struggling to complete sentences when speaking to you.

What ventilatory support would you consider for this patient?

A. Nasal cannula with 4 litre flow
B. Oxygen 30% via facemask
C. Oxygen 100% via reservoir mask
D. CPAP with a pressure of 5 cmH_2O
E. BiPAP with pressures of 5 cmH_2O and 15 cmH_2O

6. A 72-year-old man was admitted to the cardiac intensive care unit 4 hours ago, following a coronary artery bypass graft procedure. He remains intubated but is awake and alert and is breathing spontaneously. The nursing staff want to know if he is suitable for extubation at this point.

Which of the following parameters would make you consider delaying extubation?

A. Temperature 37.4°C
B. Noradrenaline is running at a rate of 3 ml/hr
C. FiO_2 is 0.45
D. Patient has received three bolus doses of morphine (total 6 mg) in the past 20 minutes
E. Chest drain output is 100 ml for the past 2 hours

7. A 79-year-old patient has returned to the coronary care unit after having a transcatheter aortic valve insertion (TAVI), performed under conscious sedation with the patient spontaneously breathing. You have been asked to review them as their blood pressure is reading 192/97 mmHg. They have a known history of hypertension, which was controlled prior to the procedure on losartan and which they received this morning. Their other medications include furosemide, atorvastatin, and aspirin.

What would be the most appropriate management of this patient?

A. Give a repeat dose of losartan at their usual dose
B. Start an intravenous infusion of glyceryl trinitrate
C. Start an intravenous infusion of dopamine
D. Give an oral calcium channel blocker
E. Give an oral calcium channel blocker combined with a beta-blocker

8. A patient has returned to the cardiac intensive care unit following an aortic valve replacement and aortic root repair. Since returning from theatre 2 hours previously they have remained persistently hypotensive, with systolic blood pressure reading below 85 mmHg. They have received four 500 ml boluses of crystalloid with no improvement seen. The drain output has been 25 ml for the past 2 hours.

Which of the following would not be appropriate to consider?

A. Starting an intravenous infusion of noradrenaline
B. Performing a passive leg raise test
C. Performing transoesophageal echocardiography
D. Stopping the sedation and waking the patient
E. Sending ACT and clotting screen

9. A 69-year-old patient returned to the cardiac intensive care unit 4 hours ago following an aortic valve replacement. They have been persistently hypotensive with a systolic BP below 85 mmHg. There has been minimal output from the surgical drain. You have taken steps to manage this situation and resuscitate the patient. Crystalloid boluses were given initially and when the haematocrit reached 23, one unit of red blood cells was given. The patient responds briefly to each fluid challenge, but this is short-lived. However, the CVP has risen steadily. Noradrenaline infusion has been started. A transthoracic echocardiogram was performed and showed no evidence of pericardial fluid. The urine output has remained acceptable at 0.5 ml/kg/hr.

What do you think is the underlying diagnosis?

A. Tamponade
B. Inadequate analgesia
C. Oversedation
D. Dehydration
E. Ventilatory asynchrony

10. A patient has returned to the cardiac intensive care unit following a pulmonary valve repair. They are known to have impaired right ventricular function.

Which of the following treatment strategies should be considered first?

A. Enoximone / milrinone infusion
B. Adrenaline infusion
C. Permissive hypoxia
D. Permissive hypercarbia
E. Increased PEEP

11. A patient has had epicardial pacing wires in situ for 4 days following an aortic valve replacement; however, pacing has not been required and they are due for removal.

Which of the following factors would make you consider delaying removal of the epicardial pacing wires?

A. The patient remains on an insulin infusion
B. The patient is receiving therapeutic heparin
C. The patient is on warfarin and the INR is 2.0
D. The patient is on levothyroxine for hypothyroidism
E. The patient was on aspirin and clopidogrel pre-operatively

12. You have been called to review a 75-year-old man who is on the coronary care unit 2 days after an angiogram and stent insertion. He is 68 kg with a background history of hypertension, hypercholesterolaemia, and gout. The nurse is concerned as he has only passed 250 ml of urine in the past 12 hours. His baseline creatinine was 74. A repeat sample has been sent and his serum creatinine is now 154.

What RIFLE criteria does this patient fall into?

A. Risk
B. Injury
C. Failure
D. Loss of kidney function
E. End-stage kidney disease

13. A 45-year-old patient post-op following repair of a thoracic aortic dissection now has reduced urine output and a slight rise in his potassium level.

Which of the following parameters are NOT indications for renal replacement therapy?

A. Urine output < 200 ml/12hrs
B. pH < 7.1
C. Urea > 25 mmol/l
D. Potassium > 6.5 mmol/l
E. Sodium > 160 mmol/l

14. You are called at 2am to review a 76-year-old patient on the cardiac intensive care unit who is 2 days post-op following a coronary artery bypass graft procedure. The nurses are concerned that he is confused and stating that he wishes to leave the hospital right now. You perform a neurological examination and determine that he is orientated in person, but not time or place. His gross motor function and cranial nerves are intact.

What is the most likely diagnosis?

A. Acute stroke
B. Post-operative cognitive dysfunction
C. Delirium
D. Hypertension
E. Pain

15. A 64-year-old man has been in intensive care for 4 days following a cardiac arrest. His sedation was stopped this morning and he was successfully extubated in the mid-afternoon. He was initially awake, alert, obeying commands, and moving all limbs. It is now evening time and he is becoming confused, pulling at his support lines, and trying to climb out of bed. You are concerned that he is endangering himself.

Which of the following pharmacological treatments would it NOT be appropriate to consider?

A. Haloperidol
B. Quetiapine
C. Risperidone
D. Clonidine
E. Lorazepam

16. A patient had a cardiac arrest 7 days ago and has been managed on the intensive care unit since this time. Sedation was discontinued 3 days ago and they have not regained consciousness.

Which of the following investigations would you consider in this patient?

A. Computerized tomography
B. Magnetic resonance imaging
C. Electroencephalography
D. Somatosensory evoked potentials
E. All of the above

17. You are called to review a 68-year-old patient on the cardiac intensive care unit who is 2 days after a mitral valve repair. He is reporting sternal wound pain.

Which of the following drugs would you avoid in this patient?

A. Paracetamol
B. Tramadol
C. Diclofenac
D. Morphine
E. Clonidine

18. You are reviewing a post-operative patient on the evening ward round. They underwent a coronary artery bypass graft and aortic valve replacement and returned to the intensive care unit 6 hours ago.

What level of surgical drain output would make you concerned that there is ongoing bleeding?

A. 200 ml/hr for the past 2 hours
B. 75 ml/hr for the past 2 hours
C. 75 ml/hr for the past 3 hours
D. 50 ml/hr for the past 4 hours
E. 50 ml/hr for the past 6 hours

19. An 86-year-old patient underwent a redo operation for mitral valve replacement, having had a repair performed in the past. The procedure was complicated and the cardiopulmonary bypass time was prolonged. Pre-operatively the patient was receiving aspirin and clopidogrel.

Which of the following factors is NOT as recognized risk factor for post-operative bleeding?

A. Younger age
B. Procedures requiring cardiopulmonary bypass
C. Redo procedure
D. Prolonged cardiopulmonary bypass time
E. Emergency surgery

20. A patient has returned to the cardiac intensive care unit following an aortic valve replacement and aortic root repair. The procedure was technically difficult and there was a long cardiopulmonary bypass time. There has been continuous high output from the drain and you are concerned that there is ongoing bleeding from the operative site. The haemoglobin is reading 76 g/dL. You have called the cardiothoracic surgeon to urgently review the patient.

Which of the following blood products would you considering administering to this patient?

A. Red blood cells
B. Platelets
C. Fresh frozen plasma
D. Fibrinogen concentrate
E. All of the above

21. Many cardiac surgical patients are receiving antiplatelet and anticoagulant medications for their underlying cardiac pathology.

Which of the following statements are true in relation to antiplatelet and anticoagulant management of cardiac surgical patients?

A. Aspirin and clopidogrel must be discontinued in patients presenting for cardiac surgery
B. All patients for cardiac surgery should be commenced on aspirin pre-operatively and this should be continued in the post-operative period
C. DOACs should be stopped for 1 week prior to cardiac surgery
D. INR should be below 1.5 prior to cardiac surgery
E. All patients on warfarin should have bridging therapy peri-operatively

22. Stress ulcers are gastric erosions which can develop in critically ill patients.

Which of the flowing statements is false in relation to stress ulcers?

A. Patients who are mechanically ventilated for >48 hours are at risk of developing stress ulcers
B. Patients receiving clopidogrel should not receive stress ulcer prophylaxis with a proton pump inhibitor
C. An INR >1.5 is associated with an increased risk of stress ulcer prophylaxis
D. The routine use of stress ulcer prophylaxis is associated with an increased risk of pneumonia
E. Stress ulcers are of concern as they can result in significant gastrointestinal haemorrhage

23. A 64-year-old man has been admitted to the cardiac intensive care unit following a coronary artery bypass graft procedure. He has a history of type 2 diabetes mellitus for which he takes metformin 500 mg bd, however this has not been given for 24 hours pre-operatively. On his initial arterial blood gas his blood glucose reads 11.2 mmol/l. The patient remains intubated and has a nasogastric tube in place.

What action would you take?

A. Give metformin 500 mg via the NG tube
B. Give metformin 1000mg via the NG tube
C. Give 10 IU of subcutaneous insulin
D. Start an intravenous insulin sliding scale
E. Repeat the blood glucose in 2 hours

24. A 72-year-old man has developed a sternal wound infection post-operatively. He is a smoker and has a history of type 2 diabetes mellitus, rheumatoid arthritis, hypercholesterolaemia, and chronic obstructive pulmonary disease. The operative course was complicated by bleeding and required transfusion of red blood cells and platelets. He has remained on an insulin infusion post-operatively as it has been difficult to keep his blood glucose under control.

The following are all risk factors for sternal wound infection except which one?

A. Smoking
B. Steroid use
C. Hypercholesterolaemia
D. Blood transfusion
E. Diabetes

25. A patient presented to the emergency department following an out of hospital cardiac arrest during which they were intubated and ventilated by the pre-hospital team. They are transferred to the intensive care unit where infusions of noradrenaline and adrenaline are started. The following day the patient is anuric and their potassium is 6.7 (unresponsive to treatment) and renal replacement therapy is commenced.

Which of the following statements correctly described the level of care required by this patient along their clinical course in the intensive care unit?

A. Level 0 on admission to ICU, now Level 3
B. Level 2 on admission to ICU, now Level 3
C. Level 3 on admission to ICU, now Level 0
D. Level 3 on admission to ICU, now Level 3
E. Level 1 on admission to ICU, now Level 2

chapter 6.1 ACUTE CARDIOVASCULAR CARE

ANSWERS

1. C. As the normal range for respiratory rate in an adult is 12–18 breaths per minute, a respiratory rate of 32 bpm represents a concerning deviation from normal. Furthermore, the significance of this measurement is exacerbated by the fact the patient is receiving supplemental oxygen. Both of these factors considered together suggest that a patient is critically unwell with high potential for deterioration if further management and support are not instituted in a timely fashion. The parameters listed for heart rate, blood pressure, and temperature are all within normal limits. A GCS of 14, while not normal, is not in isolation indicative of a critical state and may have a number of underlying causes.

2. D. Glasgow Coma Scale (https://www.glasgowcomascale.org/) is used to determine level of consciousness and is calculated using best response in three domains: eye opening, verbal and motor. The maximum score in a fully responsive patient is 15, with a score of 3 indicating a patient is totally unresponsive.

3. A. Targeted temperature management is implemented to potentially improve neurological outcome after cardiac arrest. While there has been considerable debate on the most effective specific protocol for this, it has been widely accepted that maintaining body temperature below 36°C for a minimum of 24 hours may provide some benefit and should be considered in this group of patients

4. C. Hypothermia is defined as a core temperature of <36°C and is a common finding following cardiac surgery. Hypothermia lasting for less than 24 hours is not associated with an impact on mortality. Hypothermia lasting for longer than 24 hours is associated with increased mortality in this group of patients and as such active steps should be taken to avoid and correct this situation. Meta-analysis has shown that hypothermia during surgery significantly increases blood loss and the need for transfusion. The proposed underlying pathophysiology is that hypothermia impairs platelet function, reduces clotting factor enzyme function, and increases fibrinolysis. Hypothermia may contribute to increased pain scores in post-operative patients and this, combined with shivering, results in decreased patient satisfaction. Myocardial infarction is an important cause of post-operative morbidity and mortality in all surgical populations. Hypothermia results in hypertension, tachycardia, increased catecholamine levels, and a left shift in the oxygen–haemoglobin dissociation curve; it is believed that these factors combine to increase the risk of ischaemia and arrhythmias. Post-operative hypothermia contributes to impaired wound healing due to a combination of impaired immune system function and vasoconstriction resulting in impaired oxygen delivery.

5. E. This patient is in type 2 respiratory failure, with hypoxia, hypercapnia, and an increased respiratory rate. Given that the patient's GCS is 15, the most appropriate choice of increased support in this case would be BiPAP (bilevel positive airway pressure), which is a form of non-invasive ventilation that provides supplemental oxygen with pressure support. BiPAP is effective in improving lung volumes by opening areas of atelectasis. It also increases alveolar ventilation and reduces the work of breathing. Of note, it is contra-indicated in the presence of a pneumothorax or broncho-pleural fistula.

6. E. Chest drains are left in place following cardiac surgery to allow collection of any blood that may ooze from the operative site in the initial post-operative period. The output from these should be monitored as this can indicate a developing problem. It is recommended that the output should be <100 ml/hr for 2 consecutive hours before a patient is extubated.

7. B. It is not uncommon for patients to develop hypertension following a TAVI. It has been shown that approximately half of this patient population develop new hypertension or have an exacerbation of pre-existing hypertension in the post-procedure phase and that this has been associated with improved cardiac function and increased short-term survival. In the immediate post-procedure period, the use of a glyceryl trinitrate infusion is recommended as it allows relatively rapid and short-term manipulation of the blood pressure. In addition, it can be easily titrated as changes occur or when oral long-term antihypertensive therapy is commenced.

8. D. This patient is not clinically stable and therefore it would be inadvisable to attempt to wake them at this point. It would be essential to concurrently implement measures to both stabilize their condition and also determine the underlying cause of this instability. Hypotension is common in the post cardiac surgery population and is often caused by a combination of reduced pre-load, reduced contractility, and vasodilatation. A passive leg raise and a transoesophageal echo would assist with determining the pre-load and contractility status of the patient. Noradrenaline could be helpful to provide a vasoconstrictive effect. An ACT and clotting screen would be useful to determine if there is coagulopathy present and a risk of ongoing bleeding. It would be crucial to optimize all of these factors prior to considering reducing this patient's sedation.

9. A. Given that tamponade is a common and specific complication after cardiac surgery, a high degree of clinical suspicion should be maintained for this complication. The clinical features of persistent hypotension, tachycardia and raised CVP are typical. In the post cardiac surgery period, transthoracic echocardiography has a negative predictive value of 41%, therefore the absence of pericardial fluid with this imaging modality should not provide reassurance. Further imaging should be performed—transoesophageal echocardiography has a sensitivity approaching 100% and would be the investigation of choice in this clinical situation. Tamponade in the post cardiac surgical population can be small and localized (usually over the right atrium) and therefore clinical suspicion should prompt a return to theatre.

10. A. The management of right ventricular impairment is clinically challenging and measures taken should aim to optimize preload, maintain perfusion pressure, maintain contractility, and reduce afterload. While the RV wall is thin with a smaller number of contractile fibres and thus difficult to augment, inodilators such as enoximone and milrinone which act by phosphodiesterase inhibition can enhance contractility and cause pulmonary vasodilatation. Other factors which raise pulmonary vascular resistance should be avoided—these include hypoxia, hypercarbia, acidosis, and increased PEEP. Adrenaline is an α and β agonist and causes increased contractility and increased systemic vascular resistance and may be considered in the management of fulminant RV failure, although would not be first line treatment.

11. B. Epicardial pacing wires are removed on day 3–6 post cardiac surgery, if pacing is not required. One of the major risks associated with removal is bleeding, which could result in the development of cardiac tamponade. It is advisable to stop therapeutic heparin 4 hours prior to wire removal. INR should be less than 2.5 for patients on warfarin therapy. Where direct oral anticoagulant therapy is indicated, starting this should be delayed until the wires have been removed and at least 12 hours should elapse after removal before taking the first dose.

12. B. The RIFLE Criteria are used to classify kidney status in terms of potential or actual damage. Categories are defined by changes in serum creatinine, eGFR, and urine output occurring within 7 days and are described as Risk/Injury/Failure/Loss of kidney function/End stage kidney disease. Injury suggests a twofold increase in serum creatinine, greater than or equal to 50% decrease in eGFR or a decrease in urine output to less than 0.5 ml/kg/hr for 12 hours.

13. C. The following are considered indications for renal replacement therapy:

- Anuria or oliguria (urine output <200 ml/12 h)
- Urea >30 mmol/l
- Potassium >6.5 mmol/l refractory to treatment
- pH <7.1
- Clinically significant oedema
- Symptomatic uraemia – pericarditis, neuropathy, myopathy, encephalopathy, bleeding
- Na >160 or <115 mmol/l refractory to treatment
- Mg >4 mmol with absent tendon reflexes
- Hyperthermia
- Overdose with a substance that can be removed with dialysis

14. C. Post-operative cognitive dysfunction is the most common neurological aberration following cardiac surgery and is a well-recognized but poorly defined state in which memory and executive functions deteriorate post-operatively. It is usually self-limiting, but may persist for up to three months following a procedure. In contrast, delirium occurs 24–96 hours post-operatively and is an acute, reversible state of mental confusion with disordered attention and cognitive function and reduced environmental awareness, with a fluctuating course. It is common in the post cardiac surgical population, with an incidence of 26–52%. It may be hyperactive, hypoactive, or mixed, with the latter being the most common form, encompassing features of both the others. Features of hyperactive delirium include motor agitation, restlessness, and sometimes aggressiveness. One important factor contributing to delirium is pain, therefore adequate analgesia is a cornerstone of management of this condition.

15. **E.** This patient has delirium, which is common in patients following cardiac arrest and in intensive care patients. Lorazepam is a benzodiazepine and this class of drug should not be used to treat delirium, as it has not been shown to provide any benefit and indeed may even cause harm. The only exception to this is patients with alcohol withdrawal, in whom benzodiazepine therapy is the mainstay of treatment. Atypical antipsychotics (quetiapine, risperidone) and the alpha-agonist clonidine are commonly used to manage delirium, although the evidence is unclear regarding their efficacy. Haloperidol is a typical antipsychotic that should be used only as required as it causes sedation and prophylactic administration has been shown to have no impact on the incidence of delirium. Of note, quetiapine, risperidone, and haloperidol all cause QT prolongation and this side effect should be monitored for in this group of patients.

16. **E.** Following cardiac arrest with failure to regain consciousness it is important to investigate and quantify the extent of the brain injury sustained by the patient in order to plan further management. It is vital that any reversible causes of decreased conscious level are considered and excluded, particularly sedation, paralysing medication, metabolic or electrolyte abnormalities, and ongoing subclinical seizures. Following this, all of the investigations listed above would be helpful in providing information to assist clinical decision making in this complex situation.

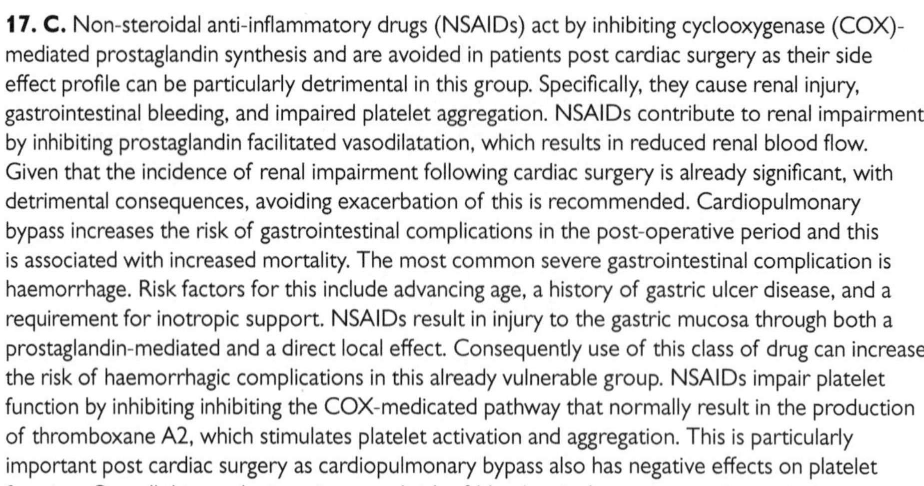

17. C. Non-steroidal anti-inflammatory drugs (NSAIDs) act by inhibiting cyclooxygenase (COX)-mediated prostaglandin synthesis and are avoided in patients post cardiac surgery as their side effect profile can be particularly detrimental in this group. Specifically, they cause renal injury, gastrointestinal bleeding, and impaired platelet aggregation. NSAIDs contribute to renal impairment by inhibiting prostaglandin facilitated vasodilatation, which results in reduced renal blood flow. Given that the incidence of renal impairment following cardiac surgery is already significant, with detrimental consequences, avoiding exacerbation of this is recommended. Cardiopulmonary bypass increases the risk of gastrointestinal complications in the post-operative period and this is associated with increased mortality. The most common severe gastrointestinal complication is haemorrhage. Risk factors for this include advancing age, a history of gastric ulcer disease, and a requirement for inotropic support. NSAIDs result in injury to the gastric mucosa through both a prostaglandin-mediated and a direct local effect. Consequently use of this class of drug can increase the risk of haemorrhagic complications in this already vulnerable group. NSAIDs impair platelet function by inhibiting inhibiting the COX-medicated pathway that normally result in the production of thromboxane A2, which stimulates platelet activation and aggregation. This is particularly important post cardiac surgery as cardiopulmonary bypass also has negative effects on platelet function. Overall this results in an increased risk of bleeding in the peri-operative period.

18. A. Surgical drain output is monitored carefully post-operatively and the following levels should raise concern that there is ongoing bleeding:

>400 ml in first hour

>200 ml in two consecutive hours

>100 ml in four consecutive hours

If the output is above these levels early consideration should be given to returning to theatre to explore the operative site; this occurs in 2–8% of patients and is associated with increased morbidity and mortality.

19. A. Increasing age has been identified as a risk factor for post-operative bleeding following cardiac surgery. Cardiopulmonary bypass has a significant impact on coagulation by activation of platelets and triggering of inflammatory pathways and longer cardiopulmonary bypass times are correlated directly with an increased risk of bleeding. Redo procedures represent a higher risk of bleeding due to the formation of scar tissue, adhesions, and more complex surgery, combined with higher rates of coagulation abnormalities.

20. E. This patient is anaemic with ongoing bleeding, therefore red blood cell transfusion would be an appropriate first step in the management of this emergency situation. The transfusion trigger for cardiac patients is 80 g/dL and in an actively bleeding patient a level of 100 g/dL should be considered to optimize clotting. This patient will have lost a considerable volume of whole blood and has had insults to the coagulation system from cardiopulmonary bypass and surgical trauma. Replacement of other blood components will be necessary. The use of thromboelastograph or thromboelastometry is useful to guide product management, although less helpful in the emergency situation due to the delay associated in obtaining results.

21. D. Aspirin should be continued prior to cardiac surgery. Clopidogrel should be discontinued in elective procedures, but this may not be achievable in emergency cases. In relation to DOACs, dabigatran should be stopped 2–3 days before surgery, rivaroxiban 2 days before surgery, and apixaban 2 days before surgery—these timeframes should be increased by 1 day in patients with renal impairment. The requirement for warfarin bridging therapy depends on the indication for which is it prescribed. In low-risk patients bridging is not required, but in high-risk patients bridging therapy with heparin should be started when the INR falls below 2.0. INR should be less than 1.5 prior to surgery.

22. A. Risk factors for the development of stress ulcers include mechanical ventilation for >48 hours and coagulopathy (INR > 1.5, platelets < 50, partial thromboplastin time (PTT) >2 times the control value). Pharmacological prophylaxis using a proton pump inhibitor (PPI) is used to prevent this complication; however, this is associated with an increased risk of developing hospital-acquired pneumonia. There is some evidence that PPIs interact with clopidogrel, although this has not been demonstrated to have an impact on the rate of complications.

23. D. The stress response to surgery can result in hyperglycaemia. While tight glucose control is not recommended (as this can result in excessive episodes of hypoglycaemia), hyperglycaemia in the peri-operative period has negative effects, including impaired wound healing, and should be avoided. Metformin is not administered in the peri-operative period due to an increased risk of developing lactic acidosis, particularly in those with impaired renal function. Subcutaneous insulin 10 IU is not appropriate in this circumstance as this patient is nil by mouth and subcutaneous administration is not easily titratable. An intravenous variable rate insulin infusion with frequent blood glucose monitoring would be the most appropriate therapy for this patient.

24. C. There is no evidence that hypercholesterolaemia contributes to an increased rate of surgical site infection. The other factors listed above have an association with increased sternal wound infection. Steps taken in the peri-operative period to decrease the risk of wound infection include the use of nasal mupirocin for *Staphylococcus* spp. decontamination, skin preparation with 2% chlorhexidine gluconate/70% isopropyl alcohol, and the administration of antibiotic prophylaxis prior to skin incision.

25. D. There are nationally agreed levels of care which describe the amount of support required by patients admitted to hospital and intensive care. Level 0 describes a patient who requires admission to an acute hospital but can be managed on a normal ward. Level 1 describes a patient at risk of clinical deterioration or who has recently been discharged from a higher level of care but may be managed on a normal ward. Level 2 describes a patient who requires single organ support or is stepping down from level 3 care and may be managed in a high dependency unit. Level 3 describes a patient who requires advanced respiratory support (mechanical ventilation) or support of two or more organ systems and requires management in an intensive care unit.

chapter

6.2

CARDIAC ARREST, RESUSCITATION, AND SUDDEN CARDIAC DEATH

QUESTIONS

1. A 24-year-old female presents to the Emergency Department after an episode of palpitations and presyncope whilst running. She has had several previous episodes but this one was the most severe. After further questioning, she says her maternal uncle died of a suspected heart attack at 36. Her ECG shows Q-waves in the inferolateral leads with large QRS voltage. There is no delta wave.

Which of the following is not a risk factor for sudden death at 5 years in this condition?

A. Increased septal wall thickness (>30 mm)
B. Multifocal ventricular ectopics
C. Left atrial enlargement
D. Young age
E. Family history

2. Which of the following is NOT true of arrhythmogenic right ventricular cardiomyopathy (ARVC)?

A. Family members that test positive for a familial variant have a greater risk of SCD than the proband
B. Abnormal late potentials on the signal averaged ECG are a minor Task Force criteria
C. Electrophysiology studies may be helpful in differentiating benign right ventricular outflow tract (RVOT) VT from ARVC
D. 2/3 of patients with ARVC will have ventricular arrhythmias on prolonged ECG monitoring
E. ARVC makes up less than 5% of sudden death in athletes

3. A 35-year-old female suddenly collapsed in a park. She had prompt bystander CPR and 1 shock was delivered from an automated external defibrillator (AED) for ventricular fibrillation (VF). She had transient ST elevation on the AED ECG strip and was transferred to nearest primary PCI centre. She had unobstructed coronary arteries at angiography. However, the left coronary artery (LCA) appeared to originate from the right coronary cusp.

Which of the following is NOT true of this condition?

A. It is an important cause of SCD in athletes
B. Most variations in coronary arteries origin are benign
C. A coronary arterial course between the pulmonary artery (PA) and the aorta is associated with increased risk of SCD
D. The most common subtype is an anomalous right coronary artery (RCA) arising from the left coronary cusp
E. Ischaemia stress testing is helpful in assessing risk of SCD

4. A 30-year-old male presents with palpitations and presyncope. A 12-lead ECG shows a QTc of 510 ms. He has no medical history and takes no regular medication.

Which of the following is NOT true of managing sudden cardiac death in long QT (LQT) syndrome?

A. Beta-blockers may reduce risk of SCD
B. ICD implant is recommended in survivors of cardiac arrest
C. Electrophysiology study can be helpful in determining risk of SCD
D. ICD implant should be considered in those who experience ventricular arrhythmias whilst on beta-blockers
E. Sodium channel blockers may be helpful in LQT3

5. Which of the following is true of catecholaminergic polymorphic ventricular tachycardia (CPVT)?

A. Beta-blockers are recommended for all patients with CPVT
B. Left cardiac sympathetic denervation (LCSD) is not helpful
C. Both documented arrhythmia and a positive genetic test are needed to make a diagnosis
D. ICD therapy is recommended for all patients
E. Strenuous exercise is allowed in moderation

6. **A 29-year-old footballer collapses on the pitch and is successfully resuscitated from a VF cardiac arrest. His 12-lead ECG shows an elevated J point in the inferior leads. A CT coronary angiogram, treadmill test, and cardiac MRI are unremarkable. He additionally has an ajmaline test which is also normal.**

   Which of the following is the most likely diagnosis?

   A. Brugada syndrome
   B. Catecholaminergic polymorphic VT (CPVT)
   C. Long QT syndrome
   D. Early repolarization syndrome
   E. Idiopathic VF

7. **Which of the following is NOT true regarding valve disease and sudden cardiac death?**

   A. Mitral annular disjunction (MAD) is a rare cause of SCD
   B. Mitral regurgitation associated with MAD is usually severe
   C. Pickelhaube sign is associated with an increased risk of SCD
   D. VT in a patient with endocarditis and aortic regurgitation is an indication for valve surgery
   E. Syncope associated with severe aortic stenosis is an indication for valve surgery

8. **Which of the following is NOT part of the management of a patient in cardiac arrest according to European Advanced Life Support (ALS) guidelines?**

   A. A shockable rhythm should be initially defibrillated with at least 150 J
   B. A regular broad complex tachycardia during cardiac arrest should be treated with 300 mg IV amiodarone after the third shock
   C. Polymorphic VT is treated with 2 g of magnesium IV
   D. In VT/VF give adrenaline 1 mg IV on the first cycle of CPR
   E. The use of waveform capnography is recommended

9. **A 74-year-old female presents with pulmonary oedema. Her ECG shows complete heart block. Her blood pressure is 75/40 mmHg and she appears drowsy.**

   Which of the following is the first step in the management of haemodynamically unstable bradycardia according to the European Advanced Life Support bradycardia Algorithm?

   A. Intravenous atropine
   B. Temporary pacing wire implant
   C. Subcutaneous adrenaline
   D. Transcutaneous pacing
   E. Percussion pacing

10. Which of the following is NOT true regarding sudden cardiac death?

A. Sudden arrhythmic death syndrome (SADS) can only be diagnosed when a heart is shown to be morphologically and histologically normal at autopsy
B. The yield of molecular autopsy after unexplained SCD is less than 25%
C. Family screening should be performed in specialized inherited cardiac conditions clinics
D. Coronary artery disease is an uncommon cause of sudden cardiac death in the under 50s
E. An autopsy may be inconclusive in up to half of cases

11. A 41-year-old presents with syncope. He has no past medical history and no family history of note. He is on no regular medication. His ECG shows a QRS duration of 115 ms and an echocardiogram shows moderate LVSD. A coronary angiogram reveals unobstructed coronaries. A cardiac MRI shows extensive myocardial fibrosis. Whilst on coronary care he is seen to have runs of second degree Mobitz II AV block. His serum ACE is significantly elevated and a CT chest shows mediastinal lymphadenopathy.

Which of the following is true?

A. The patient should have a dual chamber ICD
B. The patient should have a subcutaneous ICD (S-ICD)
C. ACE inhibitors and beta-blockers have no effect on LV function in this setting
D. Steroids will improve his cardiac involvement
E. The patient needs an endomyocardial biopsy

12. A 44-year-old gentleman with type2 diabetes and hypertension is retrieved by paramedics after complaining of chest pain and diaphoresis. He has ST elevation in V2-V5 on his ECG. During transfer, he suffers VF arrest and receives one shock which restores sinus rhythm. He has successful primary PCI to his proximal left anterior descending artery. There is no other significant coronary artery disease. His echocardiogram shows moderate LV systolic impairment (ejection fraction 40%).

Which of the following is NOT an appropriate management strategy?

A. Up titration of ACE inhibitor therapy to maximum tolerated dose
B. ICD implant
C. Bisoprolol
D. High dose statin therapy
E. Dual antiplatelet therapy

13. Which of the following drugs is recommended as an adjunct in catecholaminergic polymorphic ventricular tachycardia (CPVT) to prevent ventricular arrhythmias?

A. Flecainide
B. Amiodarone
C. Quinidine
D. Mexilitine
E. Diltiazem

14. Which of the following is incorrect regarding drugs used in the prevention of sudden cardiac death (SCD)?

A. Amiodarone may cause torsades de pointes
B. Bisoprolol may cause erectile dysfunction
C. Mexilitine and ranolazine can be used in LQT3
D. Verapamil can be used in LV fascicular VT
E. Quinidine may be used for refractory VT following ACS

15. Which of the following is NOT true of anti-tachycardia pacing (ATP)?

A. Monomorphic VT can be interrupted with appropriately timed pacing stimuli delivered into the excitable gap of a re-entrant circuit
B. Beta-blockers may increase the likelihood of successful ATP
C. Torsades de pointes and VF are likely to be interrupted by ATP
D. ATP may accelerate a ventricular arrhythmia
E. ATP delivered to the atria may terminate atrial flutter

16. A 16-year-old girl had a cardiac arrest whilst swimming. Her ECG showed a QTc of 520 ms and she has a normal echocardiogram and cardiac MRI.

What is likely diagnosis?

A. Catecholaminergic polymorphic VT (CPVT)
B. Long QT1
C. Long QT2
D. Long QT3
E. Andersen-Tawil syndrome

17. An asymptomatic 25-year-old man has an ECG (Figure 6.2.1). He has a past medical history of anxiety and depression.

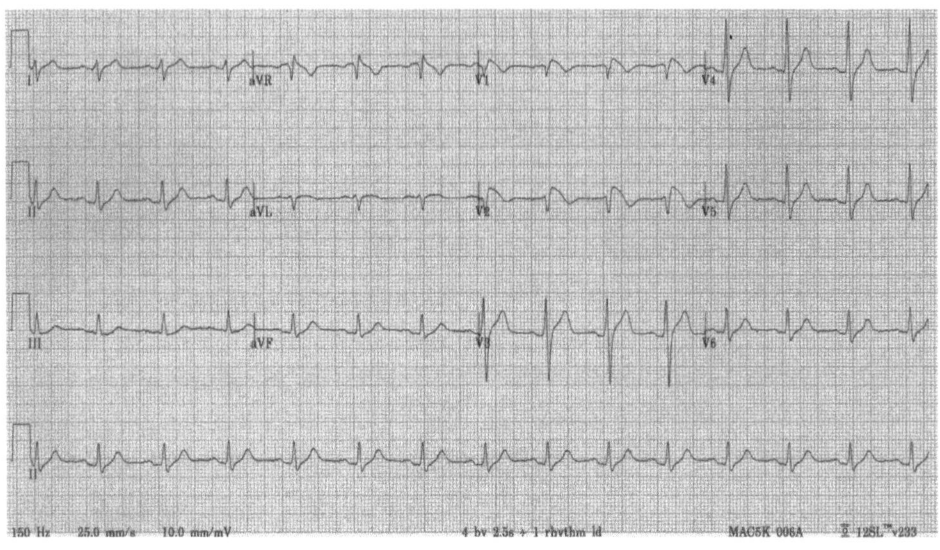

Figure 6.2.1

Which of the following is true?

A. He should have an ICD
B. He should be started on beta-blockers
C. He should have quinidine
D. He should avoid amitriptyline for his depression
E. Genetic testing is positive in >80% of cases

18. A 49-year-old female has idiopathic VT. She has a normal resting 12-lead ECG and normal cardiac MRI.

Which of the following is NOT true about the management of idiopathic VT?

A. Catheter ablation is the first-line treatment
B. Beta-blockers are a treatment option
C. Verapamil is a treatment option
D. Flecanide is a treatment option
E. ICD implantation should be considered

19. Which of the following ECG findings are NOT associated with sudden cardiac death?

A. Prolonged QT interval
B. QRS fragmentation
C. Isolated first-degree AV block
D. T-wave alternans
E. Blunted heart rate variability

20. Which of the following is NOT true regarding prevention of SCD in patients taking psychotropic medication?

A. A QT interval >500 ms warrants a change of medication to reduce QT interval
B. A QT interval that increases 60 ms on the introduction of medication warrants a change of medication to reduce the QT interval
C. Macrolides are the preferred antibiotic for treating community-acquired infections
D. Tricyclic antidepressants prolong the QT interval more than selective serotonin reuptake inhibitors
E. Avoidance of hypokalaemia is recommended

chapter

6.2

CARDIAC ARREST, RESUSCITATION, AND SUDDEN CARDIAC DEATH

ANSWERS

1. B. The HCM-SCD risk study found an association between sudden cardiac death (SCD) and the following observations.

- Younger age
- > 3 beats of VT (non-sustained VT)
- LV wall thickness >30mm
- Family history of SCD <40 in the absence of HCM diagnosis, or any age with an HCM diagnosis
- Syncope
- Enlarged left atrial diameter
- LVOT obstruction
- Failure to increase systolic pressure by at least 20 mmHg from rest to peak exercise or a fall of >20 mmHg from peak pressure

In patients with a 5-year risk of SCD <4% (using the HCM-SCD risk calculator, e.g. as shown here: https://qxmd.com/calculate/calculator_303/hcm-risk-scd), an ICD is generally not indicated, in patients with a risk of 4 to less than 6%, an ICD may be considered and in patients with a 5-year risk ≥6%, an ICD should be considered.

Populations in which the calculator should not be used include: patients under 16 years old, competitive athletes, HCM associated with metabolic diseases (e.g. Fabry disease), syndromes (e.g. Noonan syndrome), and patients with a previous history of aborted SCD or sustained ventricular arrhythmia who should be treated with ICD implant as secondary prevention.

O'Mahony C, Jichi F, Pavlou M, et al. A novel clinical risk prediction model for sudden cardiac death in hypertrophic cardiomyopathy (HCM Risk-SCD). Eur Heart J. 35, 2010–20 (2014).

2. A. Family members who also have ARVC are at lower risk of SCD than the proband. B is a class 1B ESC recommendation and C is a class IIb B ESC recommendation in the assessment of ARVC. In the US, the National Registry of Sudden Death in Athletes was established at the Minneapolis Heart Institute in the 1980s and has reported on 1866 sudden deaths in individuals <40 years of age during a 27-year observational period. Their data show that 36% of all sudden deaths in this registry are attributed to confirmed cardiovascular causes, of which the most frequent are HCM (36%), congenital anomalies of the coronary arteries (17%), myocarditis (6%), ARVC (4%), and channelopathies (3.6%). Avoidance of competitive sports is an ESC 1 C recommendation.

3. A. Anomalous coronary arteries were seen in 17% of cases of SCD in the US National Registry of Sudden Death in Athletes, although the vast majority of individuals who have anomalous coronary origins are unaffected. An interarterial course (between PA and aorta) of the left coronary artery is associated with the greatest risk of SCD. This may be due to coronary artery compression during exercise and ischaemia-driven malignant arrhythmia formation.

Finocchiaro G, Behr ER, Tanzarella G, Papadakis M, Malhotra A, Dhutia H, et al. Anomalous Coronary Artery Origin and Sudden Cardiac Death: Clinical and Pathological Insights From a National Pathology Registry. JACC: Clinical Electrophysiology. 2019 Apr;5(4):516–22.

4. C. Electrophysiology studies are not recommended (class IIIC). Beta-blockers and ICD implant are recommended after cardiac arrest (Class 1B recommendation), whilst D is a IIaB recommendation and sodium channel blockers may be used as adjunct therapy in LQT3 (Class IIb C recommendation).

5. A. Beta-blockers are recommended for all patients—particularly nadalol if available. LCSD can be helpful but there is limited long-term data. CPVT is diagnosed in the presence of a structurally normal heart, normal ECG and exercise or emotion-induced bidirectional or polymorphic VT (IC recommendation), or in those who are carriers of a pathogenic variant(s) in the genes RyR2 or CASQ2 (IC recommendation). Strenuous exercise should be avoided (IC recommendation). ICD implantation in addition to beta-blockers with or without flecainide is recommended in patients with a diagnosis of CPVT who experience cardiac arrest, recurrent syncope or polymorphic/bidirectional VT despite optimal therapy (IC recommendation).

6. D. The J point elevation in the inferior leads on the resting ECG, combined with otherwise negative investigations, suggests a diagnosis of early repolarization (ER) syndrome in this patient. J point elevation is sometimes also seen in the lateral leads. It is likely to be a polygenic condition—an accumulation of multiple single nucleotide variants to produce a phenotype. Early repolarization is a common and benign finding in the vast majority of patients. ER syndrome is diagnosed in the presence of J-point elevation ≥1 mm in ≥2 contiguous inferior and/or lateral leads of a standard 12-lead ECG in a patient resuscitated from otherwise unexplained VF/polymorphic VT.

7. B. Mitral annular disjunction is a rare cause of SCD and is often present without significant MR. It is defined as a detachment of the roots of the annulus from the ventricular myocardium producing a gap of 2–10 mm during systole. Pickelhaube sign is a high-velocity mid-systolic spike in the tissue Doppler assessment of the lateral mitral valve annulus. It is so named after the German military helmet. This should not be confused with spiked helmet sign on the ECG which refers to a characteristic QRS-ST morphology that also mimics the Pickelhaube helmet and is a pseudo STEMI pattern seen in critical illness. VT in the context of aortic regurgitation (AR) and endocarditis is an indication for surgery (Class 1C recommendation), and symptomatic severe aortic stenosis is also an indication for aortic valve surgery/intervention.

8. D. In shockable rhythms, amiodarone 300 mg and adrenaline 1 mg IV are given after the third shock and then every 3–5 minutes.

9. A. According to European ALS guidelines, the most appropriate initial treatment in an unstable patient is 500 mcg IV atropine. However, atropine is only effective in increasing the heart rate when there is a nodal escape rhythm. Atropine is ineffective with escape rhythms distal to the AV node. Isoprenaline is a beta agonist and can temporarily restore AV nodal conduction, or increase the rate of the escape rhyhthm.

10. D. Coronary artery disease is the most common cause of sudden cardiac death in those aged over 35. Survivors of an unexplained sudden cardiac arrest, where there is a suspicion of an inherited cardiac disease, should be referred to a specialist inherited cardiac disease clinic where the following tests are routinely performed: ECG (including signal averaged ECG and high leads ECG for Brugada syndrome), prolonged ECG monitoring for ventricular arrhythmias, treadmill test for exercise induced arrhythmias, and an echocardiogram.

11. A. This patient has sarcoidosis with cardiac involvement. With extensive fibrosis seen on cardiac MRI this patient is at high risk of SCD and given that he has an indication for pacing he should be considered for an ICD. His AV block is likely due to sarcoid involvement of the AV node. Although young, this patient is not a candidate for an S-ICD because it will not treat his bradyarrhythmias. Steroids have not been shown to have any improvement on LV function in randomized controlled data, but they are frequently used despite this. They may work in some patients but evidence is very limited.

12. B. In the presence of a reversible cause of ventricular arrhythmia (STEMI) and no persistent severe LVSD, there is no indication for ICD implantation. All other therapies are appropriate secondary prevention in the context of STEMI and impaired LV function.

13. A. Flecainide should be considered in addition to beta-blockers in patients with a diagnosis of CPVT who experience recurrent syncope or polymorphic/bidirectional VT while on beta-blockers when there are risks/contraindications for an ICD, or an ICD is not available or is rejected by the patient (Class IIa C recommendation).

14. E. Quinidine is used largely in Brugada syndrome and has Ito blocking properties. It has been shown to normalize the epicardial action potential dome and hence reduces phase two re-entry and ventricular arrhythmias. It is avoided after ACS.

15. C. Torsades de pointes and VF are unlikely to be successfully terminated by ATP. Beta-blockers may increase the size of the excitable gap of a re-entry circuit which is the site of action where ATP can act to terminate the arrhythmia.

16. B. CPVT typically causes syncope or palpitations, classically caused by bidirectional VT in young patients with structurally normal hearts. It usually presents before adulthood. It does not cause a prolonged QT interval but rarely some patients may have both conditions. Long QT syndrome is defined by a QT interval > 480 ms on repeated ECGs (after provoking factors have been excluded/treated) or a long QT score of >3 (Class 1C recommendation). Importantly, long QT syndromes have different triggers for ventricular arrhythmias and different ECG morphologies (Table 6.2.A1). Andersen-Tawil syndrome refers to LQTS associated with *KCNJ2* variants, periodic paralysis, characteristic dysmorphic facial features and mild learning difficulties.

Table 6.2.A1

Type	Gene	% of LQT patients[a]	Triggers	ECG pattern
LQTS1	*KCNQ1*	35%	Exercise, especially swimming	Broad based early onset T-wave
LQTS2	*KCNH2*	30%	Emotion and noise (particularly at night)	Low amplitude late T wave
LQTS3	*SCN5A*	5%	Sleep	Late onset normal looking T wave

[a]In some patients a pathogenic variant will not be identified.

17. D. ICD therapy is reserved for survivors of cardiac arrest, those with documented ventricular arrhythmias, or those with unexplained syncope with a Type 1 Brugada ECG. The risk of SCD in those without symptoms is <1% per year. Quinidine has been shown to be helpful in a large case series but lacks randomized control data. It is not a guideline-recommended first-line treatment at present. Genetic testing is positive in only 20% of cases.

Only SCN5A variants have strong data regarding pathogenicity. Lifestyle advice is recommended in all patients with Brugada syndrome:

- Abstaining from heavy meals prior to sleep
- Avoidance of excessive alcohol intake
- Avoidance of certain drugs (www.brugadadrugs.org) including amitriptyline as a class II recommendation
- Prompt treatment of any fever with antipyretic drugs

18. E. Catheter ablation by experienced operators is recommended as a first-line treatment in symptomatic patients with idiopathic left-sided VTs (Class IB recommendation). When catheter ablation is not available or desired, treatment with beta-blockers, verapamil, or sodium channel blockers (class IC agents) is recommended in symptomatic patients with idiopathic left VT, papillary muscle tachycardia, or mitral/tricuspid annular tachycardia (Class IC recommendation). ICD therapy is generally not indicated in patients with normal heart VT.

19. C. Only C has not been associated with an increased risk of SCD. Prolonged QT intervals are associated with development of polymorphic ventricular tachycardia due to R on T events, either in inherited LQTS or acquired cases due to drugs or electrolyte derangement. QRS fragmentation represents conduction system disarray usually due to scar formation which acts as a substrate for ventricular arrhythmias. A blunted heart rate variability on prolonged ECG monitoring is associated with an increased risk of SCD. T-wave alternans is an abnormal finding at rates <100bpm and has been associated in some populations with an increased risk of SCD. First-degree AV block is very common and may represent conduction disease, particularly in the elderly, but also may represent enhanced vagal tone.

20. C. Antipsychotic drug use is associated with a 1.53-fold increased risk of ventricular arrhythmia and/or SCD. A and B are class IC recommendations, whilst macrolides (such as erythromycin) prolong the QT interval and thus may be pro-arrhythmogenic in the context of psychotropic medication (IV administration is associated with high serum levels and more QT prolongation).

12/20

chapter 7

PREVENTION, REHABILITATION, AND SPORT

chapter 7.1

SPORTS CARDIOLOGY

QUESTION

1. **Which of these is an abnormal finding on an athlete's ECG?**
   A. Ectopic atrial rhythm
   B. Mobitz type II second-degree atrioventricular block
   C. Early repolarization
   D. Sokolow–Lyon criteria for left ventricular hypertrophy
   E. Left atrial enlargement

2. **Which of these findings on an athlete's ECG would warrant further investigations?**
   A. Sinus bradycardia <30 bpm
   B. Q-waves
   C. QTc >470 ms (male athlete)
   D. Prolonged PR interval >400 ms
   E. All of the above

3. **Which of the following situations warrants further investigations?**
   A. White female cyclist with LV wall thickness of 11 mm
   B. White male cyclist with LV cavity size of 60 mm
   C. White female sprinter with LV wall thickness of 10 mm
   D. Black male footballer with LV wall thickness of 12 mm
   E. White female tennis player with LV wall thickness 13 mm

4. You have been referred an 18-year-old black athlete who plays football at an elite level. He is asymptomatic with no family history of sudden cardiac death. His ECG is shown in Figure 7.1.1.

What further investigations, if any, are required?

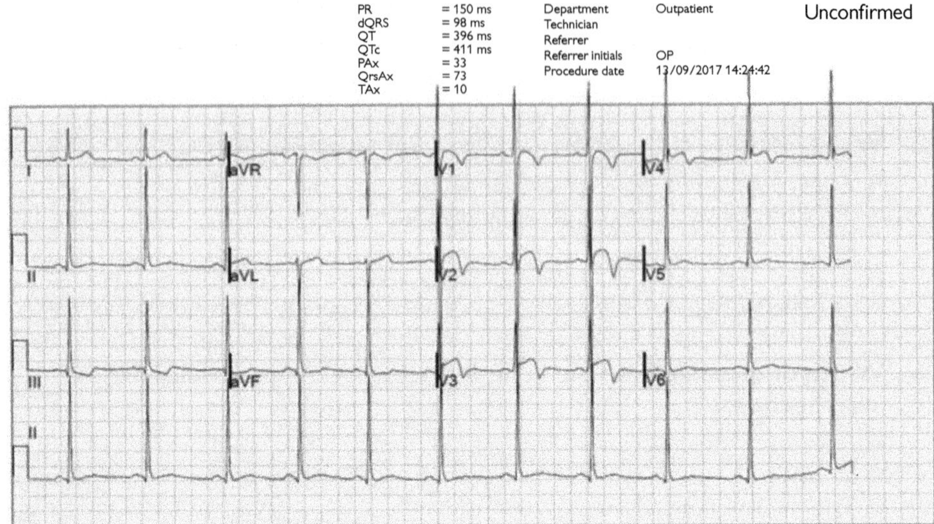

Figure 7.1.1

A. No further investigations
B. Repeat at 1 year.
C. Echocardiogram, Holter monitoring, and exercise testing
D. Cardiac MRI
E. Screening of first-degree relatives

5. A 34-year-old black footballer presents with dyspnoea. His father has a history of dilated cardiomyopathy secondary to a viral infection. An ECG performed shows T-wave inversion in leads V1 and V2 and a single premature ventricular ectopic. Further investigations including an echocardiogram and cardiopulmonary exercise testing are carried out.

Which of the following is not in keeping with a possible diagnosis of dilated cardiomyopathy?

A. S′ 5 cm/s
B. Mild diastolic dysfunction
C. Improvement of LV function on exercise echocardiography by 15%.
D. Negative genetics
E. Late gadolinium enhancement on MRI.

6. A 21-year-old international tennis player presents to your clinic as her father has recently been diagnosed with hypertrophic cardiomyopathy. She is asymptomatic. Her ECG and echocardiogram are normal. An exercise tolerance test, 24-hour Holter monitor, and MRI are also unremarkable. She has been genetically tested and has been found to be positive for a myosin-binding protein C mutation.

What would you advise regarding her participation at an elite level?

A. Recommend no higher than moderate intensity activity only.
B. Participation in low intensity activity only.
C. Participation in competitive sports with annual follow-up.
D. Participation in competitive sports with 5 yearly follow-up.
E. Should not participate in competitive sports.

7. A 30-year-old male international cyclist has been incidentally found to have moderate mitral regurgitation on routine screening through his cycling club. He is asymptomatic, with normal LV function and a peak $V0_2$ of 130% of predicted.

Which of the following criteria need to be fulfilled to allow this cyclist to compete?

A. LV end diastolic dimension <60 mm
B. LV end diastolic dimension <35.3 mm/m^2
C. Resting pulmonary artery pressures <50 mmHg
D. LVEF>60%
E. All of the above

8. A 30-year-old professional cyclist presents with palpitations and shortness of breath on exertion. He has a family history of premature cardiovascular disease in his father who had a myocardial infarction at the age of 49 years. His ECG demonstrates atrial flutter at a rate of 55 bpm. His echocardiogram is normal and his 24-hour tape confirms rate-controlled atrial flutter. He is not keen to take any medications as he is concerned it may limit his athletic performance.

How would you proceed regarding his management?

A. No competitive sports
B. Bisoprolol, anticoagulation, continue to compete
C. Anticoagulation, continue to compete
D. Recommend ablation and if successful resume competitive sports after 1 month
E. Flecainide, continue to compete

9. A 50-year-old man presents to your clinic. He has been participating in marathons and would like a letter for his insurance company to say that he is fit for an elite event abroad. He is asymptomatic. You investigate him with a resting ECG which is normal. However, you calculate his risk of a cardiovascular event over 10 years as > 5% using the global SCORE system.

What would you advise regarding his level of sporting participation?

A. No restrictions
B. Perform a CTCA
C. Perform exercise stress testing, if this is normal then he can participate in competitive sports
D. Perform a coronary angiogram
E. Restrict from all competitive sports

chapter

7.1

SPORTS CARDIOLOGY

ANSWERS

1. B. Mobitz type II atrioventricular block is not a routine finding on an athlete's ECG and requires further investigation. An ectopic atrial rhythm can often be seen in athletes due to increased vagal tone. Sinus rhythm normally resumes on exercise. Early repolarization as demonstrated by J point elevation ≥1 mm at the junction between the termination of the QRS complex and the beginning of the ST segment is common in athletes. Athletes may demonstrate remodelling of their left ventricle including an increase in wall thickness which can manifest on the ECG as evidence of LVH (S-wave in V1 + R-wave in V5/6 >35 mm). This may also be present without objective evidence of LVH but is not pathological in isolation. Isolated left atrial enlargement is not indicative of pathology unless ≥2 of the following are present; left atrial enlargement, right atrial enlargement, left axis deviation, right axis deviation, complete right bundle branch block.

2. E. Sinus bradycardia and first-degree heart block can be normal in an athlete. However, a heart rate <30 bpm or a PR interval of >400 ms raises the possibility of conduction disease. In those with profound bradycardia (<30 bpm), one should exercise the athlete (running on the spot/climbing stairs) and repeat the ECG. If there is no increase in heart rate then further evaluation should be considered based on clinical suspicion. A QTc of >470 ms in a male athlete is prolonged and should be investigated with a repeat ECG on a separate day initially. If the QT interval remains prolonged full evaluation with exercise stress testing; 24-hour Holter monitor; electrolyte assessment; family screening; and genetic testing when clinical suspicion is high should be considered. In those with pathological Q-waves that are persistent consideration should be given to echocardiography for investigation for coronary disease / cardiomyopathy.

3. E. LVH in white female athletes is not associated with physiological adaptation to sports and requires further investigations.

4. A. Findings within normal limits in a black athlete's ECG include concave ST elevation and T-wave inversion in leads V1-V4. A juvenile ECG pattern, T-wave inversion V1-V3, would not be expected to persist beyond the age of 16 years, therefore repeating an ECG beyond this age would not usually demonstrate resolution of T-wave inversion.

5. C. S′ can be reduced. It is very unusual for an athlete to demonstrate diastolic dysfunction. In cases of dilated cardiomyopathy ejection fraction would not be expected to improve significantly from baseline on exercise stress testing (<11%). A negative genetics panel does not mean that an athlete does not have DCM as there are many causes of DCM including: viral, bacterial, and fungal causes; nutritional causes such as vitamin B1 deficiency; metabolic causes including hemochromatosis; hormonal causes including hypothyroidism and phaeochromocytoma, in addition to hereditary causes. In addition, there may be pathogenic genes that are yet to be identified. A cardiac MRI may demonstrate late gadolinium enhancement in cases of DCM.

6. C. There is no evidence of any phenotypic manifestations of hypertrophic cardiomyopathy in this tennis player. Although, according to recent 2020 ESC guidelines there should be no restriction with regards to competitive sports participation, follow-up should be considered annually to assess for development of the hypertrophic cardiomyopathy phenotype.

7. E. The ESC 2020 guidelines state that individuals with mild mitral regurgitation may compete in all competitive sports. Those with asymptomatic moderate mitral regurgitation may participate in competitive sports if their LV end diastolic dimension is <60 mm (35.3 mm/m^2 in men and <40mm/m^2 in women), LV ejection fraction is ≥60%, resting pulmonary pressures <50 mmHg and the individual has a normal exercise test. Individuals with asymptomatic severe mitral regurgitation may only compete in low-moderate intensity recreational sports if their LV end diastolic dimension is <60 mm (35.3 mm/m^2 in men and <40 mm/m^2 in women), LV ejection fraction is ≥60%, resting pulmonary pressures <50 mmHg, and the individual has a normal exercise test.

8. D. An ablation in this case is recommended due to the athlete's symptoms and the risk of 1:1 conduction of atrial flutter. After successful ablation, if no reoccurrence of symptoms then competitive sports can be resumed after 1 month. This athlete does not need routine anticoagulation based on his CHA_2DS_2-Vasc score of 0. A beta-blocker would not be required as the athlete is rate controlled and beta-blockers are often poorly tolerated in the athletic population. Flecainide alone would increase the risk of 1:1 conduction of the atrial flutter.

9. C. Over the age of 35 years the most common cause of SCD during exercise is IHD. Asymptomatic athletes with increased cardiovascular risk should undergo exercise testing. If this is normal, there should be no restriction for competitive sport. If the exercise test is borderline, an additional stress test is recommended (exercise echocardiography, stress echocardiography, MRI perfusion, SPECT/PET). If there is no evidence of inducible ischaemia the athlete should not be restricted from participation in competitive sports. If the exercise test is positive then a CT or invasive coronary angiogram should be performed.

chapter

7.2

PRIMARY PREVENTION AND DYSLIPIDAEMIA

QUESTIONS

1. **A 49-year-old male presents to you in general cardiology clinic with no known history of cardiovascular disease but he has a diagnosis of hypertension for which he is taking an ACE-inhibitor. His bloods reveal an eGFR of 40 ml/min/1.73m^2 (which is stable) and a low density lipoprotein (LDL) of 2.9 mmol/L.**

   What would you recommend?

   A. Address lifestyle changes and calculate a SCORE2 (Systematic Coronary Risk Estimation 2) percentage risk and if elevated to proceed to drug therapy
   B. Address lifestyle changes only
   C. Address lifestyle changes and commence drug therapy immediately
   D. Address lifestyle changes but he is too young for the SCORE2 risk chart to be used but an alternative age adjusted one should be used and if the percentage risk is elevated to proceed to drug therapy
   E. Initiate drug therapy only

2. **The surgical team have asked your advice regarding a patient admitted under their care with acute pancreatitis as they would like to review his current medications. A lipid profile is pending.**

   Which pharmacological agent may make the clinical situation worse?

   A. HMG-Co A reductase inhibitor
   B. PPAR alpha agonist
   C. Niemann-Pick C1 like transporter inhibitor
   D. PCSK9 inhibitor
   E. CETP inhibitor

3. You are reviewing a 72-year-old male in the general cardiology clinic who has recently suffered a myocardial infarction (MI). At the time he underwent percutaneous coronary intervention (PCI) to his left circumflex artery and was commenced on appropriate secondary prevention medications. He now complains of myalgia and some difficulty mobilizing as a result.

Which of the following medications is least likely to be responsible for the impaired metabolism of a statin?

A. Amlodipine
B. Amiodarone
C. Clarithromycin
D. Atenolol
E. Ranolazine

4. A 54-year-old male is seen in clinic. Within your assessment you note an LDL-C of 6.2 mmol/L and tendon xanthoma.

Given the suspected clinical diagnosis, which of the following is the guideline recommended LDL-C level that such patients should aim to be achieving?

A. LDL-C <2.2 (mmol/L)
B. LDL-C <2.0 (mmol/L)
C. LDL-C <1.8 (mmol/L)
D. LDL-C <1.6 (mmol/L)
E. LDL-C <1.4 (mmol/L)

5. A 54-year-old male presents following a non-ST elevation myocardial infarction (NSTEMI). He is found to have a very elevated blood cholesterol level. He is diagnosed with familial hypercholesterolaemia (FH) and commenced on therapy.

Which of the following is the guideline recommended LDL-C target for this patient?

A. LDL-C < 2.0 (mmol/L)
B. LDL-C < 1.8 (mmol/L)
C. LDL-C < 1.6 (mmol/L)
D. LDL-C < 1.4 (mmol/L)
E. LDL-C < 1.2 (mmol/L)

6. A 75-year-old male is seen in cardiology clinic and you commence statin therapy. Which of the following is not true?

A. Statin therapy in those over the age of 75 is effective in preventing cardiovascular disease
B. Statin therapy is associated with a small increased risk of developing Alzheimer's disease
C. Simvastatin is a prodrug
D. Patient response to statin therapy is variable and not dose dependent
E. The absolute risk for a given cholesterol level in those >75 years of age is greater

7. A 40-year-old female is seen in clinic with a triglyceride level of 5.5 mmol/L (normal < 1.7 mmol/L). She is already on a statin due to her risk profile.

What is the next best agent to recommend?

A. PCSK9 inhibitor
B. Nicotinic acid
C. Fibrate
D. N-3 fatty acids
E. Add in an additional statin

8. Which particles have the highest concentration of triglyceride?

A. Chylomicrons
B. LDL
C. HDL
D. IDL
E. Lp(a)

9. Which of the following risk profiles and lipid targets are correctly matched when assessing a patient <70-years-of-age in the primary prevention setting?

A. Very high risk without familial hypercholesterolaemia (FH) and a LDL-C target of <1.4 mmol/L and ≥ 50% reduction from baseline
B. Very high risk with familial hypercholesterolaemia and a LDL-C target of <1.2 mmol/L and ≥ 50% reduction from baseline
C. High risk and a LDL-C target of <1.6 mmol/L and ≥ 50% reduction from baseline
D. Low risk and a LDL-C target of < 3.5 mmol/L and ≥ 50% reduction from baseline
E. Intermediate risk and a LDL-C target of <1.5 mmol/L and ≥ 50% reduction from baseline

10. A 50-year-old male in seen on coronary care having suffered an anterior MI. His cholesterol is elevated and you suspect familial hypercholesterolaemia.

Which of the following could potentially be used for diagnostic purposes?

A. Patients with premature coronary artery disease (men aged <55 years and women <60 years), cerebral or peripheral vascular disease
B. Mutation in the LDL-R gene
C. An LDL-C of 4–4.9 mmol/L
D. All of the above
E. None of the above

11. A 48-year-old male is seen in clinic with a total cholesterol of 7.6 mmol/L. He has tendon xanthomas and you suspect a diagnosis of familial hypercholesterolaemia.

Which of the following is the most likely underlying aetiology?

A. Loss of function of the LDL-R gene
B. Gain of function of the LDL-R gene
C. Loss of function of the PCSK9 gene
D. Gain of function of the PCSK9 gene
E. None of the above

12. A 65-year-old man is seen in clinic with severe chronic kidney disease (CKD), hypertension and an LDL-C of 1.6 mmol/L. He is currently on atorvastatin 40 mg daily, ramipril 10 mg daily, and amlodipine 10 mg daily.

Which of the following is the most appropriate next step?

A. Add in ezetimibe
B. Increase the statin dose
C. Add in a PCSK 9 inhibitor
D. Change to a more potent statin
E. None of the above, he has an adequate LDL-C level

13. A 65-year-old man is seen in the general cardiology clinic. He has severe chronic kidney disease (CKD) and hypertension with an LDL-C of 1.6 mmol/L. He has tried to use a multitude of different statins at differing doses but has not tolerated them due to muscle symptoms and is not keen to try them anymore.

Which of the following is the most appropriate next step?

A. Continue with statin therapy as the benefit far outweighs the relatively trivial muscle symptoms
B. Add in a PCSK9 inhibitor
C. Add in ezetimibe
D. Add in nicotinic acid
E. Add in mipomersen

14. A 65-year-old comes to see you in clinic and you undertake a cardiovascular risk assessment. Which of the following is correct?

A. A body mass index (BMI) <18.5 kg/m^2 is considered an ideal weight
B. A body mass index 20–30 kg/m^2 is a normal range for a male
C. Men should target a waist circumference of 95–105 cm
D. Women should target a waist circumference of 75–85 cm
E. Body mass index and waist circumference are both associated with cardiovascular disease (CVD) and type 2 diabetes

15. Which of the following is regarded as the best predictor of coronary artery disease amongst the cardiovascular risk scores?

A. Smoking status
B. Systolic blood pressure
C. Diabetes mellitus
D. LDL cholesterol
E. Age

16. A 28-year-old female comes to see you in clinic. She has type 1 diabetes, which is poorly controlled though she has no evidence of end organ damage. She is a current smoker. Her GP has commenced her on statin therapy. She is planning to get pregnant and wants advice regarding her medications.

A. Stop the statin
B. Continue the statin due to her cardiovascular risk profile during pregnancy
C. Check her cholesterol level and if <5 mmol/L stop the statin
D. Continue statin and add in aspirin
E. Stop the statin but add in aspirin

17. A 72-year-old male is currently on ezetimibe and simvastatin and is due to begin dialysis due to his deteriorating renal function.

Which of the following is the correct course of action?

A. Stop the statin but continue the ezetimibe
B. Stop the ezetimibe but continue the statin
C. Stop both medications due to the risk of drug accumulation
D. Stop the ezetimibe and change the simvastatin to pravastatin
E. Continue both medications

18. A 76-year-old male is taking a statin for secondary preventative purposes. He was asymptomatic but a creatine kinase (CK) level was checked. This returned as 500 U/L (normal= 40–320 U/L). What is the most appropriate action?

A. Stop treatment
B. Continue treatment
C. Stop treatment recheck CK in 1 month
D. Continue treatment and recheck CK in 1 month
E. Switch to an alternative statin

chapter 7.2

PRIMARY PREVENTION AND DYSLIPIDAEMIA

ANSWERS

1. C. ESC 2021 guidance on cardiovascular disease prevention recommends a global cardiovascular risk assessment is undertaken on anyone above 40 years of age unless they are automatically deemed high-risk or very high-risk. High risk individuals would include those with moderate renal impairment (eGFR 30–59 ml/min/1.73 m^2). Those patients would likely benefit from an LDL of <1.8 mmol/L. Lifestyle changes and a holistic approach to a patients cardiovascular risk profile should always be addressed.

2. B. Fibrates (PPAR alpha agonists) are associated with a small risk of pancreatitis and should be stopped in the setting of pancreatitis, unless the cause of the pancreatitis is secondary to significantly elevated triglycerides.

3. D. Appropriate secondary prevention after an MI will nearly always involve a high potency statin (unless significant contraindications). Statin therapy is associated with myalgia and very rarely rhabdomyolysis. Interaction with other medications metabolized by the P450 3A4 system can lead to elevated levels and thus to an increased risk of myopathy. Atenolol and nadolol appear to be the only beta-blockers that are excreted unchanged by the kidneys. Amlodipine, amiodarone, clarithromycin, and ranolazine are all metabolized by the P450 3A4 system and so can potentially interact with statin therapy.

4. C. Given the clinical stigmata of hypercholesterolaemia and LDL-C result, the patient meets the Dutch Lipid Clinic Network diagnostic criteria for a diagnosis of familial hypercholesterolaemia (FH). In line with the 2019 ESC dyslipidaemia guidelines, in the absence of established atherosclerotic disease or another major cardiovascular risk factor then treatment should be initiated with high intensity statin therapy and a LDL-C target of <1.8 mmol/L.

5. D. In patients with FH and atherosclerotic disease or any patient with documented atherosclerotic CVD then a level of <1.4 mmol/L is the recommended target.

6. B. There has been no conclusive evidence to support this statement. High cholesterol levels is associated with coronary artery disease (CAD) amongst all age groups. The absolute risk of CAD in the elderly is higher so for a given cholesterol level the risk is greater. Unsurprisingly few of the trials recruit patients >75 years of age so the evidence base for their use is less. Statin therapy for primary prevention is dictated by risk and may be considered in older people (aged >70) if at high risk or above.

7. D. In those patients who are high risk or more (according to ESC dyslipidaemia guideline assessment), a triglyceride level above 1.5 mmol/L warrants an additional agent. N-3 polyunsaturated fatty acids are the agent of choice if the patient has already been established on statin therapy (IIa B), whilst the addition of a fibrate could also be undertaken (weaker recommendation from the ESC–IIb B).

8. A. Chylomicrons contain about 95% triglycerides. LDL about 5%, HDL about 5%, IDL about 25%, and Lp(a) about 5%.

9. A. According to 2021 ESC cardiovascular disease prevention guidelines, for 'very high risk' patients without FH, a LDL-C target of <1.4 mmol/L should be considered. For very high risk with FH, an LDL-C <1.4 should be considered. High risk individuals <1.8 mmol/L should be considered. For moderate risk, a goal of <2.6 mmol/L and for low risk, an LDL-C of <3 mmol/L.

10. D. The Dutch Lipid Clinic Network diagnostic criteria, Simon Broome register, or the WHO criteria are often used to try and identify these patients via a scoring mechanism. The Dutch Lipid Clinic Network diagnostic criteria has five categories: Family history, clinical history, physical examination, LDL-C levels, and DNA analysis and provides a probabilistic approach to patient diagnosis.

11. A. FH is a monogenic disease caused by loss of function mutations (of which there are more than 1000 identified) or a gain of function in the PCSK9 gene (but much less commonly).

12. B. This patient with severe CKD is automatically placed in the very high risk profile when it comes to primary prevention. As such they would have an ideal LDL-C of <1.4 mmol/L and a reduction from baseline LDL-C of >50%. It is recommended that a high intensity statin (e.g. atorvastatin or rosuvastatin) should be utilized and titrated to their maximum tolerated doses to achieve this goal.

13. C. Muscle symptoms associated with statin use is well documented and care needs to be taken to explore such patient concerns. Changing to different agents and/or altering the dose may achieve the desired effect. Given the enormous benefit of these treatment regimes, abandoning statin therapy altogether without an adequate trial may not be in the patient's best interests. However, in this case multiple different agents/doses have been tried so it is reasonable to trial another agent. The second line agent is ezetimibe.

14. E. BMI is an easy and reproducible method that correlates with waist circumference, and when significantly raised marks patients at risk of CVD and type 2 diabetes. A waist circumference of <94 cm in men and <80 cm in women are recommended targets.

15. E. It is important to recognize the risk in those over 65 years of age based on scoring systems alone. Even those with no cardiovascular risk factors may still a high percentage risk based on age alone.

16. A. Statins should be avoided in pregnancy. Contraception advice should be given to women of child-bearing age on a statin. They should ideally be stopped 3 months prior to trying to conceive. Aspirin is safe in pregnancy but has no indication for primary prevention purposes for this patient.

17. E. CKD patients with moderate to severe renal dysfunction are considered high risk to very high risk from a cardiovascular perspective. Statin therapy and additional ezetimibe therapy may well be indicated. In those patients who become dialysis dependent who are already on these medications then continuation should be considered.

18. D. If CK is elevated but less than 10 times the upper limit in an asymptomatic individual it is reasonable to continue the treatment but to monitor the CK in 2–6 weeks.

chapter 7.3

ARTERIAL HYPERTENSION

QUESTIONS

1. **An anxious 49 year-old gentleman attends his GP for a routine blood pressure check. This is recorded diligently on three occasions, 1–2 minutes apart with the readings as follows: 142/90 mmHg, 134/86 mmHg and 140/88 mmHg.**

   This gentleman's blood pressure should be regarded as?

   A. Normal
   B. High normal
   C. Grade 1 hypertension
   D. Grade 2 hypertension
   E. Isolated diastolic hypertension

2. **A 65 year-old man is found to have an office blood pressure of 149/80 mmHg on a routine health check. The doctor decides to perform a 24-hour ambulatory blood pressure to confirm the diagnosis.**

   Which of the following blood pressure recordings on a 24-hour monitor would confirm this diagnosis based on the ESC definition of hypertension?

   A. A 24-hour mean blood pressure of 134/76 mmHg
   B. A 24-hour mean blood pressure of 130/80 mmHg
   C. A daytime (awake) blood pressure of 130/80 mmHg
   D. A daytime (awake) blood pressure of 135/85 mmHg
   E. A night-time asleep blood pressure of 119/64 mmHg

3. An anxious 72 year-old women with an increased BMI being treated for hypertension with amlodipine has recently been diagnosed with obstructive sleep apnoea. She has started to experience dizzy spells. Office blood pressures are elevated at 147/90 mmHg.

Based on ESC guidelines, the doctor decides to perform ambulatory blood pressure monitoring because?

A. They want to establish whether there is nocturnal hypotension related to the history of obstructive sleep apnoea

B. They want to confirm a diagnosis of possible 'white-coat' hypertension

C. They want to establish whether there are periods of hypotension to explain the dizzy spells

D. In a 72 year-old with elevated office blood pressures, the diagnosis of hypertension should be confirmed with an ambulatory monitor.

E. Ambulatory blood pressure monitoring can be useful in patients with resistant hypertension

4. A 73 year-old Afro-Caribbean male with a history of type 2 diabetes and hyperlipidaemia is found to have a clinic blood pressure of 142/78 mmHg and LVH by voltage criteria on his resting ECG. He is otherwise fit and well, takes no regular anti-hypertensive medication, and continues to smoke. You recommend:

A. Ambulatory blood pressure monitoring

B. Lifestyle advice and clinic review at 3 months

C. Lifestyle advice and angiotensin receptor blocker

D. Lifestyle advice, initiation of SGLT2 inhibitor and statin with review at 3 months

E. Lifestyle advice and calcium channel blocker therapy

5. A 59 year-old woman is found by her GP to have grade 1 hypertension at her clinic appointment. She has a calculated 10-year SCORE of <1% with no significant cardiovascular risk factors.

What is the next most appropriate step in her management?

A. Organize ambulatory blood pressure monitoring

B. Suggest lifestyle advice and commence on drug therapy for hypertension

C. Arrange a period of home blood pressure monitoring

D. Assess for evidence of hypertension-mediated organ damage with an ECG, urinary albumin:creatinine ratio, and fundoscopy before deciding on further management

E. Suggest lifestyle advice

6. You record a blood pressure of 156/86 mmHg in an 82 year-old gentleman who was referred to the general cardiology clinic with an elevated NT pro-BNP. The 12-lead ECG showed LVH by voltage criteria but the transthoracic echocardiogram was normal.

What would you recommend?

A. Check lying and standing blood pressure
B. Ambulatory blood pressure monitoring
C. Lifestyle modification and initiation of low dose calcium channel blocker
D. Referral for cardiac MRI
E. No intervention is required

7. A 63 year-old male attends routine cardiology follow-up. He has a past medical history of ischaemic heart disease, hypertension, and hyperlipidaeamia. His current medical therapy includes aspirin, atorvastatin, bisoprolol and ramipril. He has chronic stable angina but is otherwise well and does not complain of any treatment side effects. His blood pressure is recorded as 134/80 mmHg.

What should his target blood pressure be?

A. <140/90 mmHg
B. 130–139/90 mmHg
C. 130–139/<80 mmHg
D. <130/80 mmHg
E. <120/80 mmHg

8. An 87 year-old lady attends clinic and is diagnosed with hypertension. Her past medical history includes paroxysmal atrial fibrillation for which she takes warfarin and bisoprolol 5 mg once daily.

What should be her target blood pressure after starting anti-hypertensive medication?

A. A systolic BP of 130–139 mmHg with close monitoring for adverse effects
B. A systolic BP of 120–129 mmHg with close monitoring for adverse effects
C. 150–159/90 mmHg
D. 140–149/90 mmHg
E. Patients >80 years of age should not be commenced on treatment primarily for hypertension.

9. A 25 year-old woman with a strong family history of hypertension is found to have grade 2 hypertension after having had a pregnancy complicated by preeclampsia.

Which of the following would not prevent you from using ACE inhibitor therapy to control her blood pressure?

A. She is currently trying to get pregnant again
B. There is a concern she may have fibromuscular dysplasia
C. She is not using reliable contraception
D. Hyperkalaeamia (>5.5 mmol/L)
E. A previous history of angioneurotic oedema.

10. You review a 52 year-old female, lifelong smoker with no significant past medical history in follow-up clinic. The results of her initial ambulatory blood pressure monitor (ABPM) confirmed a mean 24-hour blood pressure of 136/82 mmHg. She subsequently had a 3 month trial of lifestyle modification and clinic blood pressure today is 148/90 mmHg. Bloods revealed an eGFR of 65 ml/min/1.73m^2 and a total cholesterol of 4.3 mmol/L. Urinalysis showed trace proteinuria.

What is the most appropriate next step?

A. A further 3 months of lifestyle modification
B. Ramipril monotherapy
C. Single pill combination therapy with ACEi and calcium channel blocker
D. Repeat the ABPM
E. Bendroflumethiazide monotherapy

11. You review a 70 year-old woman with a clinical diagnosis of angina for which she takes aspirin and GTN as required. She is found to have a clinic blood pressure of 175/100 mmHg with a heart rate of 88 bpm.

What is the most appropriate initial treatment strategy?

A. Initial monotherapy with ACEi or angiotensin receptor blocker
B. Initial combination therapy with ACEi or angiotensin receptor blocker and beta-blocker
C. Outpatient echocardiogram and CTCA with lifestyle modification and review in 3 months
D. Initial combination therapy with ACEi or angiotensin receptor blocker and calcium channel blocker
E. Initial monotherapy with bisoprolol

12. You are asked to review the antihypertensive treatment of a 60 year-old woman with essential hypertension as well as stable angina and chronic kidney disease whose blood pressure remains elevated at 158/88 mmHg despite medical therapy. Her current medications include aspirin 75 mg once daily, simvastatin 40 mg once daily, ramipril 5 mg twice daily, bisoprolol 3.75 mg twice daily, and indapamide 2.5 mg once daily. Her echocardiogram shows mild concentric left ventricular hypertrophy with an ejection fraction of 50%. The most recent blood results are as follows; creatinine 83 umol/L, urea 6.3 mmol/L sodium 139 mmol/L, potassium 5.0 mmol/L, eGFR 58 mmol/L.

What is the most appropriate next step?

A. Addition of spironolactone 25 mg once daily
B. Increase the bisroprolol to 5 mg twice daily
C. Add doxazosin 2 mg once daily
D. Stop the ramipril and after 48 hours commence sacubitril/valsartan 51/49 mg twice daily
E. Addition of amlodipine 5 mg once daily

13. An 80 year-old white man with obesity attends clinic for review of his very difficult to control hypertension. He suffers from sleep apnoea and is taking cyclosporin for rheumatoid arthritis.

Which of the following statements is not true about refractory hypertension?

A. Resistant hypertension is more common in people aged >75 years
B. Cushing's syndrome is an uncommon cause of hypertension
C. White people more commonly suffer with resistant hypertension
D. Cyclosporin can contribute to raised blood pressure
E. Sleep apnoea is a common cause of hypertension

14. A 36 year-old woman is diagnosed with Liddle's syndrome. You review her medical records and blood biochemistry.

What would you not expect to see in someone with Liddle's syndrome?

A. She has a metabolic acidosis
B. She has normal aldosterone levels
C. She has a low plasma renin activity
D. She has hypokalaemia
E. She has severe hypertension

15. A 32 year-old woman develops new onset severe hypertension during pregnancy and requires escalating treatment to gain blood pressure control.

Which of the following is not true?

A. ACE inhibitors, angiotensin receptor blockers, and direct renin inhibitors cannot be used because they are contraindicated during pregnancy
B. The recommended treatment for hypertensive crisis is intravenous hydralazine
C. First-line therapy for severe hypertension includes oral methyldopa or nifedipine
D. A systolic blood pressure of >/= 170 mmHg or diastolic blood pressure of >/= 110 mmHg in a pregnant woman is an emergency and admission to hospital is recommended
E. The mother's choice of feeding post-natally needs to be considered as all antihypertensive medications taken by the breast feeding mother are excreted into breast milk.

16. A 44 year-old black Afro-Caribbean man has been newly diagnosed with hypertension and sees you in clinic to get further advice about which medication they should start on.

Which advice is not correct?

A. A greater blood pressure reduction tends to be seen with thiazide diuretics than RAS-blocker monotherapy in black patients
B. Angiotensin receptor blockers are preferred to ACE inhibitors in black patients due to the increased risk of angioedema
C. Although hypertension is more common in white European people than in Afro-Caribbean people, treatment resistance is more common in black people.
D. Salt restriction leads to a greater reduction in blood pressure in black patients
E. Black hypertensive patients see a similar reduction in cardiovascular and renal events in response to BP-lowering treatment to white patients

17. A 69 year-old male with a prior history of hypertension presents with a transient ischaemic attack. On arrival his blood pressure is 184/110 mmHg. His current medication includes amlodipine 10 mg od.

Which is the most appropriate next step?

A. Commence intravenous labetalol to achieve a 15% reduction in blood pressure over the first 24 hours
B. Perform fundoscopy, urinalysis, ECG, and transthoracic echocardiography
C. Target a long-term blood pressure of <140/80 mmHg
D. Antiplatelet therapy should be withheld until the blood pressure is better controlled
E. Restart his antihypertensive therapy immediately, make the addition of a RAS blocker and target a systolic blood pressure of 120–130 mmHg.

18. Mr Jones is a 57 year-old gentleman who has been referred to the cardiology clinic for assessment of palpitations. He has a history of type 2 diabetes on oral therapy, hyperlipidaemia, and peripheral vascular disease with previous femoral-popliteal bypass grafting. Serial blood pressure recordings demonstrate a mean clinic blood pressure of 168/102 mmHg and routine clinical examination is normal. His resting ECG is unremarkable.

Which of the following investigations is least relevant in this patient's management?

A. Ultrasound of the carotid arteries
B. Measurement of serum creatinine and eGFR
C. Urine albumin:creatinine ratio
D. Transthoracic echocardiography
E. Fundoscopy

19. A 68 year-old man with newly diagnosed type 2 diabetes and hypertension attends your clinic because his blood pressure does not appear to be responding to medication. He would like some further advice about what level of blood pressure he should be trying to achieve.

Which of the following pieces of advice is not correct?

A. Achieving a systolic blood pressure of <135 mmHg as compared with ~140 mmHg has been demonstrated to reduce cardiovascular and all-cause mortality
B. A lower target blood pressure of <130/80 mmHg has not been demonstrated to correspond with any further reduction in cardiovascular events or stroke
C. In patients over the age of 65 years the target systolic blood pressure is 130 to 140mmHg.
D. Variation in visit-to-visit blood pressure should be given attention as this is associated with increased risk of cardiovascular and renal disease
E. Diabetic patients are at higher risk of multi-drug resistant hypertension.

20. A 30 year-old woman is found to be hypertensive during a health check while taking the oral contraceptive. She has been investigated for secondary causes including a normal echo and scan of the aorta, as well as endocrine investigations, and has a normal BMI. She is still worried she may have a secondary cause for hypertension and would like some more information about why she has developed hypertension and her risk of future disease.

What information would be incorrect to give to the patient?

A. Around 5% of women will develop hypertension whilst taking oestrogen containing oral contraceptive pills
B. Cardiovascular risk is often underestimated in younger patients with hypertension
C. The prevalence of secondary hypertension is only 10% in young people
D. Obstructive sleep apnoea can be present in patients with a normal BMI
E. In young adults aortic coarctation can be difficult to identify because changes in the aorta alter the typical Doppler characteristics

21. You are asked for an opinion on a 58 year-old Afro-Caribbean man who on serial office blood pressure measurements has a mean blood pressure of 154/102 mmHg. He is overweight with a BMI of 32 kg/m^2, drinks 20 units of alcohol per week, and has diet-controlled type 2 diabetes. ECG is normal and urine dipstick is negative.

What management would you suggest?

A. Lifestyle advice with particular attention to salt restriction
B. Lifestyle advice plus initiation of pharmacological therapy with a calcium channel blocker and angiotensin receptor blocker.
C. Lifestyle advice plus initiation of pharmacological therapy with a calcium channel blocker and ACE inhibitor.
D. Lifestyle advice plus initiation of pharmacological therapy with a calcium channel blocker.
E. Lifestyle advice plus initiation of pharmacological therapy with a calcium channel blocker and a thiazide diuretic.

22. A 78 year-old lady with a past history of ischaemic heart disease, chronic obstructive pulmonary disease (COPD) and heart failure attends the outpatient clinic. On examination her heart rate is 68 bpm, Sp0$_2$ 95% on room air and blood pressure is 142/88 mmHg. She is clinically euvolaemic. ECG shows sinus rhythm with left ventricular hypertrophy and echocardiogram demonstrated an ejection fraction of 43% with moderate calcific aortic stenosis (AVA 1.2 cm^2). Current medical therapy includes aspirin 75 mg once daily, atorvastatin 80 mg at night, Ramipril 5 mg twice daily and furosemide 40 mg once daily.

In addition to lifestyle advice, what is the most appropriate next step in her management?

A. Addition of spironolactone 25 mg once daily
B. Stop ramipril and add doxazosin aiming for a target BP <140/90 mmHg
C. Commence bisoprolol 2.5 mg once daily and up-titrate to maximum tolerated dose.
D. Add doxazosin aiming for a target BP <140/80 mmHg
E. Increase furosemide to 80 mg once daily

23. You review a 60 year-old Afro-Caribbean woman with a mean 24-hour blood pressure of 136/80 mmHg. She is morbidly obese and has insulin dependent type 2 diabetes with proteinuria. Resting 12-lead electrocardiogram shows LVH by voltage criteria. Her current medical therapy includes amlodipine 10 mg once daily, metformin 1 g twice daily and insulin.

What is the next appropriate step in her management?

A. Lifestyle advice and repeat ambulatory blood pressure monitor in 3–6 months
B. Lifestyle advice and addition of a bendroflumethiazide
C. Lifestyle advice and addition of spironolactone
D. Lifestyle advice and addition of angiotensin receptor blocker
E. Lifestyle advice and addition of bisoprolol and bendroflumethizide in a single-pill combination.

24. You are called by the orthopaedic foundation year doctor about a 66 year-old man who is due to have a hip replacement the following day. He has recently been diagnosed by his GP with hypertension and was commenced on amlodipine and perindopril. He also takes regular propranolol for an essential tremor which was discontinued on admission due to first-degree heart block and left axis deviation. Evening observations demonstrated a blood pressure of 162/98 mmHg. He is overweight with a BMI of 36 kg/m^2 and in addition to hypertension has a history of diabetes.

What would you tell them with regards to the management of his hypertension?

A. His operation does not need to be cancelled because of the hypertension
B. The beta-blocker should be recommenced.
C. The anaesthetist may consider suspending his perindopril
D. They should ensure he is screened for hypertension mediated organ damage to assess his cardiovascular risk pre-operatively
E. All of the above

chapter 7.3

ARTERIAL HYPERTENSION

ANSWERS

1. B. Blood pressure measurements should be made with the patient sitting comfortably for at least 5 minutes in a quiet environment. The cuff should be positioned at the level of the heart with the back and arm supported to avoid muscle contraction. The blood pressure should be recorded on three occasions 1–2 minutes apart (further measurements should only be made if there is >10 mmHg variation between readings) and the average of the last two readings recorded.

The ESC classification of blood pressure is recorded in Table 7.3.A1:

Table 7.3.A1

Category	Systolic (mmHg)		Diastolic (mmHg)
Optimal	<120	and	<80
Normal	120–129	and/or	80–84
High Normal	130–139	and/or	85–89
Grade 1 Hypertension	140–159	and/or	90–99
Grade 2 Hypertension	160–179	and/or	100–109
Grade 3 Hypertension	>180	and/or	>110
Isolated systolic hypertension	>140	and	<90

2. D. The ESC definitions of hypertension, depending on the setting in which they are recorded, are listed in Table 7.3.A2. Levels should be greater than these thresholds to make a diagnosis of hypertension. Expected levels averaged over 24 hours are lower than expected levels during daytime or on office measures. Therefore the high systolic recorded in answer D exceeds thresholds for diagnosis.

Table 7.3.A2

Category	SBP (mmHg)		DBP (mmHg)
Office BP	>140	and/or	>90
Ambulatory BP:			
Daytime (or awake) mean	>135	and/or	>85
Night-time (or asleep) mean	>120	and/or	>70
24hr mean	>130	and/or	>80
Home BP mean	>135	and/or	>85

Box 7.3.A1 Clinical indications for home blood pressure monitoring or ambulatory blood pressure monitoring

Considerations in which white-coat hypertension is more common, e.g.
- Grade 1 hypertension on office BP measurement
- Marked office BP elevation without HMOD

Conditions in which masked hypertension is more common, e.g.:
- High-normal office BP
- Normal office BP in individuals with HMOD or at very high total CV risk

Postural and post-prandial hypotension in untreated and treated patients

Evaluation of resistant hypertension

Evaluation of BP control, especially in treated higher-risk patients

Exaggerated BP response to exercise

When there is considerable variability in the office BP

Evaluating symptoms consistent with hypotension during treatment

Specific indications for ABPM rather than HBPM:
- Assessment of nocturnal BP values and dipping status (e.g. suspicion of nocturnal hypertension, such as in sleep apnoea, CKD, diabetes, endocrine hypertension, or autoimmune dysfunction)

3. C. The ESC indications for ambulatory or home blood pressure monitoring are listed in Box 7.3.A1. For the patient in this question, ABPM could be used to determine whether there is nocturnal hypertension related to obstructive sleep apnoea, but hypotension would not be expected. The patient already has a diagnosis of hypertension so it is not required to diagnose hypertension or establish whether she has 'white coat' hypertension. As the patient is only on one medication, by definition, she does not yet have resistant hypertension. Therefore the correct answer is C as her presenting problem is dizziness while on treatment for hypertension.

4. C. This gentleman is in the very high-risk group and has grade 1 hypertension with evidence of LVH on resting ECG and therefore requires drug therapy in addition to lifestyle intervention. Given his ethnicity, history of diabetes, and LVH on ECG an ARB is the most appropriate choice.

5. E. In patients such as this who present with grade 1 hypertension and are at low to moderate risk lifestyle advice is advised initially. If the patient remains hypertensive after a period of lifestyle intervention BP-lowering drug treatment is recommended. In higher risk patients, or patients with hypertensive mediated organ damage, with grade 1 hypertension, and all patients with grade 2 or 3 hypertension, drug therapy should be initiated simultaneously with lifestyle interventions, regardless of CV risk. In patients with high-normal blood pressure, drug treatment may be considered when the cardiovascular risk is very high.

6. E. Current ESC guidelines advise that no further action is needed in patients aged >80 years with isolated systolic blood pressure elevation less than 160 mmHg and no other compelling indication for antihypertensive therapy. If treatment is required then it may be appropriate to initiate monotherapy, or combination therapy at the lowest possible dose with very careful monitoring for side effects. A target blood pressure of 130–139/<80 mmHg is reasonable so long as therapy is well tolerated. A summary of office blood pressure thresholds for treatment is in Table 7.3.A3:

Table 7.3.A3

Age group	Office SBP treatment threshold (mmHg)					Office DBP treatment threshold (mmHg)
	Hypertension	+ Diabetes	+ CKD	+ CAD	+Stroke/TIA	
18–65 years	≥140	≥140	≥140	≥140	≥140	≥90
65–79 years	≥140	≥140	≥140	≥140	≥140	≥90
>80 years	≥160	≥160	≥160	≥160	≥160	≥90
Office DBP treatment threshold (mmHg)	≥90	≥90	≥90	≥90	≥90	

7. D. Office blood pressure targets in hypertensive patients:

- The first objective of treatment should be to lower BP to <140/90 mmHg and provided treatment is well tolerated BP values should be targeted to 130/80 mmHg or lower in most patients
- In patients <65 years old receiving BP lowering drugs, it is recommended that SBP should be lowered to a BP range of 120–129 mmHg in most patients.
- In older patients (>65 years old) receiving BP-lowering drugs:
- It is recommended that SBP should be targeted to a BP range of 130–139 mmHg
- Close monitoring of adverse effects is recommended
- These BP targets are recommended for patients at any level of CV risk and in patients with and without established CVD

A DBP target of <80 mmHg should be considered for all hypertensive patients, independent of the level of risk and comorbidities.

8. A. According to the ESC guidelines, BP lowering medications and lifestyle advice should be offered to fit older patients (including those >80 years old) when systolic blood pressure is over 160 mmHg. A systolic BP of 130–139 mmHg should be targeted with close monitoring for adverse effects regardless of the level of cardiovascular risk.

9. C. A list of potential contraindications to the use of specific antihypertensive drugs is listed in Table 7.3.A4. If she is not planning a pregnancy then personal choice of contraceptive does not exclude use of ACE inhibitors although she should be advised to seek medical advice about stopping the ACE inhibitor, and finding an alternative antihypertensive, if she unexpectedly becomes pregnant.

Table 7.3.A4

Drug	Contraindications	
	Compelling	Possible
Diuretics (thiazides/ thiazide-like, e.g. chlorthalidone and indapamide	- Gout	- Metabolic syndrome - Glucose intolerance - Pregnancy - Hypercalcaemia - Hypokalaemia

Table 7.3.A4 Continued

Drug	**Contraindications**	
	Compelling	**Possible**
Beta-blockers	- Asthma - Any high-grade sinoatrial or atrioventricular block - Bradycardia (heart rate <60bpm)	- Metabolic syndrome - Glucose intolerance - Athletes and physically active patients
Calcium antagonists (dihydropyridines)		- Tachyarrhythmias - Heart failure (HFrEF, class III/IV) - Pre-existing severe leg oedema
Calcium antagonists (verapamil, diltiazem)	- Any high-GRADE sinoatrial or atrioventricular block - Severe LV dysfunction (EF < 40%) - Bradycardia (heart rate <60 bpm)	- Constipation
ACE inhibitors	- Pregnancy - Previous angioneurotic oedema - Hyperkalaemia (potassium >5.5 mmol/L) - Bilateral renal artery stenosis	- Women of child-bearing potential without reliable contraception
Angiotensin receptor blockers		- Women of child-bearing potential without reliable contraception

10. B. This lady has grade 1 hypertension on clinic BP measurement and confirmed with ABPM. There is no evidence that the BP has improved with a reasonable period of lifestyle modification and so it is appropriate to initiate medical therapy. Given her 10-year SCORE risk is <1% (low-risk European countries chart) and Grade 1 hypertension with BP <150 mmHg systolic she should be started on monotherapy. Given the mildly reduced eGFR and trace proteinuria ACEi should be used in preference to thiazide diuretics.

11. B. The suggested treatment algorithm (ESC) for patients with hypertension and coronary artery disease is shown in Figure 7.3.A1:

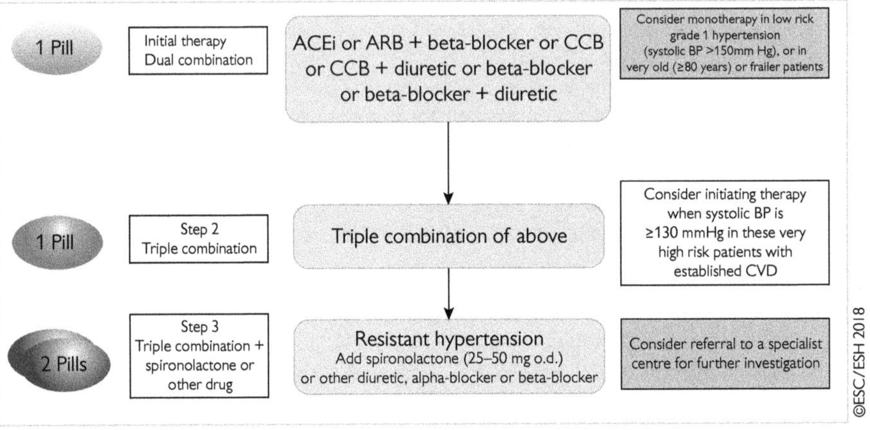

Figure 7.3.A1

Reproduced from Williams B, Mancia G, Spiering W, et al; ESC Scientific Document Group. 2018 ESC/ESH Guidelines for the management of arterial hypertension. Eur Heart J. 2018 Sep 1;39(33):3021–3104. doi: 10.1093/eurheartj/ehy339. © European Society of Cardiology. With permission from Oxford University Press.

12. E. This lady has resistant hypertension and underlying coronary disease. She is already on triple therapy with an ACEi, beta-blocker, and indapamide. Given that she is already on a diuretic, does not have another indication for spironolactone, and already has a potassium result at the upper limit of normal, addition of a calcium channel blocker is the most appropriate next step.

13. C. Refractory hypertension is much more common in black people, as well as older people and those with obesity, excess dietary sodium intake, high baseline blood pressure, and concomitant disease including diabetes, atherosclerotic vascular disease, and aortic stiffening. Cushing's disease as an underlying cause for his obesity leading to hypertension is uncommon, as are phaeochromocytoma, fibromuscular dysplasia, aortic coarctation, and hyperparathyroidism. Primary hyperaldosteronism, sleep apnoea, and CKD are more common secondary causes. A number of drugs and substances can also contribute to hypertension. These include oral contraceptives, decongenstants, NSAIDs, cyclosporin, erythropoietin, excessive liquorice, steroids, cocaine, and amphetamines.

14. A. Liddle's syndrome is a genetic disorder with autosomal dominant inheritance that is characterized by early, and frequently severe, high blood pressure associated with low plasma renin activity, metabolic alkalosis, low blood potassium, and normal to low levels of aldosterone. It typically responds well to treatment with a low sodium diet and potassium sparing diuretics such as amiloride.

15. B. Intravenous hydralazine is no longer the drug of choice as it is associated with more perinatal adverse effects than other drugs. Where necessary ACE inhibitors, angiotensin receptor blockers, and direct renin inhibitors can be used to control blood pressure. Most antihypertensive medications are excreted into breast milk at very low concentrations except for propranolol and nifedipine which have breast milk concentrations similar to those in maternal plasma.

16. C. Hypertension is both more common and more resistant to treatment in black populations. ACEi and ARBs are less effective in black populations and are associated with a higher rate of angioedema. There tends to be a better response to treatment with thiazide-like diuretics and calcium-channel blockers.

17. E. Multiple meta-analyses have demonstrated that ischaemic stroke is the one major CV event that is reduced with lower achieved BP levels. For this reason the ESC suggest a target blood pressure range of 120–130 mmHg in patients with prior ischaemic stroke/TIA. Antihypertensive medication should be recommenced immediately for patients with TIA and after several days in acute stroke. Patients receiving thrombolysis should have BP lowered to <180/105 mmHg for at least 24 hours after thrombolysis; however, BP lowering early after acute ischaemic stroke in patients not undergoing thrombolysis showed a neutral effect on the prevention of death or dependency. A reasonable goal in those with a BP >220/120 mmHg may be to reduce BP by 15% during the first 24 hours.

18. D. Measurement of renal function and eGFR, urine albumin:creatinine ratio, and ECG is recommended in all patients with hypertension. Fundoscopy should be performed in diabetic patients or those with grade II/III hypertension. Ultrasound of the carotid arteries may be considered in patients with documented evidence of vascular disease, but echocardiography is only recommended routinely when the resting ECG is abnormal or when the detection of LVH will alter the treatment strategy. Additionally renal ultrasound should be considered where there is evidence of chronic kidney, albuminuria, or suspected secondary hypertension. Neuroimaging should be considered if there is evidence of cognitive decline or other neurological symptoms to detect brain infarctions, microbleeds, and white matter lesions.

19. B. The ADVANCE trial demonstrated a significant reduction in cardiovascular and all-cause mortality when a systolic blood pressure of <135 mmHg was achieved as opposed to ~140 mmHg. The ACCORD trial showed an overall reduction in CV events with intensive systolic blood pressure lowering to <130 mmHg, whilst the ONTARGET study demonstrated an incremental reduction in stroke risk with lower blood pressure. ONTARGET also found better CV protection was associated with less visit-to-visit variation in blood pressure.

20. E. Around 5% of women do develop hypertension while taking oestrogen-containing oral contraceptive pills and obstructive sleep apnoea can be present in those with a normal BMI. A secondary cause of hypertension is present in around 10% of patients under 50 year of age with hypertension but is more common in those with severe hypertension. Cardiovascular risk is underestimated in younger patients. However, although the diastolic tail on Doppler measures can disappear with aortic stiffening, this only becomes a problem in older adults when the stiffening is more marked.

21. E. This gentleman has grade 2 hypertension and is at high risk given his history of diabetes. Lifestyle advice is clearly important and salt restriction is of particular benefit in people of Afro-Caribbean descent; however, given his BP values and his risk profile, he should also be commenced on pharmacological therapy. Black patients tend to show a reduced response to RAS-blocker monotherapy, and additionally angioedema is more common with ACEi therapy. Conversely there is often a better response to calcium channel blockers and thiazide diuretics. For this reason the ESC guidelines advocate initial two-drug combination therapy, preferably with a single-pill combination.

22. C. This lady has heart failure with reduced ejection fraction and so, regardless of blood pressure, should be on a beta-blocker, which should be titrated to the maximum tolerated dose. The presence of COPD should not be used as a contraindication unless there is known intolerance in which case a more cardioselective beta-blocker may be considered. Aortic stenosis is not a contraindication to the use of ACE inhibitors.

23. D. Although there is often a better blood pressure response to thiazide diuretics in Afro-Caribbean people, in this case the presence of significant diabetic nephropathy with proteinuria warrants the addition of a RAS-blocker.

24. E. Non-cardiac surgery need not be deferred because of grade 1 or 2 hypertension, but deferral should be considered if the blood pressure is >180/110 mmHg and the surgery is not an emergency. Abrupt discontinuation of beta-blockers should be avoided as it may result in blood pressure or heart rate rebounds, which may be harmful. A recent prospective study demonstrated a significant reduction in cardiovascular events in patient who had peri-operative discontinuation of RAS-blockade awaiting non-cardiac surgery. Hypertensive patients should be screened for hypertension-mediated organ damage prior to non-cardiac surgery in order to assess and plan for their cardiovascular risk.

chapter

7.4

DIABETES

QUESTIONS

1. **A 55-year-old woman reported 6 months history of polydipsia and polyuria. You suspect this patient has diabetes.**

   Which of the following investigation would help you to confirm the diagnosis of diabetes mellitus?

   A. An HbA1c of 43 mmol/mol
   B. A fasting plasma glucose of 6.8 mmol/L
   C. A 2-hour glucose value of 12.0 mmol/L following an oral glucose tolerance test
   D. A random plasma glucose value of 9.3 mmol/L in the absence of relevant symptoms
   E. None of the above

2. **Your patient wants to know if he should have an oral glucose tolerance test to find out if he has diabetes.**

   Which of the following can you tell him?

   A. It is the most widely used test for the diagnosis of diabetes
   B. It remains the gold standard test for the diagnosis of diabetes, but it is laborious
   C. A 2-hour glucose value of 10.2 mmol/L confirms the diagnosis of diabetes according to the WHO criteria
   D. A 2-hour glucose value of 7.5 mmol/L confirms impaired glucose tolerance according to the WHO criteria
   E. None of the above

3. **Your patient is diagnosed with type 1 diabetes at the age of 35 years old.**

   What can you tell him regarding his new diagnosis?

   A. Type 1 diabetes only occurs in patients below the age of <60 years
   B. It accounts for approximately a quarter of all diabetes in the UK
   C. It is characterized by failure of the pancreatic beta cells
   D. In certain cases, measurement of autoantibodies such as glutamic acid decarboxylase (GAD) can be useful in differential diagnosis with other types of diabetes
   E. It can sometimes be treated with oral hypoglycaemic agents alone

4. A 44-year-old man has taken part in a healthy volunteer research study and has been found to have raised glucose levels 10 mins after having eaten a meal and he has relatively low insulin levels. Based on what you know about insulin secretion which of the following statements might be relevant to his post-prandial hyperglycaemia?

A. As insulin release is monophasic, this suggests he is going to be hyperglycaemic throughout the day
B. This indicates a problem with first phase insulin release as this typically controls glucose levels for 3–4 hours after a meal
C. This suggests he has a problem with second phase insulin release as the first phase controls background insulin levels
D. The stages of insulin release are only affected in patients with type 1 diabetes so this patient should start treatment for type 1 diabetes
E. Reduced first phase insulin release may be an early sign of type 2 diabetes

5. A 35-year-old patient was concerned about his recent diagnosis of type 2 diabetes mellitus.

What can you tell him?

A. Insulin deficiency and pancreatic beta-cell dysfunction are the cardinal features
B. There is a steady trend towards an onset at younger age
C. It is of autoimmune origin
D. It accounts for approximately 75% of all diabetes in the UK
E. The International Diabetes Federation predicts a small reduction in prevalence of type 2 diabetes by 2030

6. A 58-year-old patient has had type 2 diabetes for 20 years and has background diabetic retinopathy, and more recently reported intermittent numbness in his toes. You are trying to explain microvascular complications of diabetes to him with one of the following:

A. Their severity is not related to the glycaemic control
B. They have an earlier onset compared to macrovascular complications
C. Their clinical manifestation may not be apparent until frank diabetes appears
D. The triad of retinopathy, nephropathy, and neuropathy is often seen in other conditions apart from diabetes
E. The direct glucose-mediated endothelial damage is the only causative mechanism

7. A 27-year-old patient with type 1 diabetes attended annual retinal screening and was told he has background diabetic retinopathy.

What can you advise him to help delay and/or prevent deterioration of his retinopathy?

A. It is an uncommon cause of visual loss in working-age adults in the developed world
B. The existing treatments can cure the disease
C. Once diabetic retinopathy has been established, glycaemic control cannot delay its progression
D. Routine screening for diabetic retinopathy is offered only to patients with type 1 diabetes due to longer exposure to the disease
E. Smoking and hyperlipidaemia are important risk factors for the condition

8. A 66-year-old patient has had type 2 diabetes for 30 years and is worried about developing diabetic nephropathy.

What can you advise him?

A. It can only be diagnosed in the presence of macroalbuminuria
B. Good glycaemic control helps delay diabetic nephropathy progression
C. It is an uncommon cause for end-stage renal failure (ESRF) in the UK
D. The identification of microalbuminuria should prompt clinicians to manage aggressively all cardiovascular risk factors
E. Beta-blockers are the first line treatment for management of hypertension and albuminuria in people with diabetes

9. A 27-year-old patient had type 1 diabetes for 15 years and reported tingling, numbness, and intermittent pain in his toes. You think he has diabetic neuropathy.

What can you tell him?

A. The most common form is a proximal sensory neuropathy
B. The neuropathic pain typically responds to simple analgesia
C. Autonomic dysfunction is not a manifestation of diabetic neuropathy
D. It is always symptomatic
E. Multidisciplinary team input is often required

10. A 45-year-old woman has been newly diagnosed with diabetes and is concerned about her risk of cardiovascular disease.

Which of the following is true?

A. About 25% of the mortality in people with diabetes is related to cardiovascular disease
B. About 60% of patients with type 2 diabetes are either overweight or obese
C. The release of free fatty acids from adipose tissue impairs insulin sensitivity results in hyperinsulinaemia
D. Free fatty acids-induced impairment of the PI3K pathway results in increased production of nitric oxide that predicts increased CVD
E. Ventricular dysfunction in patients with type 2 diabetes is always associated with coronary atherosclerosis

11. A 65-year-old patient with type 2 diabetes and no previous cardiovascular disease developed cardiomyopathy.

Which of the following is true?

A. It is associated with coronary atherosclerosis and hypertension
B. Impairment of the PI3K/Akt pathway plays a key role in cardiac dysfunction in type 2 diabetes
C. Hyperglycaemia does not seem to directly affect the myocardial contractility
D. Thiazolidinediones are the first-line treatment for the condition
E. Interstitial fibrosis is an unusual feature of the condition

12. A 45-year-old woman has been newly diagnosed with diabetes and wants to understand what evidence there is that glucose control is going to be important for her long-term health. You explain there have been several landmark studies that have shaped our understanding of diabetes and its related complications including the Diabetes Control and Complications Trial (DCCT) and the United Kingdom Prospective Diabetes Study (UKPDS) are landmark trials.

Which of the following would be correct to tell her about the findings from these trials?

A. Early glucose control is important (metabolic memory)
B. Intensive glycaemic control reduces the long-term microvascular complications, but not the macrovascular ones
C. Tighter glycaemic control is not clearly associated with improved microvascular outcomes
D. Intensive treatment does not affect the outcomes of progression of retinopathy
E. The increased cost of intensive diabetes management outweighs the financial benefits of reduction in diabetes-related complications

13. Your 67-year-old patient was recently started on metformin (biguanide) to manage his type 2 diabetes.

What can you tell him about metformin?

A. It is often associated with hypoglycaemia
B. It should be discontinued if the e-GFR drops below 45 ml/min/1.73m^2
C. Its mode of action is by release of insulin (insulin provider)
D. It is associated with an increase in cardiovascular events
E. It can be associated with mild weight loss in most cases

14. You are considering sulfonylureas for your 72-year-old patient with type 2 diabetes.

Which of the following is true?

A. They are insulin sensitizers
B. The newer agents, like gliclazide, are associated with increased cardiovascular risk
C. They often cause mild weight gain
D. They cannot be used in addition to metformin
E. They do not cause hypoglycaemia

15. Your 54-year-old patient heard about a new diabetes medication, glucagon-like peptide 1 (GLP-1) agonists (exenatide, liraglutide, albiglutide) but is worried about potential side effects.

What can you tell him?

A. Their commonest side effect is lactic acidosis
B. They usually cause weight gain
C. They often cause hypoglycaemia
D. They are linked with an increase in the risk of cardiovascular disease
E. They can cause arrhythmias

16. Your 54-year-old patient has been started on a sodium-glucose co-transporter-2 (SGLT-2) inhibitor and would like to understand why there are cardiac benefits associated with their use of in patients with diabetes.

What is the possible mechanism?

A. Their mode of action is through inhibition of glucose absorption in the bowel
B. They are associated with preload reduction due to diuresis
C. They are associated with a paradoxical rise in the blood pressure
D. Their commonest side effect is lower respiratory tract infections
E. They often cause hypoglycaemia

17. A 68-year-old man with diabetes has recently been found to have elevated cholesterol levels despite treatment.

According to the guidelines of the European Society of Cardiology on the management of cardiovascular disease in diabetes (2023), which of the following statements regarding hyperlipidaemia and diabetes is true?

A. The aim should be to keep LDL <4.0 mmol/l
B. Fibrates are usually the first-line treatment given the beneficial effect on retinopathy as well
C. In very high-risk patients the target is to achieve a LDL of <1.4 mmol/l
D. In patients with documented cardiovascular disease by invasive testing, the target is to achieve a LDL of <1.8 mmol/l
E. Ezetimibe is contraindicated in patients with diabetes

18. A 35-year-old patient weighs 120 kg, BMI 35kg/m^2, had been asked to aim for a modest weight loss (5% of body weight) in the first instance at the diabetes clinic. He is worried 5% is too little and asks for your advice.

Which of the following is true?

A. It is not clinically significant
B. It is associated with reduction in HbA1c but not in blood pressure
C. It is associated with a 5 mmHg reduction in systolic blood pressure and neutral effect on diastolic blood pressure
D. It does not affect the rate of progression to diabetes from impaired glucose tolerance
E. It is associated with a clinically significant reduction in triglycerides

19. A 30-year-old man with diabetes with a BMI of 55 kg/m^2 is keen to consider bariatric surgery to achieve weight loss. Choose a correct statement from below to advise him.

A. Most of the patients have regained their pre-operative body weight at 10-year follow-up
B. There is resolution of diabetes in a small proportion of patients following successful bariatric surgery
C. The overall mortality is not affected
D. The antidiabetic effect is sustained even up to 15 years
E. Consensus guidelines suggest bariatric surgery is indicated for any patients with a BMI over 25 and type 2 diabetes

20. Your 73-year-old patient has diabetes and had a myocardial infarction 5 years ago.

She researched anti-platelet therapy for people with diabetes, and asked if any of the following statements is true?

A. Primary prevention with aspirin 75 mg once daily is recommended in all adults >40 years old with diabetes
B. Dual anti-platelet therapy with aspirin and clopidogrel is recommended in adults with diabetes and microalbuminuria
C. Post-prandial hyperglycaemia has been shown to cause platelet activation
D. Platelet activation plays a key role in atherothrombosis only towards late phases of type 2 diabetes
E. Fasting and persistent hyperglycaemia is unrelated to platelet activation

21. A GP colleague contacted you for advice on blood pressure treatment in diabetes patients. Advise him with one of the following:

A. The treatment target is to lower SBP to less than 130 mmHg in all patients with diabetes
B. Beta-blockers are the first-line treatment for patients with diabetes and hypertension
C. In patients with diabetes and chronic kidney disease, a SBP <130 mmHg is desirable if tolerated
D. The angiotensin receptor blockers should be avoided in patients with diabetes
E. Blood pressure control does not affect the rate of progression of diabetic retinopathy

22. A 67-year-old retired GP with type 1 diabetes attends your clinic wanting to know her cardiovascular risk and how to use QRISK3 cardiovascular assessment tool and the scores.

Which of the following is true?

A. It can be used in patients with type 1 diabetes to assess cardiovascular risk
B. It can be routinely used for monitoring of treatment of patients with established cardiovascular disease
C. It should be avoided in patients with familial hypercholesterolaemia
D. A QRISK3 of 5 (5% risk of CVD event over the next 10 years) indicates that primary prevention with lipid lowering therapy should be considered
E. A QRISK3 over 20 (20% risk of CVD event over the next 10 years) indicates that primary prevention with dual-lipid-lowering therapy (such as statin and ezetimibe) should be considered

23. A 66-year-old woman with diabetes develops severe chronic kidney disease.

Which of the following statements about diabetes and severe chronic kidney disease with eGFR <30 ml/min/1.73m^2 is false?

A. The metformin should be discontinued
B. The ACE-inhibitor should be discontinued
C. The treatment target for lipid control should be for a LDL <1.8 mmol/l
D. Albuminuria is a driver for ongoing renal damage in these patients
E. A significant proportion of these patients will require renal replacement therapy

24. A 58-year-old woman with type 2 diabetes has recently been diagnosed with heart failure.

How would you optimize her anti-diabetic medication?

A. Newer agents of sulfonylureas (such as gliclazide) have been shown to increase risk for heart failure
B. Sodium-glucose co-transporter-2 (SGLT-2) inhibitors increase the preload and the risk of heart failure
C. In patients who developed heart failure, saxagliptin, and alogliptin should be stopped for monitoring
D. Pioglitazone should be continued in a patient admitted to the hospital with acute heart failure
E. Treatment with metformin is associated with heart failure

25. Your 67-year-old patient has recently heard that new NICE guidelines have been releases for management of people with type 2 diabetes. He attends your clinic to discuss what might need to change in his care.

What would be correct to tell him from the list below?

A. The general treatment target should be an HbA1c of 48–52

B. Treatment with oral hypoglycaemic agents can be intensified to a maximum of two agents at the same time

C. Failure to achieve an HbA1c of 53 on two oral hypoglycaemic agents is an indication for insulin treatment in all cases

D. Individualized approach is recommended

E. All patients with type 2 diabetes should be followed up in secondary care

chapter 7.4

DIABETES

ANSWERS

1. C. Diagnosis of diabetes mellitus is defined by guidelines from WHO and ADA with one of the following criteria: HbA1c>48, fasting blood glucose ≥7 mmol/L, random blood glucose ≥11.1 mmol/L with symptoms, or positive oral glucose tolerance test. In this question, only C fits the criteria.

2. B. The trick of answering this question is to remember the diagnostic criteria (listed in explanation for question 1). Based on the criteria, we can exclude answer C and D. The oral glucose tolerance test takes 2 hours, is laborious, and practically difficult for wide used. Therefore, the correct answer is B.

3. D. Type 1 diabetes is characterized by insulin deficiency due to destruction of pancreatic beta-cells and treated by lifelong insulin injection. Typically, it occurs in younger people, but a small proportion of people develop type 1 diabetes later on in life. It accounts for up to 10% of the total population of people who have diabetes in the UK. The presence of autoantibodies, such as GAD and ZnT8, can be useful to differentiate type 1 diabetes and other types of diabetes.

4. E. Insulin secretion is biphasic, with an immediate first phase release after eating lasting about 10 minutes followed by a sustained release of insulin in the second phase that reaches a steady state at 2–3 hours. Reduced first phase insulin release may be the earliest detectable beta-cell defect predicting onset of type 2 diabetes with the main clinical manifestation in post-prandial hyperglycaemia.

5. B. Type 2 diabetes is characterized by a combination of insulin resistance and progressive beta-cell failure and accounts for up to 90% of the all patients of diabetes in the UK. It is not autoimmune in nature. Insulin deficiency is the cardinal feature of type 1 diabetes. With increasing global obesity affecting children and those under the age of 40, there is a steady tread towards type 2 diabetes onset at much younger age. The international diabetes federation predicts an increase in prevalence of type 2 diabetes by 2030.

6. B. The microvascular triad of retinopathy, nephropathy, and neuropathy is unique to diabetes. Landmark clinical trials have established a clear relationship between microvascular disease and glucose control. Direct glucose-mediated endothelial damage is one of the mechanisms that chronic hyperglycaemia leads to organ dysfunction. Individuals with hyperglycaemia and insulin resistance may show microvascular damages before frank diabetes.

7. E. Diabetic retinopathy is one of the commonest causes of visual loss in working-age adults in the UK and the developed world. Good glycaemic control delays the presentation and slows down the progression of diabetic retinopathy but does not cure the disease. Routine retinal screening in the UK is offered to people with all type of diabetes. DM duration, glycaemic control, blood pressure, and lipid management and smoking are the strongest risk factors for its development and progression.

8. B. Diabetic nephropathy is diagnosed with the presence of microalbuminuria. The identification of microalbuminuria should prompt clinicians to manage all CV risk factors aggressively. Good controls in blood glucose and hypertension are part of the treatments to delay disease progression. ACE-inhibitors and angiotensin receptor blockers are preferred first-line treatment for management of hypertension and albuminuria in patients with diabetes.

9. E. The most common form of diabetic neuropathy is a distal, symmetrical sensorimotor neuropathy and can be asymptomatic in up to 50% of patients. It includes a wide range of clinical syndromes including autonomic dysfunction. Neuropathic pain is extremely common and difficult to treat and often does not respond to simple analgesia. Multidisciplinary team input is often required.

10. C. Diabetes doubles the age-adjusted risk for CVD in men and triples it in women. Between 80–90% of patients with type 2 diabetes are either overweight or obese. The release of free fatty acids and cytokines from adipose tissue impairs insulin sensitivity leading to hyper-insulinaemia and hyperglycaemia. Free-fatty-acid-induced impairment of the PI3K pathway results in decreased production of nitric oxide which is an important predictor of CVD development. Ventricular dysfunction in patients with type 2 diabetes maybe associated with diabetic cardiomyopathy in the case of coronary atherosclerosis and hypertension.

11. B. The diagnosis for this patient is diabetic cardiomyopathy. Ventricular dysfunction in patients with type 2 diabetes maybe associated with diabetic cardiomyopathy in the absence of coronary atherosclerosis and hypertension. Impairment of phosphatidylinositol 3-kinases (PI3K)/Akt pathway is critically involved in cardiac dysfunction in type 2 diabetes. Additionally, hyperglycaemia directly contributes to cardiac and structural abnormalities leading to myocardial hypertrophy and fibrinolysis with ventricular stiffness and chamber dysfunction. Thiazolidinediones increases the risk of heart failure in patients with diabetes and should not be used as a first line or in those with existing history of heart failure.

12. A. These large landmark clinical trials have shown that early glucose control is important due to its metabolic memory. Intensive glycaemic control reduces the long-term microvascular complications including retinopathy, nephropathy, and neuropathy, and when started early, tight glycaemic control can also reduce macrovascular risks.

13. E. Metformin is an insulin sensitizer and improves insulin sensitivity. It is not associated with hypoglycaemia and should be discontinued if eGFR drops below 30 ml/min/1.73m^2. Metformin has shown to lower the cardiovascular events in the diabetes patients and that it has a protective effect on coronary arteries beyond its hypoglycaemic effects. It can be associated with mild weight loss in most cases.

14. C. Sulfonylureas promote insulin secretion and can lead to hypoglycaemia. It can be used with metformin and other anti-diabetic medications. Newer agents of sulfonylureas have shown to have neutral cardiovascular risks.

15. E. GLP-1 RA may promote arrhythmias but not associated with atrial fibrillation (possible exception of albiglutide). Its use has demonstrated reduced cardiovascular events and mortality. It does not lead to hypoglycaemia. It is associated with weight loss. Lactic acidosis is a rare side effect and likely avoidable if not used in patients with renal and liver failure.

16. B. SGLT2 inhibitors works via inhibition of glucose reabsorption in the proximal tubule of the nephrons. It does not cause hypoglycaemia with potential side effects of low blood pressure and genitourinary tract infections.

17. C. Both 2023 CVD management in diabetes 2019 ESC/EAS guidelines recommend both a ≥50% LDL-C reduction from baseline and an absolute LDL-C treatment goal of <1.4 mmol/L (<55 mg/dL) for very high-risk patients. For patients at high risk, a ≥50% LDL-C reduction and an LDL-C goal of <1.8 mmol/L (<70 mg/dL) are recommended. Statins remains the first-line treatment unless there are contraindications.

18. E. Modest weight loss of approximately 5% of body weight is clinically significant as it associated with a 0.5% point reduction in HbA1c, a 5-mmHg decrease in diastolic BP, a 5-mmHg decrease in systolic BP, a 0.13 mmol/L increase in HDL cholesterol, and a 0.45 mmol/L decrease in triglycerides.

19. B. Bariatric surgery is effective at improving glycaemic control and can lead to diabetes resolution in a high percentage of patients with significant weight loss being maintained at 10 years, and sustained glycaemic control up to 16 years and a reduction in mortality in patients with diabetes.

20. C. Platelet activation plays a key role in the initiation and progression of atherothrombosis. Both post-prandial and persistent hyperglycaemia have been shown to cause platelet activation in the early and late phases of the progression of type 2 diabetes. Aspirin 75 mg once daily may be considered in patients with no previous CVD and diabetes.

21. C. Target SBP is 120–129mmHg in patients aged <65 years old, but rises to an SBP of 130–139 mmHg in those aged >65. In patients with nephropathy lower BP (SBP <130 mmHg) is desirable if tolerated. All available blood pressure lowering agents can be used, but evidence strongly supports an inhibitor of the RAAS (ACEi/ARB).

22. E. CV risk assessment tools are used to assess CVD risk in people with type 2 diabetes, including SCORE2-Diabetes and QRISK3 (used in UK NICE guidelines). The QRISK3 tool should not be used in patients with type 1 diabetes, patients with established CVD or those at high risk of developing CVD because of familial hypercholesterolaemia or other inherited disorders of lipid metabolism. For primary prevention of CVD should be considered for people who have a 10% greater 10-year risk of developing CVD.

23. C. 2023 CVD in diabetes guidelines and 2019 ESC/EAS Guidelines recommend both a ≥50% LDL-C reduction from baseline and an absolute LDL-C treatment goal of <1.4 mmol/L (<55 mg/dL) for very high-risk patients. For patients at high risk, a ≥50% LDL-C reduction and an LDL-C goal of <1.8 mmol/L (<70 mg/dL) are recommended. Statins remains the first-line treatment unless there are contraindications.

24. C. Metformin is an insulin sensitizer and improves insulin sensitivity. It is not associated with hypoglycaemia and should be discontinued if eGFR drops below 30 mls/min/1.73m^2. Metformin has shown to lower the cardiovascular events in the diabetes patients and that it has a protective effect on coronary artery beyond its hypoglycaemic effects. It can be associated with mild weight loss in most cases. Sulfonylureas promote insulin secretion and can lead to hypoglycaemia. It can be used with metformin and other anti-diabetic medications. Newer agents of sulfonylureas have shown to have neutral cardiovascular risks. SGLT2 inhibitors works via inhibition of glucose reabsorption in the proximal tubule of the nephrons. It does not cause hypoglycaemia with potential side effects of low blood pressure and genitourinary tract infections. Thiazolidinediones increases the risk of heart failure in patients with diabetes and should not be used as a first line or in those with existing history of heart failure.

25. D. The treatment for patients with type 2 diabetes can be intensified aiming for an HbA1c of 53 mmol/mol (7%) or less; an individualized approach should be adopted with involvement of the patient in the decision-making about their individual HbA1c targets.

chapter

7.5 CARDIAC REHABILITATION

QUESTIONS

1. **You are asked to refer a 39-year-old woman, who has recently survived a cardiac arrest, to an appropriate cardiac rehabilitation programme. She has had an ICD inserted and has now returned to work as a checkout staff in her local super market. She lives with her husband and her hobbies include knitting and cooking.**

   What is the most appropriate management and rationale at this stage?

   A. Refer to an exercise-based cardiac rehabilitation as it will significantly reduce her sedentary time at home
   B. Refer to an exercise-based cardiac rehabilitation programme as it will significantly reduce cardiac-related hospital readmissions
   C. Refer to an education-only cardiac rehabilitation programme as it will lead to significant improvements in cardiovascular mortality
   D. Do not refer to cardiac rehabilitation as it is contraindicated post-ICD insertion
   E. Defer cardiac rehab for 6 months

2. **A 60-year-old male patient has had urgent revascularization for NSTEMI with PCI. There is no significant bystander disease and his left ventricular function is normal. He is a father of two primary school children and responsible for driving them to school every day. He is asking for your advice on when he can restart driving after the procedure.**

   What advice would you give him?

   A. 1 week
   B. 2 weeks
   C. 4 weeks
   D. 6 weeks
   E. No restriction to driving

A 56-year-old diabetic patient (type II) is about to start an outpatient cardiac rehabilitation programme (phase III) 2 weeks after elective PCI.

What advice would you give before starting the exercise programme?

A. Check blood glucose levels before and after exercise and optimize diet
B. Check blood pressure before and after exercise and increase protein intake
C. Check blood glucose levels just before exercise and increase hydration
D. Check blood glucose levels just after exercise and avoid carbohydrates
E. Check blood glucose only if feeling unwell before exercise

4. **Which of the following statements is true for cardiac rehabilitation?**

A. Cardiac rehabilitation refers only to the outpatient exercise-based programme
B. Cardiac rehabilitation reduces cardiovascular mortality
C. Cardiac rehabilitation is not cost-effective when considering modern medical methods
D. Cardiac rehabilitation has limited effect on cardiac readmissions
E. There is no evidence that cardiac rehabilitation reduces rehospitalization

5. **A typical phase III cardiac rehabilitation programme runs at least twice weekly for a total duration of:**

A. 8–12 weeks
B. 4–6 weeks
C. 2–4 weeks
D. 14–16 weeks
E. 0–2 weeks

6. **During your multidisciplinary team meeting, the cardiac nurses mention that only 30% of the patients that are referred to the hospital's cardiac rehabilitation programme actually attend the classes. The team discuss possible strategies to improve uptake.**

Which of the following strategies is least likely to improve uptake?

A. Ensure that the acute cardiology team initiates referral to cardiac rehabilitation
B. Offer more follow-up medical appointments post-discharge to all patients
C. Create additional women-only cardiac rehabilitation classes
D. Offer additional choice for a home-based programme
E. Improve access to outpatient programmes at various times

7. **Which of the following health professionals are not usually part of a cardiac rehabilitation programme (phase III)?**

A. Occupational therapist
B. Psychologist
C. Exercise trainer
D. Pain management team
E. Dietician

8. A 75-year-old patient had elective CABG surgery 4 days ago. He is a retired chef and lives at home with his 69-year-old wife in a two-storey house. He usually does most of the cooking and his main physical activity is light gardening. During the early rehabilitation period in the hospital, you and your team focus on improving his physical function in preparation for his return at home.

Which of the following exercise options would you least advise in this early phase?

A. Walking 30 meters in a flat corridor
B. Walking up a flight of stairs (10)
C. Upper limb stretching exercises
D. Upper limb strength training exercises
E. Walking 50 metres on the flat outside

9. A 70-year-old female patient is being discharged following an admission with a large anterior STEMI. She has successful PCI to the LAD. There is no residual coronary artery disease. LVEF is 38%.

After how long can she resume driving her car (Group 1) following discharge?

A. After 1 week
B After 2 weeks
C No restriction, can immediately resume driving.
D After 3 weeks
E After 4 weeks

chapter

7.5

CARDIAC REHABILITATION

ANSWERS

1. B. Exercise-based cardiac rehabilitation reduces cardiac-related hospital readmissions but evidence shows that it does not have an effect on sedentary or sitting time in everyday life. This is why patients with cardiovascular disease need to be advised to both increase their activity levels as well as reduce sitting/sedentary time when at home. Education-only programmes do not have an effect on cardiovascular mortality. Patients post-ICD insertion can engage with cardiac rehabilitation exercise programmes (having an ICD is not a contraindication for participation to such programmes).

2. A. Driving a private car can resume after 1 week according to current DVLA advice.

3. A. Patients with type-II diabetes who begin cardiac rehabilitation exercise classes are advised to monitor their own blood sugar levels before and after exercise and to adapt their diet accordingly. Refer to specialized diabetes team for diet optimization if patients have not had advice or if diet is not well controlled.

4. B. Cardiac rehabilitation has been shown by a number of systematic reviews and meta-analyses to reduce cardiovascular mortality. The rest of the statements are false. There is good evidence that cardiac rehabilitation reduces cardiac related hospitalization and that it is highly cost-effective even considering modern medical management (post 2010). Also, cardiac rehabilitation refers to the multidisciplinary interventions for prevention and rehabilitation throughout the cardiac pathway, not just an outpatient-based exercise programme.

5. A. The most common duration of phase III outpatient-based cardiac rehabilitation programmes in the UK is 8 weeks and in Europe 12 weeks.

6. B. Follow-up medical appointment may be good for reviewing the patient's status and it is a good opportunity to discuss concerns, but such discussion is unlikely to increase uptake of cardiac rehabilitation classes in itself. All other options could be considered either on their own or in combination as they have been shown to improve uptake.

7. D. Psychologists, dietitians, and occupational therapists are involved in the education sessions that are part of the programme. Exercise trainers can be part of the team that delivers the exercise component if certified for cardiac rehabilitation.

8. D. Strength training upper limb exercises especially involving weights should be avoided for approximately 6 weeks post operation.

9. E. Driving may resume after 1 week after successful coronary intervention if:

- No other urgent revascularization planned (within 4 weeks of acute event)
- LVEF at least 40% before hospital discharge
- There is no other disqualifying condition

If any of the above points are present then driving may resume only after 4 weeks form the acute event.

chapter 8

CARDIAC PATIENTS IN OTHER SETTINGS

chapter

8.1

AORTIC DISEASE AND TRA
TO THE AORTA OR HEAR

QUESTIONS

1. **A 60-year-old lady with a background of moderately well-controlled hypertension, who is otherwise fit and well, is reviewed in the cardiology clinic following her CTCA which was done after a couple of episodes of atypical chest pain (Figure 8.1.1). This shows minimal coronary artery disease, but an incidental finding of a dilated aortic root is noted.**

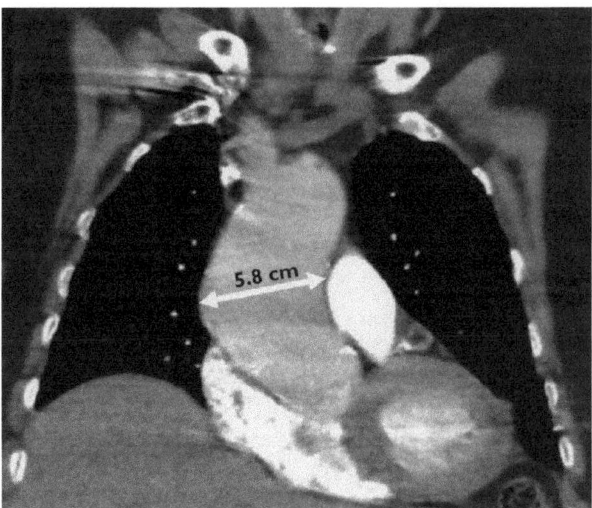

Figure 8.1.1

A. Surgical intervention is indicated
B. Surgical intervention is indicated if she is symptomatic
C. Surgical intervention would be indicated if there is evidence of severe aortic regurgitation
D. Surgical intervention is indicated if there is an increase of >0.5 cm on her follow-up CT scan in 12 months
E. Surgical intervention is indicated once the diameter is ≥6 cm

68-year-old man presents with acute tearing pain in the centre of his back. An aortic dissection is identified.

Aortic vessel weakness is typically due to weakness of which layer?

A. Tunica intima
B. Tunica media
C. Tunica adventitia
D. Endothelium
E. All of the above

3. **A 32-year-old lady with Marfan syndrome and a strong family history of thoracic aortic aneurysms is referred to the joint obstetric cardiology clinic as she plans to have a baby. She is asymptomatic. A transthoracic echocardiogram shows a tricuspid aortic valve with mild aortic regurgitation and an aortic root diameter of 46 mm. This is confirmed on the CT scan of her aorta.**

   What is the best management approach with this patient?

   A. Continue annual surveillance and refer for thoracic aortic surgery once the aortic root diameter exceeds 50 mm
   B. Advise against pregnancy in the future and commence beta-blockers and contraception
   C. Commence on a beta-blocker and refer to the multi-disciplinary team meeting for consideration of thoracic aortic surgery
   D. Commence on a beta-blocker and follow up in 1 year with a cardiac MRI scan
   E. Follow up in 1 year with a cardiac MRI scan and recommend pregnancy if aortic dimensions remain stable

4. **A 56-year-old-year-old lady has undergone aortic surgery for an aneurysm. She attends clinic to ask what her risk of needing a re-operation might be as she has heard 10–20% of patients who undergo aortic surgery for aneurysms require re-operation by 10–20 years.**

   Of the following which is not a risk factor for re-operation?

   A. Valve-preserving surgery
   B. Atrial fibrillation
   C. Marfan syndrome
   D. Annulus diameter of >2 cm
   E. Mitral valve prolapse

5. A 68-year-old gentleman is incidentally found to have an abdominal aortic aneurysm (AAA) measuring 47 mm in diameter.

Which of the following is most likely to have an effect on the rate of expansion of his AAA?

A. Blood pressure control with an ACE inhibitor
B. Blood pressure control with a beta-blocker
C. Smoking cessation
D. Statin therapy
E. Antiplatelet therapy with aspirin

6. An 82-year-old man is admitted with a suspected acute aortic syndrome. The admitting team have requested a set of blood tests including D-dimers. Which of the following is untrue with regards to the use of D-dimers in the assessment of all patients with suspected acute aortic syndromes (AAS)?

A. D-dimers have a high negative predictive value and should be routinely tested in all patients with suspected AAS
B. When the clinical probability of AAS is low, a negative D-dimer should be considered a rule out of the diagnosis
C. D-dimers may be helpful in some cases
D. D-dimer testing is not recommended in patients with a high probability of having an AAS
E. If a patient with an intermediate probability of an AAS has a positive D-dimer, further imaging should be arranged

7. A 64-year-old lady is brought into hospital after developing sudden onset, severe central chest pain radiating to the back. She has had intermittent chest pains in the past and an angiogram was done 3 years ago which showed normal coronary arteries. At the time of review, she has mild epigastric pain. On examination, her heart rate is 85 bpm, blood pressure is 128/86 mmHg, and she has a soft systolic and diastolic murmur. There is no blood pressure difference between the two arms. Her admission ECG shows normal sinus rhythm without any ischaemic changes and blood results show a troponin of 13 ng/L (normal <5 ng/L), and raised D-dimers of 1025 ng/ml (normal <500 ng/ml). Chest x-ray (AP film) shows a widened mediastinum.

What is the next most appropriate investigation?

A. Serial troponins and ECGs
B. Transthoracic echocardiogram
C. CT pulmonary angiogram
D. CT aorta
E. Trans-oesophageal echocardiogram

8. **Below is the CT scan of an 88-year-old lady who presented with an aortic dissection (Figure 8.1.2). It is seen starting at the aortic arch, beyond the origin of the left subclavian artery and does not involve the ascending aorta.**

   Which of these classifications best describes this?

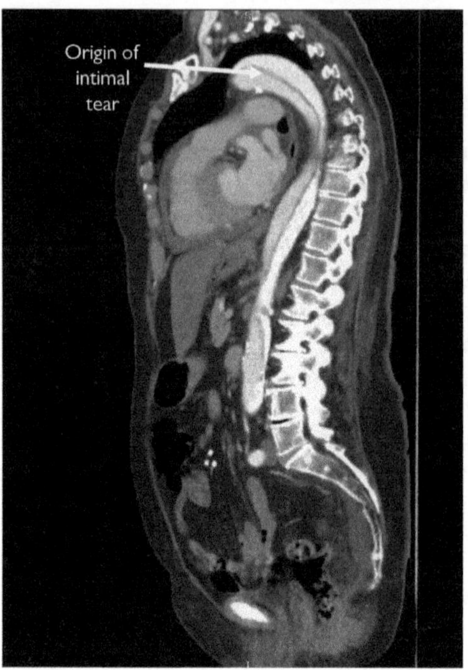

Figure 8.1.2

   A. Stanford Type A
   B. Stanford Type B
   C. DeBakey Type I
   D. DeBakey Type II
   E. DeBakey Type III

9. **You are reviewing a 76-year-old woman who has had a dissection of the descending aorta. She asks which area of the aorta is most at risk of dissection.**

   Which of the following is at the highest risk of dissection?

   A. Ascending aorta
   B. Aortic arch
   C. Descending aorta
   D. Thoracic aorta
   E. Abdominal aorta

10. A 52-year-old female with a background of Loeys-Dietz syndrome, hypercholesterolaemia and previous TIAs is admitted after developing slurred speech and dense left-sided hemiparesis 2 hours ago. She is unable to give a history and fulfils criteria for thrombolysis.

Which of the following must be undertaken before thrombolysis is considered?

A. CT head
B. CT head and neck
C. CT head and aorta
D. CT head, neck and aorta
E. CT head and CT angiogram of head and neck vessels

11. A 63-year-old male who is fit and well is brought in with sudden onset chest pain resulting in loss of consciousness. A CT aorta was done on admission and shows a Stanford type A dissection. A large global pericardial effusion measuring 2.6 cm is also noted and a haemopericardium is suspected. The patient is haemodynamically unstable with a blood pressure of 85/65 mmHg and heart rate of 115 bpm.

What is the most important next step?

A. Admission to the intensive care unit for close monitoring
B. Medical therapy with analgesia to alleviate the pain
C. Urgent bedside echocardiogram to look for features of cardiac tamponade and acute severe aortic regurgitation
D. Urgent pericardiocentesis to establish some haemodynamic stability
E. Urgent cardiothoracic referral for surgical intervention

12. A 76-year-old man is under regular review in the cardiology clinic with a thoracic aortic aneurysm at the level of the ascending aorta. He has no other underlying medical problems. The most recent measurement you have shows the aneurysm is 4.3 cm in diameter.

At what point would you recommend surgical repair to him?

A. 4.0–4.5cm
B. 4.5–5.0 cm
C. 5.0–5.5 cm
D. 5.5–6.0 cm
E. >6.0 cm

13. You are reviewing a CT scan of a 63-year-old man who has presented with chest pain. You notice he has a penetrating aortic ulcer.

Which statement is not true about aortic ulcers?

A. They can lead to intramural haematoma, dissection, and acute aortic rupture
B. They are more likely to occur in the descending thoracic aorta in association with intramural haematoma
C. The mainstay of treatment for uncomplicated type B lesions is pain relief and blood pressure control
D. Surgery is usually offered if depth and width of the ulcer is >1 cm and >2 cm respectively
E. Surgery is usually considered if a penetrating aortic ulcer occurs in the abdominal aorta

14. A 46-year-old male is admitted to hospital following a road traffic accident. A trauma CT is performed which shows changes consistent with acute aortic rupture. His blood pressure is 146/72 mmHg and heart rate is 110 bpm. His haemoglobin is 124 g/L.

Which of the following is true regarding his treatment?

A. Surgical repair is not indicated as his blood pressure and haemoglobin are stable
B. Therapeutic hypotension with vasodilators is required
C. Aggressive fluid resuscitation is needed to maintain the effective circulating volume
D. Blood pressure control is the key priority, aiming for a systolic pressure of around 120 mmHg
E. Open aortic repair is preferred over endovascular repair as it avoids risk of destabilizing other traumatic lesions and resulting complications

15. A 19-year-old female has a strong family history of Ehlers–Danlos syndrome (EDS) and is concerned about the risk of aortic complications?

Which subtype of EDS is associated with aortic pathologies?

A. Type I EDS
B. Type II EDS
C. Type III EDS
D. Type IV EDS
E. Type VII EDS

16. You are reviewing a 17-year-old female in the cardiology clinic who has been identified with a dilated aorta and notice she has a short stature.

Which of the below combinations are recognized associations between clinical signs and aortopathies?

A. Tall stature and Turner syndrome
B. Wide angle stature and Marfan syndrome
C. Hypertelorism and arterial tortuosity
D. Short stature and Ehlers–Danlos Type IV
E. High arched palate and Loeys–Dietz

17. An 18-year-old man is referred for an echocardiogram after routine examination identified a systolic murmur. The echocardiogram demonstrated a bicuspid aortic valve and coarctation of the aorta.

Which of the following statements is true regarding conditions associated with aortopathies?

A. 25% of patients with aortic dissection are found to have bicuspid aortic valves
B. A Kommerell's diverticulum may result in tracheal or oesophageal obstruction
C. Difficulty in swallowing caused by an aberrant right subclavian artery is referred to as dysphagia aortica
D. Up to 80% of patients with Turner syndrome have coarctation of the aorta
E. The revised Ghent nosology is a scoring system for systemic features of Loeys-Dietz syndrome

18. A 56-year-old male with no past medical history is admitted with fatigue, shortness of breath, joint pains, and feeling hot and cold. This has been ongoing for a few weeks. He has a low-grade fever of 37.6°C, blood pressure of 129/36 mmHg, HR of 101 bpm and oxygen saturations of 96% on room air. On examination, he has a collapsing pulse, bruits over the carotid arteries with notable tenderness, and a diastolic murmur in the aortic region, but there are no peripheral stigmata of infective endocarditis. Blood results reveal raised inflammatory markers: CRP 160 mg/L (normal <10 mg/L) and ESR 95 mm/h (normal 1–30 mm/h). Blood cultures are pending. A transthoracic echocardiogram is undertaken which shows a dilated aortic root, severe aortic regurgitation with normal biventricular function. This is confirmed on the transoesophageal echocardiogram which does not show any vegetations on the aortic valve. An aortitis and associated aneurysm is suspected.

Which of the following is true regarding his presentation?

A. A diagnosis of infective endocarditis remains possible and antibiotics for infective endocarditis must be continued with serial blood cultures
B. The gold standard investigation for diagnosis of aortitis is digital subtraction angiography (DSA)
C. There is no scope for treatment with immunosuppressive therapy in this case
D. The most likely cause for an aortitis, if present, is a bacterial or fungal infection
E. The best management option for this patient is surgery, regardless of the aetiology of his aortitis

19. You are performing a transoesophageal echocardiogram on a 64-year-old man with aortic valve disease. During the procedure you notice extensive atheroma throughout the aorta.

Which of the following is true concerning atheromatous disease of the aorta?

A. Hardly affects the aortic arch
B. Is treated with anti-platelet agents or anticoagulation
C. Results in increased aortic compliance
D. Can be diagnosed using multiple imaging modalities but TOE is first-line
E. Confers an annual stroke risk of 24% once the aortic plaque is over 3.5 mm

20. A cardiology review is requested on a normally fit and well 28-year-old man who is in the resus department. He was brought in by ambulance following a road traffic accident involving a high-impact collision between two vehicles. He has multiple bruises and lacerations that are both superficial and deep on his body, with small shards of glass within the wounds. His polytrauma CT scan shows multiple rib fractures, a small left-sided pleural effusion, and a moderate circumferential pericardial effusion of 15 mm. You are asked to review him as he is persistently hypotensive, despite fluid therapy. The ITU registrar is also in attendance and has inserted an arterial line.

The patient complains of chest pain and some difficulty in breathing. On examination, he has a raised JVP, quiet heart sounds, and bilateral air entry with reduced breath sounds in the left lung base. You notice these waveforms (Figures 8.1.3 and 8.1.4) on the monitors as you are reviewing him. You perform a bedside echocardiogram which shows a moderate-sized pericardial effusion as noted on the CT scan, with fibrin scans and clots suggestive of a haemopericardium. Diastolic collapse of the right ventricle is also noted.

What is your management plan?

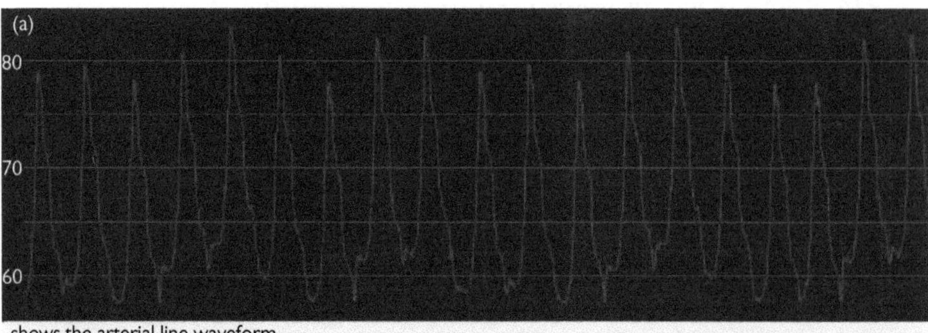

shows the arterial line waveform

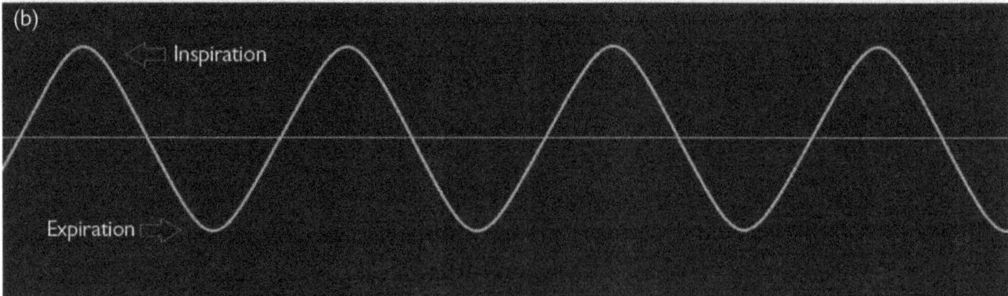

shows the corresponding respiratory waveform

Figure 8.1.3 and 8.1.4

A. Urgent referral to cardiothoracic surgery for a thoracotomy
B. Start on high dose aspirin and steroids
C. Urgent pericardiocentesis
D. Repeat CT scan to look for an evolving/loculated pericardial effusion
E. Urgent portable chest X-ray to look for a tension pneumothorax

chapter

8.1 AORTIC DISEASE AND TRAUMA TO THE AORTA OR HEART

ANSWERS

1. A. Aneurysm formation is the second most common pathology affecting the aorta, after atherosclerosis. A localized aneurysm is defined as a greater than 50% dilatation of the vessel compared to the diameter of the adjacent normal vessel. A diameter of >5.5 cm in the ascending aorta is therefore considered aneurysmal. Table 8.1.A1 shows the normal transthoracic echocardiogram (TTE) values for the proximal aorta. Once the aortic size index exceeds >4.25 cm/m^2, the risk of rupture or dissection is high and is about 20% per year. Generally, intervention is reserved for symptomatic or expanding aneurysms but as the risk of rupture increases significantly when the ascending aorta is >6.0 cm, surgery is recommended once the diameter is >5.5 cm, regardless of the presence or absence of symptoms or valvular disease. As this lady's scan shows an aortic root diameter of 5.8 cm, she should be referred for further surgical intervention immediately.

Table 8.1.A1 Normal dimensions of the proximal aorta

Aortic segment	Diameter (cm)	
	Men	**Women**
Aortic annulus	2.6 ± 0.3	2.3 ± 0.3
Sinus of Valsalva	3.4 ± 0.3	3.0 ± 0.3
Aortic root	2.9 ± 0.4	2.6 ± 0.3
Ascending aorta	2.8 ± 0.4	2.6 ± 0.4

2. B. The aortic wall is up to 4 mm thick and made up of three layers: the inner intima, middle media, and outer adventitia (Figure 8.1.A1). The ability of the aorta to provide constant pulsating blood flow to the rest of the body is determined by the elastic properties of the aortic wall. This in turn is dependent upon the elastin and collagen fibres as well as the smooth muscle cells which predominantly make up the medial layer. Cystic medial degeneration which is seen in Marfan syndrome, loss of vascular smooth muscle, loss of elastic fibres, and inflammatory responses that result in granuloma formation are all processes which lead to reduced aortic wall strength and aortic pathologies.

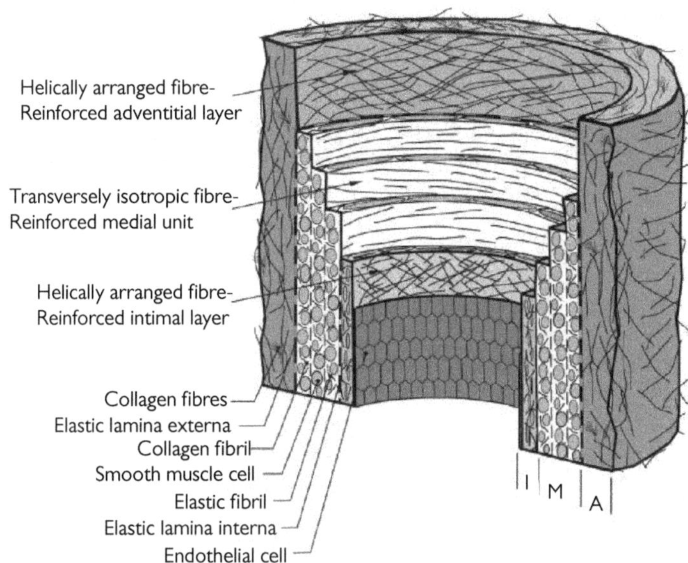

Figure 8.1.A1 Structure of the arterial wall. I= Intima, M= Media, A= Adventitia

Tasmis et al. Tsamis A, Krawiec JT, Vorp DA. Elastin and collagen fibre microstructure of the human aorta in ageing and disease: a review. *J R Soc Interface*. 2013;10(83):20121004. Published 2013 Mar 27. doi:10.1098/rsif.2012.1004 https://www.ncbi.nlm.nih.gov/pmc/articles/PMC3645409/

3. C. For patients with Marfan syndrome and thoracic aortic aneurysms, the ESC guidelines of 2014 recommend surgery once the aortic diameter is >50 mm. However, in the presence of certain risk factors, consideration of surgery is recommended at lower thresholds (Class IIa Level C). In patients with Marfan syndrome with a family history of aortic dissection, aortic size increase of >3 mm/year, severe aortic or mitral regurgitation, and/or a desire for pregnancy, surgery should be considered once the maximal aortic root diameter is > 45 mm. Hence, surgery is the best option for this lady even in the absence of other risk factors, to facilitate family planning and pregnancy. In the interim, she should be commenced on a beta-blocker such as bisoprolol or propranolol as there is evidence to suggest they can reduce aortic dilatation in Marfan syndrome. Patients should not be advised against pregnancy unless there is a significant risk of harm to their life which cannot be modified through available treatment options.

4. D. An annulus diameter of >2.5 cm (not 2 cm) is a risk factor for re-operation. The bigger the annulus, the more likely that a re-operation will be required. Other risk factors for re-operation include Marfan syndrome, mitral valve prolapse, atrial fibrillation, a valve preserving operation and having other concomitant procedures performed. Indications for a re-operation are the same as that for an initial operation. Open surgical repair carries significant risk of morbidity and mortality and the risk of surgery needs to be weighed against the risk of complications and death from an untreated aneurysm. Endovascular repair is a rapidly evolving field and is another treatment option for patients with aortic aneurysms, particularly those who may not be candidates for surgery. Current data suggests a lower risk of morbidity and peri-operative death with endovascular approaches, but higher reintervention rates compared to open repair. Long-term follow up data (from the UK EVAR trial) shows an increased aneurysm-related mortality rate in EVAR patients after 8 years, mainly due to secondary aneurysm sac rupture, necessitating lifelong follow-up in these patients. Ultimately, the approach (open vs endovascular repair) depends on several factors such as the patient's surgical risk, their anatomy, and whether it is suitable for endovascular repair and the anticipated durability of the procedure. All of this should be taken into consideration and the decision should be made using a multi-disciplinary team approach.

5. C. The main aims of medical therapy in the setting of AAAs are: 1) cardiovascular risk factor management and 2) stabilization of the aortic aneurysm. Most patients with AAAs have risk factors for cardiovascular disease, such as hypertension and hypercholesterolaemia and are more likely to die from a major cardiovascular event (such as a myocardial infarction) than rupture of the AAA. Hence, efforts must be undertaken to optimize these risk factors. ACE inhibitors and/or beta-blockers may be used for blood pressure control, statins for lowering lipid levels and for their pleiotropic effects, and aspirin for the secondary prevention of cardiovascular disease. However, there is limited/ conflicting evidence supporting the use of these drugs in the stabilization of AAAs (i.e. to influence aneurysmal growth). For patients with Marfan syndrome, there is some evidence to show that prophylactic treatment with beta-blockers, ACE inhibitors, and angiotensin receptor blockers (ARBs) may reduce progression of aortic dilatation. However, this effect has not been observed in AAA due to other aetiologies and there is no indication for these drugs for the purpose of AAA stabilization, (except in patients with Marfan syndrome). Similarly, evidence for use of statins in this context is conflicting with only small observational studies suggesting that they may inhibit aneurysmal dilatation. The ESC guidelines recommend use of statins for cardiovascular risk reduction. Studies have also failed to confirm a beneficial effect of antiplatelet therapy on AAA progression, but they may be used for other purposes such as reducing risk of thrombus. On the other hand, data from a meta-analysis including 15,475 patients with AAA showed that current smoking was associated with an increased rate of expansion of 0.35 mm/year; twice as fast compared to ex- and non-smokers. Other population studies have also identified tobacco smoking as the single most important predictor of future aortic aneurysms in the general population.

6. A. The 2014 ESC guidelines recommend the use and interpretation of D-dimers depending on the pre-test probability of the suspected AAS. Table 8.1.A2 shows their recommendations for laboratory testing in the diagnostic work-up for AAS. For those with a low probability, a negative D-dimer test has a high negative predictive value and can safely rule out an AAS. In patients with an intermediate probability, a positive D-dimer test should prompt further imaging. D-dimer testing is not recommended in patients with a high probability of AAS. Its usefulness requires further investigation in the diagnosis of intramural haematoma, penetrating aortic ulcers, and acute aortic dissections with a totally thrombosed false lumen. Therefore, it is helpful in the diagnosis of AAS in some but not all cases.

Table 8.1.A2 Recommendations for laboratory testing in the diagnostic work up for AAS

Laboratory testing		
In the case of suspected AAS, the interpretation of biomarkers should always be considered along with the clinical pre-test probability.	IIa	C
In the case of a low clinical probability of AAS, a negative D-dimer should be considered to rule out the diagnosis.	IIa	B
In the case of an intermediate clinical probability of AAS with positive D-dimer, further imaging should be considered.	IIa	B
In patients with high probability risk scores (2 or 3) of AD, testing of D-dimers is not recommended.	III	C

Reproduced from Erbel R, Aboyans V, Boileau C, ESC Committee for Practice Guidelines. 2014 ESC Guidelines on the diagnosis and treatment of aortic diseases: Document covering acute and chronic aortic diseases of the thoracic and abdominal aorta of the adult. The Task Force for the Diagnosis and Treatment of Aortic Diseases of the European Society of Cardiology (ESC). Eur Heart J. 2014 Nov 1;35(41):2873-926. doi: 10.1093/eurheartj/ehu281. © European Society of Cardiology. With permission from Oxford University Press.

7. B. The 2014 ESC guidelines propose a diagnostic algorithm for use in suspected acute aortic syndromes (AAS). Firstly, this is dependent on the patient's haemodynamic stability and secondly, their probability of having an AAS (characterized by their history/ family history, nature of the pain, and examination features). In this scenario, the patient presents with a history that is highly suspicious of an aortic dissection. Further, there are high risk examination features, such as low blood pressure and presence of a diastolic aortic murmur. These features are highly suggestive of a type A aortic dissection. Given that she is haemodynamically stable at present, the next step as per the guidelines, would be to perform a transthoracic echocardiogram (TTE) to look for a type A aortic dissection. If confirmed, urgent cardiothoracic referral is advised. If the TTE is inconclusive, a CT aorta or even a transoesophageal echocardiogram may be performed to confirm the diagnosis.

The question assesses understanding of the flow chart proposed by the ESC guidelines in the diagnosis of an acute dissection. In clinical practice, CT aorta is often undertaken preferentially due to its ready availability and diagnostic accuracy compared to TTE. Even if the diagnosis is confirmed on a TTE that is performed immediately, a subsequent CT aorta will be required prior to surgery to examine the nature and extent of the dissection. Similarly, TTE may complement findings of the CT aorta and provides additional information regarding the structure and function of the heart and aortic valve and also to enable assessment of the severity of aortic regurgitation if present. Options B, C, D, and E will all lead to the diagnosis but each of these imaging modalities vary in their characteristics and usefulness. Option A is the least useful in this setting and will not lead to the correct diagnosis.

Figure 8.1.A2 shows the flowchart for decision-making in suspected AAS, as per the 2014 ESC guidelines.

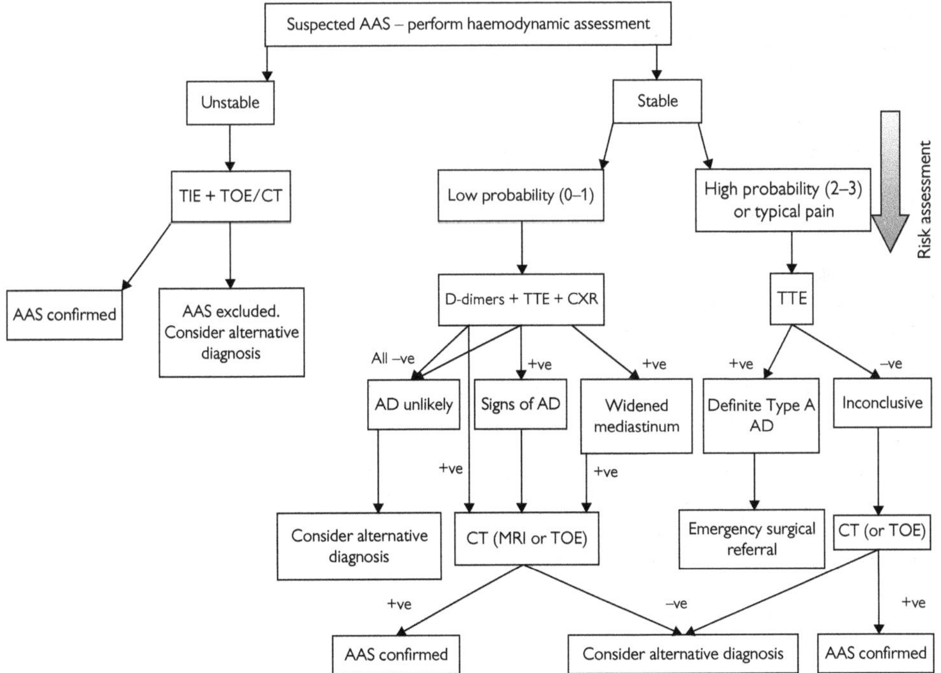

Figure 8.1.A2

Reproduced from Erbel R, Aboyans V, Boileau C, ESC Committee for Practice Guidelines. 2014 ESC Guidelines on the diagnosis and treatment of aortic diseases: Document covering acute and chronic aortic diseases of the thoracic and abdominal aorta of the adult. The Task Force for the Diagnosis and Treatment of Aortic Diseases of the European Society of Cardiology (ESC). Eur Heart J. 2014 Nov 1;35(41):2873-926. doi: 10.1093/eurheartj/ehu281. © European Society of Cardiology. With permission from Oxford University Press.

8. B. Stanford type A is used to describe dissections that involve the ascending aorta and type B, for those that do not involve the ascending aorta. The DeBakey classification is based on the origin of the intimal tear and is classified into three types; Type I which starts in the ascending aorta and extends distally to involve the entire aorta; Type II which starts in the ascending aorta and remains confined to the ascending aorta; and Type III which starts in the descending aorta. It is further classified depending on whether the dissection is limited to the descending aorta (Type IIIa) or whether it extends below the diaphragm (Type IIIb). Neither the Stanford nor the DeBakey classification specifically refers to the involvement of the aortic arch. The image shows a dissection starting at the aortic arch ruling out options A, C and D which best describe dissections starting in the ascending aorta (Figure 8.1.2). Option E (DeBakey Type III) that specifically refers to dissections starting in the descending aorta is also incorrect. Hence option B (Stanford Type B), though ambiguous regarding the involvement of the aortic arch, best describes this as it refers to any dissection that does not involve the ascending aorta. Arch tears occur in approximately 30% of patients with acute aortic dissections.

Stanford Type B dissections are generally treated conservatively with analgesia and blood pressure control (usually with intravenous beta-blockers), with a target systolic blood pressure between 110–120 mmHg. This is the approach for acute, uncomplicated Type B dissections and stable chronic Type B and isolated aortic arch dissections. However, there are circumstances in which interventional/surgical management is required. This is usually when a Type B dissection is complicated by other features such as malperfusion, critical diameter of >5.5 cm, refractory pain, and rapid expansion of >1 cm/year, when there is retrograde extension involving the ascending aorta, and when it occurs in patients with pre-existing conditions, such as Marfan and Ehlers–Danlos syndrome.

9. A. A dissection is defined as a separation in the layers of the aortic wall due to an intimal tear and the bleeding that results, along and within the wall. Most dissections are spontaneous and it is unclear whether they are initiated by a primary haemorrhage within the media leading to subsequent rupture of the intima or if it is the primary rupture within the intima that leads to dissection of the medial wall. The proximal aorta is at highest risk of dissection as it is subject to the steepest fluctuations in pressure. Blood flowing at high pressure passes through the tear and separates the intima from either the media or adventitia creating a false lumen which can extend in an anterograde or retrograde manner. This can also result in complete occlusion of the true lumen, leading to malperfusion of essential organs. For this reason, blood pressure control is an essential component in the management of acute aortic dissections. Dissections can be classified according to the pathology (Classes I–V) or the anatomy. In routine clinical practice though, an anatomical classification is generally preferred (Table 8.1.A3).

Table 8.1.A3 Anatomical classification of aortic dissection

Pathological classification	
Class I	Refers to the 'classic' aortic dissection with the intimal flap between the true and false lumens. It is subdivided into the Stanford and DeBakey classifications
Class II	Intramural haemorrhage/ haematoma
Class III	Ulcerating aortic plaque: *accounts for <5% of all aortic dissections*
Class IV	Subtle/discrete aortic bulge—typically seen in Marfan syndrome: *this can be difficult to diagnose*
Class V	Iatrogenic/ traumatic—e.g. post cardiac catheter manipulation
Anatomical classification	
Proximal	Involving the aortic root or ascending aorta (Standford Type A, DeBakey Type I and DeBakey Type II)
Distal	Beyond the left subclavian artery (Standford Type B and DeBakey Type III)

10. D. Loeys–Dietz syndrome is a rare autosomal dominant genetic syndrome that results in connective tissue abnormalities. It is characterized by the weakening and tortuosity of not just the aorta, but also other arteries in the body, increasing the risk of dissections and aneurysms (Figure 8.1.A3). Acute aortic dissection and rupture of aortic aneurysms are well known complications of this condition and are associated with a high mortality. Although an ischaemic stroke may be more likely, it is important to rule out an aortic or carotid artery dissection as a cause of the stroke, prior to thrombolysis. Hence, imaging of the aorta and neck is required in addition to that of the brain.

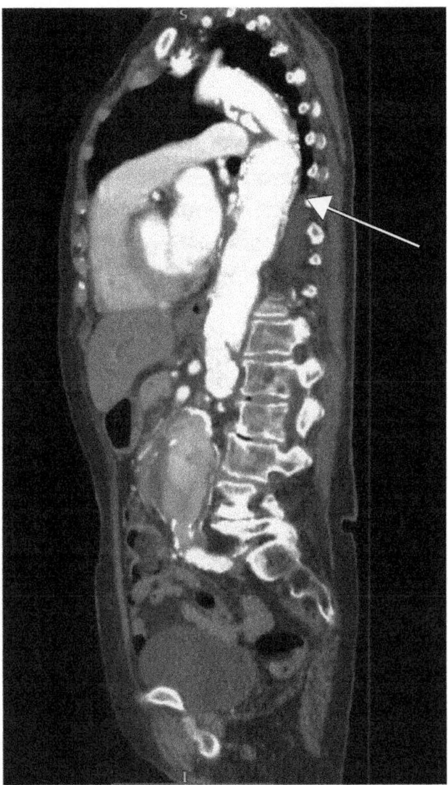

Figure 8.1.A3 The figure shows multiple contrast-filled aneurysms within the arteries as well as a descending thoracic aortic aneurysm (white arrow)

11. E. In this patient who has presented with a type A aortic dissection, urgent referral to cardiothoracic surgery for aortic repair is the most important next step. The mortality of acute type A dissection without surgical intervention is 50% in the first 48 hours. In this situation, the need for urgent surgical intervention is even more pressing, as the large pericardial effusion with haemodynamic instability may be due to aortic rupture, amongst other factors, causing cardiac tamponade. Cardiac tamponade associated with aortic rupture is a major risk factor for peri-operative mortality in patients with acute type A dissections. Pericardiocentesis in the setting of aortic dissections is generally contraindicated as aggressive drainage of pericardial blood can accelerate bleeding and worsen shock and hypotension. However, a recent paper published by the European Society of Cardiology evaluating multiple studies identified controlled pericardial drainage as an effective temporizing measure in *selected* patients with acute type A dissection complicated by critical cardiac tamponade. It may lead to improvement in the patient's pre-operative state and subsequent surgical outcomes. Nonetheless this should not be undertaken unless necessary, without confirmation of tamponade or discussion with the cardiothoracic team.

Options A, B, and C are not incorrect and should be part of the management plan. ITU involvement is necessary given the haemodynamic compromise. Medical therapy with fluid resuscitation and analgesia is essential and an echocardiogram will provide crucial information regarding the presence/ absence of tamponade as well acute severe aortic regurgitation which can cause cardiogenic shock even if there is no tamponade.

12. D. In patients with aortic aneurysms, repair is recommended if the ascending aorta is >5.5–6.0 cm and the distal aorta is >6.0 cm. This threshold is lower for patients with Marfan syndrome and bicuspid aortic valves (Table 8.1.A4)

Table 8.1.A4 Summary of the thresholds for surgery in terms of the maximal aortic diameter according to the 2014 ESC guidelines on the diagnosis and treatment of aortic disease

Patient factor	Aortic diameter thresholds for surgery
Ascending aortic aneurysms	
• Any patient	≥55–60 mm
• Marfan syndrome	≥50 mm
• Marfan syndrome and additional risk factors (family history of dissection, size increase of > 3mm/year, severe aortic regurgitation or desire for pregnancy	≥ 45 mm
• Loeys–Dietz Syndrome	Same criteria as for Marfan syndrome
• Bicuspid aortic valve	≥55 mm
• Bicuspid aortic valve and additional risk factors (family history, systemic hypertension, coarctation of the aorta, increase in aortic diameter of >3mm/year and factors such as age, body weight, other comorbidities and type of surgery)	≥ 50 mm
• Turner syndrome	≥ 27.5 mm/m^2 body surface area
Aortic arch aneurysms	
• Any patient	>55 mm
Descending aortic aneurysms	
• Any patient	≥55–60 mm
• Marfan syndrome	Lower thresholds may be considered
Abdominal aortic aneurysms	
• Male	≥55 mm
• Female	≥50–55 mm

Reproduced from Erbel R, Aboyans V, Boileau C, ESC Committee for Practice Guidelines. 2014 ESC Guidelines on the diagnosis and treatment of aortic diseases: Document covering acute and chronic aortic diseases of the thoracic and abdominal aorta of the adult. The Task Force for the Diagnosis and Treatment of Aortic Diseases of the European Society of Cardiology (ESC). Eur Heart J. 2014 Nov 1;35(41):2873–926. doi: 10.1093/eurheartj/ehu281. © European Society of Cardiology. With permission from Oxford University Press.

13. E. Penetrating aortic ulcers are more likely to occur in the middle and lower descending thoracic aorta (Type B lesions) and abdominal aorta in association with intramural haematoma. They result from progressive erosion of mural plaques penetrating the elastic lamina, leading to separation of the medial layers. This is turn can lead to other acute aortic syndromes (AAS) such as intramural haematoma, dissection, and aortic rupture. A penetrating aortic ulcer should be treated as an AAS as the adventitia is reached and acute aortic rupture may be imminent. It is usually diagnosed with CT imaging. The principles of management are similar: surgical intervention if the lesion involves the ascending aorta and medical management if the lesion involves the descending aorta. Interventions are usually undertaken if width is > 2cm and depth is >1 cm. Medical therapy encompasses blood pressure and pain control.

14. B. Nearly all patients with acute aortic ruptures are candidates for surgical repair, regardless of the blood pressure or haemoglobin. Traumatic aortic rupture usually occurs due to sudden deceleration either from head-on or side impact collisions. Although hypotension is common and regarded as a predictor for traumatic aortic injury, a small proportion of patients present with systolic hypertension. The rapid deceleration which results in torsion and shearing forces stretch the aorta and this stretching stimulus is thought to cause blood pressure elevation, mediated by the sympathetic afferent nerve fibres located in the aortic isthmus. Once the diagnosis is confirmed on the CT scan, therapeutic hypotension with vasodilators and beta-blockers are essential. Blood pressure should be maintained at around 90 mmHg with a heart rate of <100 bpm. Aggressive fluid replacement should be limited to prevent extension of the rupture, coagulopathy, and hypertension. Patients with free aortic rupture or large periaortic haematoma should be taken to theatre immediately for emergency repair which may be surgical or endovascular. Endovascular repair has become the treatment of choice for those with favourable anatomy as it reduces the risk of destabilizing other traumatic lesions in the lungs, brain, and abdomen, and peri-operative morbidity and mortality.

15. D. There are 13 sub-types of EDS. It is important to note that only EDS type IV (vascular form) is associated with pathologies of the aorta as well as that of other blood vessels. Most of the other sub-types are characterized by disorders of the joint and skin. Type I EDS refers to classical EDS which results in skin hyperextensibility, atrophic scarring and generalized joint hypermobility. Type II is classical like EDS which is is characterized by skin hyperextensibility, joint hypermobility, and easy bruising. Type III is hypermobile EDS which requires joint hypermobility, systemic manifestations of a connective tissue disease, a positive family history, and other musculoskeletal complications for diagnosis. Type VII EDS is arthrochalasia EDS which results in hypermobility with recurrent subluxations congenital bilateral hip dislocations etc.

16. C. Table 8.1.A5 summarizes the genetic syndromes associated with aortopathies, their phenotype and associated genetic abnormalities.

Table 8.1.A5 Summarizes the genetic syndromes associated with aortopathies, their phenotype and associated genetic abnormalities

Syndrome	**Phenotype**	**Associated genes**
• Marfan syndrome	- Tall stature - Cardiovascular features such as dilatation of the ascending aorta, aortic dissection, mitral valve prolapse etc. - Ocular features such as ectopia lentis - Skeletal features such as arachnodactyly, pectus carinatum/ excavatum, hypermobility of wrist or thumb joints - Spinal features such as dural ectasia	FBN1
• Turner syndrome	- Short stature - Low hair line, webbed neck, wide angle stature - Congenital cardiac defects - Aortic abnormalities such as bicuspid aortic valve - Other features: metabolic and hormonal abnormalities	45X karyoptype
• Loeys–Dietz syndrome	- Triad: Hypertelorism, bifid uvula/cleft palate, arterial tortuosity - Craniosynostosis - Aneurysms and dissections of aorta and other arteries	TGFBR1 TGFBR2

(continued)

Table 8.1.A5 Continued

Syndrome	Phenotype	Associated genes
• Ehler–Danlos syndrome (Type IV)	- Short stature, pinched and thin nose, thin lips, prominent ears, tightness of skin over the face - Bicuspid aortic valve and aortic coarctation - Other features: rupture of gravid uterus, gastrointestinal rupture, rupture of medium to large sized vessels	COL3A1
• Arterial Tortuosity Syndrome	- Elongated face, blepharophimosis and down-slanting palpebral fissures, beaked nose, highly arched palate, and micrognathia - Signs of generalized connective tissue disorders: soft, hyper-extensible skin, arachnodactyly, chest wall deformity, joint laxity, and contractures - Tortuosity, elongation, stenosis and aneurysm or aorta, other large and middle sized arteries	SCL2A10

17. B. Bicuspid aortic valves are common and affect 1–2% of the population. Around 15% of patients with dissections have a bicuspid aortic valve. A Kommerell's diverticulum can be described as a diverticular out-pouching at the origin of an anomalous subclavian artery. This can be an aberrant right subclavian artery with a left aortic arch or an anomalous left subclavian artery with a right aortic arch. In some situations, the diverticulum may compress the trachea or oesophagus, causing symptoms of dyspnoea and dysphagia respectively. The difficulty in swallowing caused by compression from an aberrant right subclavian artery is referred to as dysphagia lusoria. Dysphagia aortica refers to the difficulty in swallowing caused by extrinsic compression of the oesophagus from a dilated thoracic aorta/ thoracic aneurysm. Turner syndrome is characterized by the 45X karyotype and the classical phenotype of a webbed neck, low set ears and hairline, broad chest, and short stature. It is associated with congenital cardiac abnormalities and aortic abnormalities. About 12% of patients with Turner syndrome have coarctation of the aorta and 30% have a bicuspid aortic valve. The revised Ghent nosology is a scoring system for systemic features of Marfan syndrome.

18. A. Although there are no peripheral stigmata of infective endocarditis, the fevers, raised inflammatory markers and new murmur with echocardiographic evidence of severe aortic regurgitation raise suspicion of this condition. Further, the blood culture results are still pending. It is important to remember that the sensitivity and specificity of transthoracic (TTE) and transoesophageal echocardiography (TOE) is not 100% and a negative echocardiographic result does not rule out a diagnosis of infective endocarditis, particularly in the early stages. Antibiotics should be continued with serial blood cultures while investigating for the underlying aetiology. A repeat echocardiogram may be considered at a later stage. Aortitis may often mimic infective endocarditis and distinguishing between the two can be challenging. It can be broadly categorized into infective and non-infective aortitis. Determining the aetiology is crucial as the latter is treated with immunosuppressive therapy which may worsen infective processes. Common causes of infective aortitis include syphilis, bacteria such as *Staphylococcus aureus* and fungi such as *Candida albicans*. Common causes of non-infective aortitis include large vessel vasculitis and atherosclerosis.

The exact cause of this patient's symptoms remains unclear and we cannot definitively rule out potential for treatment with an immunosuppressive agent in case it is a non-infective aortitis. Non-infective large vessel vasculitis is the most common cause of aortitis. Diagnosis of aortitis usually requires multiple imaging modalities such as TOE/CT/MRI, each which has its own pros and cons. Digital subtraction angiography is useful in providing information regarding luminal changes. However, these changes are only seen in the later stages. PET scans can be particularly useful in detecting vascular inflammation when combined with cross-sectional imaging modalities such as CT. Surgery is usually indicated in infective non-syphilitic aortitis, alongside treatment with a prolonged course of antibiotics. Mortality for infected aneurysms treated with antibiotics alone is 90%.

19. D. Atheromatous disease tends to affect the aortic arch and descending aorta. It results in reduced aortic compliance. Risk factors for its development include hypertension, hypercholesterolaemia, diabetes, and smoking. TOE is usually the first modality for diagnosis, although CT and MRI can also be used. Management comprises risk factor modification, statin therapy, and antiplatelet medications. Statins are superior to anticoagulation and antiplatelets in those with atheromatous disease in the aorta and at high risk of emboli. An aortic plaque thickness of ≥4 mm is considered a major risk factor for stroke with an annual occurrence of 12%.

20. A. The arterial line and respiratory waveforms demonstrate pulsus paradoxus, a key feature seen in cardiac tamponade. Pulsus paradoxus is defined as a drop in blood pressure of more than 10 mmHg during inspiration which is not normally observed. Even though the bedside echocardiogram shows a moderate-sized pericardial effusion that is unlikely to cause cardiac tamponade under normal circumstances, in the acute setting (e.g. with cardiac trauma), even a small volume of fluid may be enough to cause tamponade as the pericardium does not have enough time to stretch and compensate for the rapid increase in volume.

In this case, the patient presents following a road traffic accident which would generally result in high speed deceleration injury causing blunt force trauma to the chest wall. This can damage the epicardial coronary vessels and result in a haemopericardium. However, the patient also has evidence of multiple lacerations on his torso which are superficial and deep as well as a small left-sided effusion. In the setting of trauma, this may well be a haemothorax due to penetrating chest trauma that may also be responsible for the haemopericardium. Given this possibility, an urgent cardiothoracic referral is warranted for an emergency thoracotomy so that the tamponade can be relieved through a pericardiotomy rather than pericardiocentesis. If there is no uncertainty regarding the aetiology of his haemopericardium (blunt force trauma rather than penetrating trauma), pericardiocentesis should be performed urgently.

Pulsus paradoxus is also seen in other conditions, such as asthma and obstructive lung disease (less likely in this scenario), and with tension pneumothorax. Bilateral air entry noted on auscultation of the lungs rules this out. Tension pneumothorax is a clinical diagnosis.

A repeat CT scan may provide a better quality image and show evidence of a loculated effusion but is unlikely to change management. Instead it will delay treatment which ultimately needs relief of the cardiac tamponade to achieve haemodynamic stability, regardless of the size of the effusion or presence or absence of a loculated effusion. NSAIDs should be avoided in this setting. Use of corticosteroids is recommended only in Dressler's syndrome.

chapter 8.2

PERIPHERAL ARTERY DISEASE

QUESTIONS

1. **Which of the following medical conditions is NOT associated with the development of arterial disease?**
   A. Marfan's syndrome
   B. Takayasu's disease
   C. End stage renal failure
   D. Diabetes mellitus
   E. Moderate alcohol consumption

2. **Mr. Johnson is a 65-year-old man who has Type II diabetes and hypertension. He presents with a history of gradual onset pain in his left thigh and calf when he walks more than 50 metres. He has no palpable foot pulses. His ankle brachial pressure index (ABPI) is 0.7 in the left leg.**

   What is the prevalence of PAD in people over 60 years old with one or more cardio-vascular risk factors?
   A. 10–20%
   B. 25–30%
   C. 40–50%
   D. 50–60%
   E. 60–70%

3. **Mr. Johnson (from Q2) is referred to a vascular surgeon for further assessment.**

   Which of the following examination findings is NOT indicative of a diagnosis of PAD?
   A. Ankle brachial pressure index >1.4
   B. Pallor on elevation of the limb
   C. Swelling of the limb
   D. Rubor (redness) on dependency of the limb
   E. Ankle brachial pressure index ≤0.9

4. Which of the following symptoms is NOT associated with PAD?

A. Erectile dysfunction
B. Burning foot pain in a diabetic patient
C. Reproducible pain on walking a set distance in thighs and/or calves; the distance is decreased by walking uphill
D. Pain in foot at night, relieved by hanging foot out of bed
E. Unilateral blue toe

5. Mr. Smith is a 55-year-old man who reports recent onset of pain in his right calf on walking 200 metres. He is able to continue in his job as a painter and decorator. He occasionally has to stop when walking up hills. He has smoked 10–20 cigarettes a day since the age of 18.

Which of the following interventions is rarely indicated in a patient with stable symptoms of intermittent claudication?

A. Statin therapy
B. Increased exercise, specifically walking
C. Antiplatelet therapy
D. Popliteal artery angioplasty
E. Blood pressure management

6. Mr Smith (from Q5) has a duplex ultrasound, which demonstrates a full-length (25 cm) occlusion of his right superficial femoral artery.

Which of the following statements is false regarding his best management?

A. Antiplatelet and statin therapy should be prescribed
B. Conservative (medical) therapy alone is an option
C. Surgical bypass carries a higher risk of MI or death compared to endovascular intervention
D. Endovascular treatment may have limited durability
E. Angioplasty alone will be sufficient

7. Which of the following statements regarding the use of anticoagulation and antiplatelet therapy in people with PAD is <u>TRUE</u>?

A. Oral anticoagulation should not be used for atrial fibrillation
B. Addition of low dose rivaroxaban to antiplatelet therapy increases the risk of major bleeding
C. Direct oral anticoagulant (DOAC) is preferred to warfarin (coumarin) for patients with end stage renal failure
D. Ticagrelor is superior to clopidogrel
E. Anticoagulation alone is preferable to antiplatelet therapy

8. A 75-year-old lady with Type 2 diabetes presents with a superficial ulcer on her left fourth toe. She has moderate peripheral neuropathy, and her podiatrist was unable to feel pulses in her feet. Doppler signals are monophasic and incompressible. She is already taking a statin and amlodipine. A recent HbAlc was 76 mmol/mol.

Which of the following tests provides an objective measure of tissue perfusion in this patient?

A. Ankle brachial pressure index
B. Capillary refill time
C. Transcutaneous measurement of oxygenation levels
D. Contrast enhanced CT angiogram
E. Intra-arterial digital subtraction angiogram

9. A 60-year old male presents with a 12-hour history of sudden onset pain in their left leg. Prior to this they had noticed worsening symptoms of intermittent claudication over the last 6 months. He suffered a NSTEMI 2 years previously. He started smoking again 6 months ago. On examination the leg is white with absent pulses below the femoral artery. There is profound motor and sensory impairment in the foot.

Which of the following procedures is rarely used for revascularization in acute limb ischaemia?

A. Surgical embolectomy
B. Catheter-directed thrombolysis
C. Plain old balloon angioplasty ('POBA')
D. Aspiration thrombectomy
E. Surgical bypass

10. A 25-yearold female secretary is referred electively because of worsening pain in her right shoulder and arm. She has recently noticed that her hand goes white after she has brushed her hair. On examination at rest she has no muscle wasting, no arm swelling, and palpable radial pulse. On arm abduction and external rotation her radial pulse is lost. If she then clenches her fist in this position it reproduces her upper limb pain.

Which of the following is least associated with compression at the thoracic outlet, better known as thoracic outlet syndrome?

A. Carpal tunnel syndrome
B. Upper limb DVT
C. Acute upper limb ischaemia
D. Raynaud's syndrome
E. Cervical rib

11 Mrs. Jackson is an 81-year-old lady, who is referred from the stroke clinic with a one-week history of an episode of transient visual loss in her left eye and difficulty finding her words (dysphasia). She has type 2 diabetes mellitus and hypertension. She has never smoked. She has been started on aspirin and clopidogrel by her stroke physician. She was already prescribed metformin, ramipril, and simvastatin. Carotid duplex scan shows a 50–69% stenosis of the left internal carotid artery with <50% stenosis of the right internal carotid artery.

Which of the following cerebral ischaemic events is associated with the lowest risk of subsequent stroke?

A. Minor stroke with sensory symptoms and no motor loss
B. MRI proven parietal infarct with full neurological recovery
C. Transient ischaemic attack with dysphasia
D. Transient ischaemic attack with motor dysfunction
E. Amaurosis fugax (transient unilateral visual loss)

12. Insertion of a carotid artery stent via the femoral artery might be considered in which of the following situations?

A. An internal carotid artery occlusion
B. Symptomatic carotid stenosis with previous neck radiotherapy
C. Patient with known distal aortic occlusion
D. Asymptomatic internal carotid artery stenosis in 80-year-old woman
E. After major disabling stroke (Rankin Scale Score 5) with no recovery

13. A 70-year-old male undergoes a carotid duplex after a bruit is heard in his left neck. He is a life-long smoker, hypertensive, and he has mild coronary artery disease. His scan shows a 70% left internal carotid artery stenosis with a <50% stenosis of the right internal carotid artery.

For an asymptomatic carotid stenosis, which of the following features of the carotid plaque is NOT associated with higher risk of stroke?

A. Heavily calcified smooth plaque
B. Large lipid core
C. Ulcerated plaque
D. Progressive stenosis on serial imaging
E. Intraplaque haematoma

14. Which of the following statements regarding abdominal aortic aneurysms is TRUE?

A. For a given aortic diameter, rupture is less likely in women than men
B. Repair is always indicated of an aortic aneurysm once the maximum aortic diameter reaches 5 cm
C. Local anaesthetic is preferable to general anaesthetic when performing elective EVAR (provided patient will tolerate)
D. Local anaesthetic is preferable to general anaesthetic when performing emergency EVAR (provided patient will tolerate)
E. EVAR is associated with better long-term survival than open surgical repair

15. A 78-year-old male presents to their general practitioner with a history of worsening lower back pain. He is an ex-smoker of 10 years following a single transient ischaemic attack (TIA). On examination his doctor palpates a pulsatile abdominal mass. An urgent ultrasound confirms the presence of a 5-cm diameter abdominal aortic aneurysm (AAA).

Which of the following is NOT a risk factor for AAA growth?

A. Diabetes mellitus
B. Smoking
C. Advancing age
D. Family history
E. Chronic obstructive pulmonary disease

16. Regarding population screening for abdominal aortic aneurysm, which of the following statements is TRUE?

A. Screening for AAA has been shown to be cost effective in women
B. CT angiogram is the best screening test
C. Only people who smoke need inviting for screening
D. The majority of detected aneurysms are small (3.0–4.5 cm)
E. Screened patients undergoing aneurysm surgery have a worse outcome than patients who present as an incidental finding

17. A 62-year-old lady complains of having lost 1½ stone in the last 6 months because she was finding it difficult to eat. After even a small meal she experiences severe central abdominal pain. She had a coronary artery bypass 4 years ago following an MI. She continues to smoke.

Which of the following symptoms or signs is NOT associated with chronic mesenteric ischaemia?

A. Weight loss
B. Diarrhoea
C. Severe abdominal pain brought on by eating
D. Jaundice
E. Vomiting

18. Which artery is the most important to revascularize in both acute and chronic mesenteric ischaemia?

A. Coeliac trunk
B. Superior mesenteric artery
C. Middle colic artery
D. Inferior mesenteric artery
E. Internal iliac artery

19. A 44-year old female is investigated for refractory hypertension after she presented with frequent headaches. On presentation her blood pressure was 220/140 mmHg. She has a moderately elevated BMI (27kg/m^2). Plasma cortisol and thyroid hormone levels were normal. MR angiogram showed bilateral renal artery stenosis with appearance highly suggestive of fibromuscular dysplasia (FMD).

Which of these antihypertensive medication would it be unsafe to prescribe as first-line in this patient?

A. Amlodipine
B. Bisoprolol
C. Ramipril
D. Bendroflumethiazide
E. Doxazosin

20. Which of the following statements regarding balloon angioplasty for unilateral renal artery stenosis is FALSE?

A. Is routinely performed to treat hypertension
B. Is indicated for treating flash pulmonary oedema
C. Is indicated in FMD causing renal impairment and/or hypertension
D. May not significantly improve renal function
E. When associated with end stage renal failure carries a poor prognosis

chapter 8.2

PERIPHERAL ARTERY DISEASE

ANSWERS

1. E. Moderate alcohol consumption has been shown to be protective for coronary artery disease. There is conflicting evidence as to whether there is benefit for PAD, but no evidence of harm. Marfan syndrome, an autosomal dominant gene mutation in Fibrillin-1 (FBN-1), is associated with cystic medial degeneration of the aortic wall. This can lead to aortic aneurysm or dissection. Takayasu's disease is a rare vasculitis affecting the aorta and main branches. In the acute phase this can lead to occlusion of the arteries (it is also known as 'pulseless disease'). Renal failure and diabetes are associated with higher prevalence and more rapid progression of peripheral arterial disease (PAD).

2. B. PARTNERS (PAD awareness risk and treatment: New resources for survival) reported a 29% prevalence of PAD in a high-risk patient cohort. The definition of PAD is an ABPI ≤0.9. Using this definition up to half of people are asymptomatic. PAD prevalence increases with age. Approximately one third of people with PAD have diabetes. Smoking, hypercholesterolemia, hypertension, and chronic kidney disease are other risk factors.

3. C. Swelling is not associated with PAD. Common causes of leg swelling are weight gain, venous disease, and congestive cardiac failure. An elevated ABPI indicates that there is arteriosclerosis, thickening of the lower limb arterial wall. This is associated with the subsequent development of stenotic atherosclerotic lesions. Pallor on elevation and rubor (redness) on dependency of a limb is a positive Buerger's test for critical limb threatening ischaemia (CLTI). Pallor is due to insufficient blood pressure at the ankle to maintain foot perfusion once elevated. Rubor is a sign of maximum capillary vasodilation in compensation for the chronically low tissue oxygen levels. An ABPI ≤0.9 is the diagnostic threshold for PAD.

4. B. Burning pain, or sharp pain, in the feet is typically of a diabetic peripheral neuropathy. Whilst this can occur in conjunction with PAD it is frequently present in patients with a normal arterial supply. Erectile dysfunction has a number of causes, including stress, anxiety, medication (specifically beta-blockers), and exhaustion. Leriche syndrome is the classic association between aorto-iliac occlusive disease and erectile dysfunction. Reproducible pain on walking, but not at rest, in the muscles of the calf, thigh, or buttock is typical of intermittent claudication. Walking distance is typically reduced on inclines as the effort of walking is increased. Pain on elevation of the leg which is only relieved by dependency is typical of ischaemic rest pain (i.e. CLTI). Blue toe syndrome results from either peripheral arterial disease or embolization from a more proximal source.

5. D. Popliteal angioplasty has a high re-occlusion rate, more so when a stent is used, so is rarely of clinical benefit for stable intermittent claudication. The evidence for benefit for statin therapy is largely extrapolated from coronary artery disease but is supported by findings from the HEART PROTECTION STUDY and REACH (PAD registry). Supervised exercise therapy is the 'gold standard' for symptom relief in PAD. In the CAPRIE trial patients with PAD treated with clopidogrel 75 mg had their annual risk of ischaemic stroke, MI, or vascular death reduced by 8.7% as compared with 325 mg aspirin (5.32% vs 5.83% respectively, CI 3–165, intention to treat analysis). There isn't good evidence for prescribing anti-hypertension medication specifically to patients with PAD; however, lowering blood pressure has overwhelming evidence for benefit.

6. E. When there is a long arterial occlusion (>10 cm) angioplasty alone is rarely successful and stent placement in addition is required. Even with stenting of the superficial femoral artery durability remains a concern. As per Q5 all patients with PAD should receive cardiovascular disease modifying medication with an anti-platelet therapy and statin (unless contra-indicated). Surgical bypass carries a higher risk of MI or death but is likely to be a more durable option than endovascular therapy. It is durability concerns that have moved management away from intervention towards supervised exercise therapy.

7. B. COMPASS showed higher bleeding risk from rivaroxaban and aspirin than aspirin alone. In VOYAGER PAD the addition of anticoagulation to aspirin increased bleeding on one of two outcome measure used. Patients with atrial fibrillation are at increased risk for embolic stroke and should be formally anti-coagulated provided there is no contra-indication to this. An eGFR <30 ml/mg/min is a contra-indication to the use of a direct oral anticoagulant. Ticagrelor 90 mg BD was shown to be non-superior to clopidogrel 75 mg od in EUCLID, with more patients ceasing treatment with ticagrelor due to dyspnoea and minor bleeding. In people with PAD no trials have been performed of anticoagulation alone.

8. C. Transcutaneous oxygen measurement is a non-invasive way of directly assessment of oxygen levels in the tissues below the skin. Assessing foot perfusion, ideally by measuring toe brachial index (TBI) or transcutaneous oxygen measurement is especially important in people with diabetes. However, TBI is not always possible in patients with active ulceration. People with diabetes can have a preserved lower limb arterial supply with micro-vascular disease within the digital arteries. Ankle brachial pressure index, cross-sectional imaging (CTA and magnetic resonance angiography), and angiography will show if there is macro-vascular disease (i.e. proximal arterial stenosis) but these tests are not objective measures of perfusion of the tissues in the foot. The ABPI will often be falsely elevated in people with diabetes due to arterial wall thickening and calcification.

9. C. Angioplasty alone is not a good option in acute limb ischaemia as it will often result in distal thrombus embolization and loss of the limb ('distal trash'). To fully answer this question, you need to know the aetiology of the ischaemia. For an embolus, for instance in a patient with atrial fibrillation, surgical embolectomy or aspiration thrombectomy are the correct treatment choices. For acute or chronic occlusion from atheromatous disease, catheter-directed thrombolysis and surgical bypass are both effective alternatives

10. A. Carpal tunnel syndrome may co-exist with a thoracic outlet syndrome but the two are not directly associated. Thoracic outlet syndrome is strongly associated with the presence of a cervical rib or cervical fibrous band. Thoracic outlet syndrome is also associated with Raynaud's syndrome on the affected side. Recurrent arterial trauma can result in aneurysmal degeneration; this in turn can lead to thrombosis or distal embolization with acute limb ischaemia. The subclavian vein may be similarly damaged, leading to fibrosis and acute upper limb deep vein thrombosis (Paget–Schroetter syndrome).

11. E. Of these events, amaurosis fugax carries the lowest risk of being followed by a major stroke. Minor stroke and TIA are differentiated only by the presence or absence of an ischaemic lesion on diffusion weighted cross-sectional brain imaging (MRI). When due to a significant internal carotid artery stenosis, >50% on NASCET measurement, the risk of a major stroke is highest in the following 48 hours.

12. B. Previous radiotherapy to the jugular nodes can make surgical carotid endarterectomy a challenging procedure, with a high risk of cranial nerve injury, major haemorrhage, or infection. Carotid stenting may well be a lower risk procedure for such a patient. An internal carotid artery occlusion is not amenable to treatment with a carotid stent. Aortic occlusion will prevent femoral access to stent a carotid lesion. The benefit of intervention for an asymptomatic carotid stenosis is less in women than in men. As it takes 5 years for the benefit of intervention for an asymptomatic stenosis to fully outweigh the procedural risk, this is rarely indicated for patients aged over 75 years (ASCT-1). Following major stoke there is a risk of intra-cerebral haemorrhage with reperfusion. Whilst it is no longer deemed necessary to wait 6 weeks before intervention most operators would wait 2 weeks and assess functional recovery before intervening.

13. A. Studies of carotid plaque morphology aim to better predict future embolic events in patients with asymptomatic internal carotid stenosis than the degree of stenosis alone. Calcification alone is not associated with acute ischaemic events. Smooth plaque morphology indicates an intact fibrinous 'cap' over the plaque and reduced risk of stroke. The other plaque characteristics listed have all be associated with plaque instability and a higher risk of embolic events.

14. D. In a post-hoc observational analysis of the IMPROVE trial dataset, local anaesthetic for ruptured AAA treatment with EVAR (endovascular AAA repair) was associated with lower in hospital mortality than general anaesthesia. Aortic aneurysms in women rupture at a smaller size than men. Small aneurysm surveillance up to a diameter threshold of 5.5 cm is safe (UKSAT). At this threshold a shared decision is made as to whether operative repair is indicated to prevent AAA rupture and extend life. There is no evidence of benefit for using local anaesthetic for elective EVAR. Long-term outcomes for EVAR in comparison to open surgical repair is available from OVER, EVAR 1, and DREAM trials (the French ACE trial lacked long-term data). All three trials showed no difference in all-cause survival at 10 years. The early aneurysm-related survival benefit from EVAR was lost over time due to a higher rate of reinterventions and late ruptures.

15. A. Diabetes is a risk factor for most cardiovascular diseases but is negatively associated with aortic growth. One possible explanation, yet to be tested in clinical trials, is that metformin may play a protective role against aortic growth. The most important risk factors for AAA growth are ageing and cigarette smoking. Genetics plays a part, with estimates suggesting 10% of people with AAA have some genetic component. The association between chronic pulmonary disease and aortic aneurysm is complex but appears to go beyond a simple joint association with smoking: it is postulated that there could be a common genetic, inflammatory, or remodelling pathway.

16. D. The prevalence of abdominal aortic aneurysm is highest for small aneurysms. An AAA screening programme for women, designed to be similar to that for men, is unlikely to be cost effective (SWAN collaborators). CT is inferior to ultrasound as an AAA screening test. CT can only be performed in a healthcare setting, exposes patients to ionizing radiation and will result in additional investigations for incidental findings. Ultrasound is more cost effective and with standardized training non-visualization rates <2% can be achieved. The current 30-day mortality for AAA repair for patients from the NHS AAA screening programme is 1.1%. This is lower than the UK mortality for elective AAA repair (2.3%).

17. D. Jaundice is a symptom of hepatic dysfunction or bile duct obstruction. Chronic mesenteric ischaemia, also known as 'mesenteric angina', is typified by the central abdominal pain experienced following meals. Fear of this pain leads to loss of appetite and weight loss. Disturbed eating is a frequent cause of vomiting and diarrhoea. Other common cause of pain after eating are gastro-oesophageal reflux and peptic ulcer disease. Chronic diarrhoea and vomiting may also be symptoms of irritable bowel syndrome, inflammatory bowel syndrome, or coeliac disease.

18. B. Symptoms of mesenteric ischaemia are most likely to manifest when the superior mesenteric artery is significantly stenosed. Coeliac trunk occlusion frequently occurs due to median arcuate ligament compression syndrome (MALS) without sequalae. This is explained both by portal venous supply to the liver combined and collateralization from SMA to hepatic arteries via the gastro-duodenal artery. The middle colon is rarely revascularized; most emboli that lodge that distal infarct the small bowel and require laparotomy and bowel resection. Pelvic blood supply via the superior and middle rectal arteries is important for the sigmoid colon and rectum. Whilst ligation or embolization of the internal iliac arteries may result in acute mesenteric ischaemia, these are rarely revascularized.

19. C. Prescribing an ACE inhibitor to a patient with bilateral renal artery stenosis may cause acute kidney injury. ACE inhibitors are used to treat hypertension in people with unilateral renal artery stenosis provided that renal function is carefully monitored. Calcium channel blocker, beta blocker, thiazide diuretic, and alpha-blocker are all alternative antihypertensives for people with known renal artery stenosis.

20. A. Angioplasty for renal artery stenosis is only rarely performed to treat resistant hypertension. The better indications for treating renal artery stenosis are flash pulmonary oedema and fibromuscular dysplasia (FMD) with renal impairment and/or hypertension. Atherosclerotic renal artery stenosis as a cause of renal failure has a poor prognosis. Intervention for unilateral stenosis rarely improves renal function, it is sometimes performed when there has been no improvement with medication. Even for bilateral stenosis treatment may not improve renal outcomes.

chapter

8.3

THROMBOEMBOLIC DISEASE

QUESTIONS

1. When using a 2-level Wells score for the diagnosis of DVT

A. A score of 2 points or more suggests DVT is likely
B. A score of 3 points or more suggests DVT is likely
C. A score of 4 points or more suggests DVT is likely
D. Only a score of 0 would indicate DVT is unlikely
E. Should not be used in the diagnosis of DVT

2. D-dimer testing in the diagnosis of DVT

A. Should be used in conjunction with a high Wells score
B. Has a good positive predictive value
C. Should be performed in a patient with a high Wells score but a negative duplex ultrasound
D. Has no role in the diagnosis of DVT
E. Should be performed in all patients with suspected DVT

3. A 40-year-old woman with lung cancer is diagnosed with a proximal DVT. She has a background of anxiety and has severe needle phobia. She has normal renal function and no risk factors for bleeding. The most appropriate choice for anticoagulation is:

A. Unfractionated heparin infusion
B. Low molecular weight heparin
C. Rivaroxaban
D. Aspirin
E. Warfarin

4. A 43-year-old man who is normally fit and well is found to have thrombus within the right soleal vein on compression duplex ultrasound. He presented with mild swelling of the right calf after a long-haul flight. The most appropriate course of action is:

A. Start a 3-month course of anticoagulation with a DOAC
B. Reassure and discharge him
C. Repeat the duplex at 1 week and 2 weeks
D. Repeat the duplex in 1 month
E. Perform a CTPA to exclude co-existent PE

5. A 35-year-old man is involved in a road traffic accident and suffers a fractured left femur. The fracture requires open reduction and internal fixation under general anaesthetic. He makes a good recovery and is discharged home. He re-presents 8 weeks later with a swollen left leg. He is diagnosed with a proximal left DVT. You start anticoagulation with rivaroxaban. The recommended duration of treatment should be:

A. 6 months
B. 3 months
C. Extended anticoagulation if he was deemed to have low bleeding risk
D. 4 months
E. Extended anticoagulation irrespective of bleeding risk

6. Regarding the diagnosis of pulmonary embolism

A. $S_1Q_3T_3$ pattern on ECG is commonly seen
B. On chest X-ray Fleischner's sign refers to an area of regional oligaemia distal to an occlusive pulmonary embolus
C. All patients are hypoxaemic
D. Syncope suggests high burden proximal PE
E. A large unilateral pleural effusion on chest X-ray would be typical

7. An 85-year-old lady is admitted with shortness of breath and pleuritic chest pain. She has a past medical history of COPD. You suspect she has a PE. Her blood pressure is 110/70 mmHg, her heart rate is 115 bpm and her oxygen saturation is 88% on 2 L/min oxygen via nasal cannulae. Her chest X-ray shows hyperinflated lung fields. Her troponin is elevated at 135 ng/L and her eGFR is 60 ml/min. She has a CTPA, which shows bilateral proximal pulmonary emboli with right ventricular dilatation, flattening of the intraventricular septum and reflux of contrast into the IVC.

Based on the above information her combined early mortality assessment would categorize her into which group?

A. High risk
B. Intermediate–high risk
C. Intermediate–ow risk
D. Low risk
E. Unable to determine from above information

8. Which initial treatment would be most appropriate for the above patient?

A. Systemic thrombolysis
B. Sub-cutaneous low molecular weight heparin
C. Unfractionated heparin infusion
D. Tirofiban
E. Pulmonary embolectomy

9. A 60-year-old man attends ambulatory care with pleuritic chest pain and is suspected to have a PE. His 2-level Wells score for PE is 1 hence he goes on to have a D-dimer test, which is positive. He has a CTPA, which is reported 'good opacification of the pulmonary arterial tree, no evidence of pulmonary embolism'.

What is the correct course of action?

A. Reassure and discharge him
B. Perform a V/Q scan
C. Repeat the CTPA in 1 month
D. Assess for clinical evidence of a DVT and perform a compression duplex ultrasound if clinical suspicion remains high
E. Perform an MR angiogram

10. A 70-year-old man is brought into the emergency department by ambulance. He had collapsed at home and was found by his wife. He had been complaining of breathlessness on climbing the stairs over the last 3 days. His past medical history was unremarkable, and he was on no regular medication. He was drowsy with a blood pressure of 60/40 mmHg and a heart rate of 130 bpm. His oxygen saturations were 90% on 5 L/min. His heart sounds were dual with a loud P2 and an RV heave and a pan systolic murmur. His chest X-ray is normal. His ECG shows T-wave inversion in the anterior leads and right axis deviation. You perform a bedside echocardiogram, which shows a volume loaded, dilated impaired right ventricle with a mildly elevated PAP. His left ventricle is normal. He is too unstable for transfer.

What is the most appropriate course of action?

A. 1L bolus of crystalloid
B. Immediate intubation and ventilation
C. Start a vasopressor infusion
D. Systemic thrombolysis
E. Sub-cutaneous low molecular weight heparin then CTPA when more stable

11. A 32-year-old lady who is 29-weeks pregnant is admitted with a suspected PE. Clinical examination is unremarkable other than noting a gravid uterus. Baseline blood tests, chest X-ray, and ECG are unremarkable. The most appropriate initial investigation is:

A. D-dimer test
B. MR angiography of pulmonary vessels
C. CTPA or V/Q scan
D. Compression duplex ultrasound of both lower limbs
E. Echocardiography

12. A 32-year-old lady who is 29-weeks pregnant is found to have bilateral pulmonary emboli on a CTPA. She is haemodynamically stable with a normal troponin and normal echocardiogram. The correct treatment for her pulmonary emboli is:

A. LMWH with concomitant warfarin loading
B. A DOAC
C. Unfractionated heparin infusion
D. LMWH—dose based upon current weight
E. LMWH—dose based upon booking weight

13. Regarding chronic thromboembolic pulmonary hypertension (CTEPH)

A. Should be routinely screened for in all patients following a PE
B. Is an uncommon cause of breathlessness
C. Presents with signs and symptoms of RV failure early in the disease
D. Can be diagnosed based on specific findings at echocardiography
E. There must be a prior history of venous thromboembolic disease to make the diagnosis

14. A 49-year-old man is seen with progressive exertional dyspnoea 6 months after being diagnosed with large bilateral, proximal, unprovoked pulmonary emboli. He has been taking rivaroxaban since diagnosis. He has a normal chest X-ray. His ECG shows an RV strain pattern. His echocardiogram shows an estimated RVSP of 48 mmHg with good right and left ventricular systolic function. The next most appropriate investigation to exclude CTEPH is:

A. CTPA
B. V/Q scan
C. Conventional pulmonary angiography
D. Right heart catheterization
E. MR pulmonary angiography

15. Regarding the treatment of CTEPH:

A. Medical therapy should be tried before referring for surgical treatment
B. Bosentan is licensed for the treatment of inoperable CTEPH
C. Pulmonary endarterectomy is the treatment of choice
D. Riociguat should be used after pulmonary endarterectomy in all patients for 6 months
E. In hospital mortality for pulmonary endarterectomy is around 10%

16. An 82-year-old man with a background of metastatic prostate cancer presents with exertional dyspnoea and haemoptysis. His blood pressure is 130/90 mmHg with heart rate 120 bpm, respiratory rate 20/min and oxygen saturations of 89% on air. His chest X-ray is unremarkable and his ECG shows a sinus tachycardia. The suspected diagnosis is pulmonary embolism.

What is his sPESI score?

A. 4
B. 2
C. 5
D. 3
E. 1

17. Regarding duration of anticoagulation in VTE which of the following is correct?

A. 6 months anticoagulation for an unprovoked PE
B. 2 months anticoagulation for a provoked distal DVT
C. 3 months anticoagulation for a provoked proximal DVT
D. 4 months anticoagulation for a malignancy associated DVT
E. Extended anticoagulation for provoked proximal PEs causing haemodynamic instability

18. A 45 year old man presents with pleuritic chest pain 3 weeks after a right total knee replacement. He is otherwise fit and well. On examination his heart rate is 120 bpm. There is no clinical evidence of a DVT. You feel PE is the most likely diagnosis.

What is his 2-level Wells score for PE?

A. 6
B. 5
C. 3
D. 1.5
E. 4

19. A 45-year-old man presents with pleuritic chest pain 3 weeks after a right total knee replacement. He is otherwise fit and well. On examination his heart rate is 120 bpm his blood pressure is 145/70 mmHg. There is no clinical evidence of a DVT. His renal function is normal. You feel PE is the most likely diagnosis. He is not suitable for outpatient management and a CTPA is not immediately available.

What is the most appropriate course of action?

A. Measure D-dimer level. If positive proceed to anticoagulation and CTPA
B. Rivaroxaban followed by CTPA
C. Commence warfarin followed by CTPA
D. Echocardiogram
E. Unfractionated heparin infusion followed by CTPA

20. In PE an sPESI score of ≥1 is associated with a 30 day mortality of:

A. 5.5%
B. 10.9%
C. 15.1%
D. 20%
E. 7.7%

21. Which of the following is a proximal deep vein of the lower extremity?

A. Soleal
B. Great saphenous
C. Tibial
D. Gastrocnemial
E. Popliteal

22. Chest X-ray findings which would be consistent with a diagnosis of PE include:

A. Lobar consolidation
B. Pulmonary oedema
C. Tracheal deviation
D. Pleural effusion
E. Hilar lymphadenopathy

23. A 72-year-old man is diagnosed with an unprovoked proximal DVT. He has a past medical history of pulmonary embolism 15 years ago for which no provoking risk factor was found. He was treated with a 3-month course of warfarin which was terminated due to an upper GI bleed associated with an unexplained INR of 8.

What is the most appropriate treatment option?

A. Insert an IVC filter
B. Extended therapy with warfarin
C. Extended therapy with LMWH
D. Extended therapy with a DOAC
E. Catheter directed thrombolysis

24. The estimated annual incidence of chronic thromboembolic pulmonary hypertension (CTEPH) is:

A. 0.1 per million
B. 5 per million
C. 5 per 100,000
D. 1 per 10,000
E. 1 per 1000

25. The following clinical features are associated with PE:

A. Pyrexia
B. Pleuritic chest pain
C. Syncope
D. Cough
E. All of the above

chapter

8.3

THROMBOEMBOLIC DISEASE

ANSWERS

1. A. If a DVT is suspected, a 2-level Wells score should be used. A score of 2 points or more indicates a DVT is likely and a score of 1 point or less indicates a DVT is unlikely.

2. C. There are two situations in which D-dimer testing should be used in the diagnosis of DVT. The first is in the context of a low Wells score (1 point or less) where a negative D-dimer can exclude the diagnosis of DVT. The second is in the context of a high Wells score (2 points or greater) where a leg vein ultrasound is not immediately available (within 4 hours). In this situation a positive D-dimer in conjunction with a negative leg vein ultrasound should lead to a repeat ultrasound in 6–8 days. The D-dimer test has a good negative predictive value and hence has no role in cases where a DVT is considered likely and a leg vein ultrasound is immediately available.

3. C. Traditionally, low molecular weight heparin has been the treatment of choice for VTE in the context of active cancer. However, more recently guidelines recommend a DOAC can also be used, considering drug interactions and bleeding risk. In this case the history of needle phobia would make INR monitoring with warfarin and administration of LMWH problematic. Aspirin is not indicated as first-line anticoagulation for VTE and an unfractionated heparin infusion is not required in the absence of established renal failure or high bleeding risk. The most appropriate answer is therefore rivaroxaban.

4. C. The soleal vein is a deep vein of the lower extremity. As this is not classified as a proximal DVT and there are no severe symptoms or risk factors for clot extension, anticoagulation is not required at this stage. The most appropriate course of action is to repeat the ultrasound at 1 and 2 weeks. At this stage anticoagulation should be started if the thrombus extends but remains within the distal veins or if thrombus extends into the proximal veins. In this case there are no signs or symptoms to suggest PE, hence a CTPA is not warranted.

5. B. This is classified as a provoked proximal DVT as the surgery was performed within the last 3 months. In this situation anticoagulation for 3 months is recommended. In this case there is a very clear provoking transient risk factor; however, there may be situations in which clinical judgement needs to be used to assess whether a risk factor is considered significant, particularly in the case of immobility.

6. D. In the context of suspected or proven PE, syncope is a concerning symptom. Syncope results from a transient reduction in systemic blood pressure and cerebral perfusion. This implies a clot burden large enough to impede right ventricular outflow and compromise left ventricular filling. If hypotension is persistent, the patient should be considered for thrombolytic therapy. Although frequently cited, the S1Q3T3 ECG pattern is only seen in approximately 20% of cases of acute PE. This ECG pattern is also non-specific and can be seen in other causes of right ventricular strain. Fleischner's sign refers to the appearance of an enlarged pulmonary artery on chest X-ray. A small pleural effusion can be observed on chest X-ray in PE, often in association with pulmonary infarction; however, a large pleural effusion should prompt a search for alternative diagnoses. Peripheral low-volume pulmonary emboli may not cause hypoxaemia.

7. B. When large volume PE with features of right heart strain have been identified on CTPA, the first priority is assessment for hypotension. This carries a high risk of mortality and thrombolytic treatment should be considered. In this case, hypotension is not present, however a high sPESI score of 4 (1 point scored for each of age >80, heart rate ≥110 bpm, presence of COPD, and arterial oxygen saturation <90%) together with CT features of right ventricular dysfunction and an elevated troponin put this patient in the intermediate-high risk. If the troponin was normal the risk category would be intermediate–low.

8. B. Anticoagulation is required for the treatment of an acute PE. In this case, systemic thrombolysis and unfractionated heparin infusions are not indicated as the patient is haemodynamically stable with adequate renal function. Similarly, pulmonary embolectomy is not indicated. Tirofiban is an anti-platelet agent which is not indicated in the treatment of VTE. The correct answer is therefore sub-cutaneous low molecular weight heparin. A DOAC could also be considered in this situation; however, the intermediate–high risk category would favour initial treatment with LMWH.

9. D. The high-quality imaging obtained from CTPA in this case excludes PE; there is no indication for further diagnostic imaging such as a V/Q scan, MR angiogram, or repeat CTPA. Nevertheless, the positive D-dimer should prompt a clinical assessment for the presence of DVT. If there is a clinical suspicion of DVT, a leg vein ultrasound should be performed.

10. D. In this case the combination of a history of breathlessness, and clinical findings of hypotension, hypoxaemia, and right ventricular strain are strongly suggestive of PE. This is also supported by the ECG features of right ventricular strain and findings on echocardiogram. The significant hypotension immediately categorizes this as high risk and the treatment of choice is systemic thrombolysis. Treatment with vasopressors of intravenous crystalloid will not treat the underlying problem of right ventricular outflow obstruction and may well exacerbate right ventricular strain and further compromise blood pressure. Treatment with LMWH while awaiting CTPA in this circumstance leaves the patient at high risk of cardiovascular collapse.

11. C. The investigation of choice in this scenario is a CTPA or VQ scan. CTPA is preferred to VQ scan if the chest X-ray is abnormal. The use of D-dimer testing in pregnancy is unreliable as D-dimer levels are frequently elevated as part of normal pregnancy. If there were clinical signs or symptoms of DVT, an ultrasound of both lower limbs would be a reasonable initial investigation. Echocardiography is only likely to be useful in the context of suspected large PE with haemodynamic compromise. MR angiography is not indicated as first line investigation of suspected acute PE.

12. E. Both warfarin and DOACs are contraindicated in pregnancy. LMWH is the treatment of choice and dosing should be based upon booking weight. An unfractionated heparin infusion should be considered in PE with haemodynamic instability; however, that is not indicated in this situation.

13. B. CTEPH should be suspected in a patient with persisting breathlessness or new signs and symptoms of RV failure following an acute PE having completed 3 months of anticoagulation. Although breathlessness is a common symptom of CTEPH, overall CTEPH is an uncommon cause of breathlessness. Signs and symptoms of RV failure only manifest as a late feature of CTEPH. Although echocardiography is useful in the diagnosis of CTEPH, findings are non-specific and need to be combined with supportive evidence based on imaging and right heart catheterization to make the diagnosis. CTEPH may be diagnosed in a patient without a prior history of VTE if previous thromboembolic events were unrecognized at the time.

14. B. The persisting symptom of exertional dyspnoea together with the echo findings of elevated RVSP following an acute PE with high clot burden is highly suggestive of CTEPH. The next investigation should be a V/Q san as this is the most sensitive imaging modality for excluding CTEPH. CTPA can be used in the diagnosis of CTEPH but should not be used as a stand-alone test to exclude the diagnosis. Right heart catheterization, MR pulmonary angiography, and conventional pulmonary angiography may have a role further along the diagnostic pathway but are not indicated at this stage.

15. C. Pulmonary endarterectomy is the treatment of choice for operable CTEPH. This procedure is performed in specialist centres and results in substantial symptom relief and near normalization of haemodynamics for the majority of patients. Riociguat is an oral soluble guanylate cyclase stimulator which is licenced for the treatment of inoperable CTEPH or persisting pulmonary hypertension following pulmonary endarterectomy. In Europe, in-hospital mortality for pulmonary endarterectomy is around 4.7% and lower in high-volume experienced centres. Bosentan is an endothelin receptor antagonist and is primarily used for the treatment of pulmonary arterial hypertension.

16. A. One point is scored for each of the following: age >80, cancer, heart rate ≥110 bpm and arterial oxygen saturation <90%. The total score is therefore 4.

17. C. Treatment duration of anticoagulation for a provoked proximal DVT or PE should be 3 months if the provoking risk factor is no longer present and the clinical course has been uncomplicated. Extended anticoagulation beyond 3 months should be considered for unprovoked proximal DVT and PE, taking into account the balance between bleeding risk and risk of VTE recurrence. If the decision has been made to treat a distal DVT, the duration of treatment should be the same as for proximal DVT.

18. A. The score is 3 points as PE is felt to be the most likely diagnosis. 1.5 points are scored for heart rate >100 bpm and a further 1.5 points for surgery in the previous 4 weeks. The total score is therefore 6.

19. B. In this case, the high Wells score should prompt either immediate CTPA or interim anticoagulation followed by a CTPA. As a CTPA is not immediately available, the correct choice is to start interim anticoagulation while awaiting diagnostic imaging. The most appropriate choice in this case is rivaroxaban; this has the advantage of being able to being able to be continued for longer term anticoagulation if the CTPA confirms the diagnosis of PE. A D-dimer is not indicated in the context of a high Wells score. Warfarin is not suitable as interim anticoagulation and an unfractionated heparin infusion should only be used in the context of established renal failure or high bleeding risk. Echocardiography is not recommended as a first-line investigation for acute PE without haemodynamic instability.

20. B. An sPESI score of 0 points is associated with a 30-day mortality risk of 1% and a score of ≥ 1 is associated with a 30-day mortality risk of 10.9%.

21. E. Deep veins of the lower extremity include iliac, femoral, popliteal, tibial, peroneal, soleal, and gastrocnemial. Of these, iliac, femoral, and popliteal are considered proximal.

22. D. The chest X-ray may be normal in PE. Signs which can be observed are all non-specific and should not be considered diagnostic. Signs which may be observed in PE include atelectasis, pleural effusion (typically small), enlarged pulmonary artery (Fleischner's sign), regional oligaemia (Westermark's sign), and peripheral wedge-shaped opacification (Hampton hump).

23. D. This is the second instance of unprovoked VTE which puts this patient in a high-risk category for future VTE recurrence. Extended anticoagulation is therefore recommended. The previous upper GI bleed was associated with an elevated INR and would therefore not be a contraindication to extended anticoagulation. Warfarin treatment has previously been problematic for this patient hence the most appropriate choice here is a DOAC. An IVC filter could be considered if there was an absolute contraindication to anticoagulation. Catheter-directed thrombolysis is only recommended for symptomatic iliofemoral DVT. In the absence of active cancer, extended anticoagulation with a DOAC is preferable to LMWH.

24. B. The annual incidence of CTEPH is estimated to be around 5 per million. The cumulative incidence is between 0.1 and 9.1% within 2 years of a symptomatic PE. The large variability is likely to be due to referral bias, difficulty in identifying early symptoms and difficulty in differentiating acute PE from symptoms of pre-existing CTEPH.

25. E. The broad spectrum of common clinical signs and symptoms which can be associated with PE frequently present a diagnostic challenge. In a patient with undifferentiated symptoms who is considered to be at low risk of PE, the pulmonary embolism rule-out criteria (PERC) rule can help determine whether further investigations for PE are needed.

chapter 8.4

PULMONARY HYPERTENSION

QUESTIONS

1. **A GP contacts you about a young woman in whom he believes a diagnosis of pulmonary arterial hypertension has been made. He tells you that she has had a 'range' of tests.**

   Which one of the following is essential to confirm the diagnosis?

   A. An echocardiogram demonstrated a dilated right heart and tricuspid regurgitant peak velocity of 4m/s
   B. During an exercise echocardiogram, the estimated RV systolic pressure (derived from the jet of tricuspid regurgitation) was greater than 30 mmHg at peak exercise
   C. A computed tomography pulmonary angiogram demonstrated bilateral pulmonary emboli
   D. Mean pulmonary artery pressure at rest was 32 mmHg on a right heart catheterisation and pulmonary artery wedge pressure was 8 mmHg
   E. Mean pulmonary artery pressure at rest was 32 mmHg on a right heart catheterization and normal pulmonary artery wedge pressure at 16 mmHg

2. **You are asked by a cardiac physiologist to review an echocardiogram on an elderly patient who presents with breathlessness. Estimated RV systolic pressure, as judged by the velocity of the tricuspid regurgitant jet, is moderately elevated.**

   In terms of aetiology of the pulmonary hypertension, which of the following is true?

   A. The presence of left atrial dilatation and advanced diastolic dysfunction, in the setting of diabetes and hypertension suggests a diagnosis of pulmonary hypertension due to left heart cause
   B. Lung disease is the most common cause of pulmonary hypertension
   C. Thrombus seen in the proximal pulmonary arteries confirms chronic thromboembolic disease as the cause of her pulmonary hypertension
   D. A history of rheumatoid arthritis would make connective tissue disease associated pulmonary arterial hypertension the most likely explanation
   E. Echocardiographic evidence of an old myocardial infarction is not relevant from a diagnostic perspective

3. You admit a middle-aged woman who has been investigated for breathlessness for several years. She has peripheral oedema, raised venous pressures, and other clinical features to suggest heart failure. Pulmonary hypertension is suspected. The most appropriate initial management would be:

A. Start sildenafil
B. Start warfarin if pulmonary hypertension is confirmed
C. Give diuretics in the clinical setting of symptomatic heart failure
D. Give an ACE inhibitor to benefit right ventricular function
E. Refer for cardiac catheterization

4. A 70-year-old woman with a history of an acute pulmonary embolism presents 4 months later with persistent breathlessness. She is in WHO functional class III. Her INR has been within the therapeutic range. Serial echocardiograms demonstrate persistent features of pulmonary hypertension.

Which one of the following is an appropriate next step?

A. Continue warfarin as the clot will resolve eventually
B. Commence riociguat
C. Refer to a specialist PH centre for further investigations and consideration of pulmonary endarterectomy
D. Change her anticoagulant
E. Refer her for a balloon atrial septostomy

5. You have been contacted by the infectious diseases team about a man with HIV who has become progressively more breathless over several months. He has had a CT pulmonary angiogram which has excluded pulmonary embolus. You go onto to discuss the scan with a radiologist.

From a CT perspective which one of the following statements is true?

A. If the right ventricle is of normal size this excludes pulmonary hypertension as a cause for his symptoms
B. Deviation of the interventricular septum indicates balanced pressures between right and left atrium
C. Normal lung parenchyma would make a diagnosis of pulmonary hypertension unlikely
D. If the pulmonary artery is dilated (PA > Ao), this suggests pulmonary hypertension might be present
E. A pericardial effusion if present will be unrelated to pulmonary hypertension

6. **You are managing a patient admitted with worsening heart failure symptoms. She has been diagnosed with idiopathic pulmonary arterial hypertension and receives continuous intravenous epoprostenol. An ECG shows atrial flutter with a rate of 110 bpm.**

   Which of the following is true?

   A. An interruption to the intravenous epoprostenol infusion can be tolerated for up to 6 hours
   B. Atrial flutter with a high ventricular rate may explain the deterioration and should be treated urgently, if necessary with cardioversion.
   C. Treatment with epoprostenol is only for symptomatic relief
   D. Epoprostenol cannot be used in combination with other advanced therapies
   E. If leakage from the indwelling line is suspected, you should never switch to a peripheral line.

7. **You are invited by your consultant to report the data recorded from right heart catheterization.**

   Which one of the following statements is correct?

   A. The transpulmonary gradient is mean pulmonary artery pressure − pulmonary wedge pressure
   B. The pulmonary vascular resistance is transpulmonary gradient multiplied by cardiac output
   C. Raised left atrial pressure is reflected by a pulmonary wedge pressure greater than 10 mmHg
   D. A reduction of mean pulmonary artery pressure from 65 mmHg to 50 mmHg on vasodilator testing is a positive vasoreactivity test
   E. Nitric oxide cannot be used to assess to assess vasodilatation response

8. **Which of the following are markers of poor prognosis in pulmonary hypertension?**

   A. A 6-minute walk distance less than 165 meters
   B. History of repeated syncope
   C. WHO functional class IV
   D. NT pro BNP levels > 1100 ng/l
   E. All the above

9. **Concerning the treatment of pulmonary hypertension:**

   A. Isolated lung transplant is the cornerstone of management.
   B. Sildenafil is recommended for patients with left heart failure as a treatment
   C. A majority of patients will require calcium channel blockade
   D. Sildenafil must not be given to young men as it causes priapism.
   E. Prostanoid analogues are available as oral, inhaled, and subcutaneous as well as intravenous preparations

10. With respect to pulmonary hypertension patients with congenital heart disease:

A. Pregnancy is well tolerated, making pre-pregnancy counselling unnecessary
B. Venesection is recommended for most patients to reduce hyperviscosity
C. Eisenmenger syndrome describes reversal of a left-to-right shunt due to the development of pulmonary hypertension
D. Transthoracic echocardiography inadequately images the upper septum so sinus venous defects may be missed
E. The 6-minute walk test is a gold standard measure of disease severity

11. A 35-year-old lady with history of limited scleroderma has been breathlessness for several months. On examination she has normal heart sounds and no signs of cardiovascular or respiratory pathology. An echocardiogram showed normal left ventricular function with no significant valvular pathology and a tricuspid regurgitant peak velocity of 3 m/s. The left and right atria area measured 21 cm^2 in the four-chamber view. Lung function tests show an FEV1 of 90%, FVC of 88% of predicted and a DLCO of 58% of predicted.

What would be the most appropriate next step?

A. Screening for the presence of PAH using DETECT algorithm
B. Referral to pulmonary hypertension specialist centre
C. Start treatment with calcium channel blockers
D. Reassure PH is unlikely
E. Commence an IV prostacyclin continuous infusion

12. These are the results of a cardiac catheterization performed on a 55-year-old patient as part of the work-up for breathlessness persisting for 6 months after pulmonary embolism. Anticoagulation has been continued since the initial diagnosis of pulmonary embolism.

RA pressure 10 mmHg

RV systolic pressure 50 mmHg, end diastolic 14 mmHg

PA pressure 48/18 (mean 30) mmHg

PCWP 12 mmHg

PA O_2 saturation 77%

Aortic pressure 126/78 mmHg

LV pressure 124/10 mmHg

Arterial oxygen saturation 98% (on room air)

Cardiac output by thermodilution 5.1 l/min

What is the diagnosis here?

A. Precapillary pulmonary hypertension
B. Postcapillary pulmonary hypertension
C. Pulmonary arterial hypertension
D. Pulmonary veno-occlusive disease
E. Hypoxic pulmonary hypertension

13. A 78-year-old diabetic, hypertensive woman has been referred for cardiac catheterization for assessment of exertional breathlessness. Echocardiography shows preserved LV systolic function and an enlarged left atrium. Coronary angiography shows only mild atheroma. At right cardiac catheterization her RA pressure is 8 mmHg, RV pressure 59/12 mmHg, PA pressure 57/24 (mean 38) mmHg, PCWP 22 mmHg, PA O_2 saturation of 77%, and cardiac output by thermodilution was 4.4 L/min. LV pressure is 162/23 mmHg and aortic pressure is 148/99 mmHg.

What is the underlying diagnosis?

A. Heart failure with preserved ejection fraction
B. Severe aortic stenosis with secondary pulmonary hypertension
C. Pulmonary arterial hypertension
D. No pulmonary hypertension
E. More data required to make a diagnosis

14. A 42-year-old female remains breathless since she had an acute pulmonary embolism a month ago.

Which of the following would be the most appropriate?

A. Repeat CT scanning to determine operability
B. Cardiac catheterization to determine if pulmonary hypertension has developed
C. Start sidenafil to improve prognosis
D. Start riociguat to relieve breathlessness
E. Continue anticoagulation and reassess in 2 months

15. A 28-year-old has been investigated for exertional syncope. Clinical examination reveals a loud P2 and a palpable parasternal heave. Autoantibody screen and HIV testing are negative. There is no family history of PH and she has no history of anorexigen or recreational drug intake. ECG shows RBBB and right axis deviation. On echocardiography the interventricular septum is flattened in systole with a tricuspid valve regurgitant velocity of 3.4 m/s. On CT of the chest the parenchyma is normal and the pulmonary artery is dilated at 3.8 cm with no evidence of thromboembolic disease. Cardiac catheterization shows mean PA pressure of 45 and PCWP of 11 and a PVR of 12 WU. Vasodilator test is negative.

What would be the most appropriate therapeutic first step?

A. Start sildenafil 25mg tds
B. Start IV epoprostenol
C. Refer for urgent heart and lung transplant
D. Start nifedipine at 20 mg sustained release
E. Refer for pulmonary endarterectomy

16. A 59-year-old lady presented with syncope. She has a history of limited scleroderma, pulmonary arterial hypertension, and previous pulmonary embolism. She has been on sildenafil 50 mg three times daily and IV epoprostenol continuous via ambulatory pump at 18 ng/kg/min. There is a previous intolerance to oral ambrisentan. Her husband described how she has been having trouble with the pump for a few hours and she started to be feeling acutely more breathless. The most appropriate action is:

A. Refer to pulmonary hypertension specialist centre.
B. Insert a peripheral line and start IV epoprostenol as soon as possible
C. Urgent admission to a monitored bed to rule out any arrythmogenic cause of the syncope
D. Increase the dose 20 ng/kg/min
E. Lower the dose 14 ng/kg/min

17. A 68-year-old lady with a 40-pack per year index smoking history presented with increasing breathlessness over the previous few months and falling exercise tolerance. She has past medical of limited scleroderma and type 2 diabetes. An echocardiogram revealed a dilated right atrium and ventricle with preserved left-sided ventricular size and function. A CT scan of the lungs has been done previously and showed extensive emphysematous changes. Lung function tests showed (FEV1 65%, FVC 70%, and DLCO 35% of predicted for age and sex). Cardiac catheterization showed PA pressure of 44/18 (mean 28), PCWP 8 mmHg and a PVR of 3.5 WU.

What would be the most appropriate next step?

A. Start calcium channel blockers
B. Start calcium channel blockers only after vasodilator test
C. Start sildenafil 25mg tds
D. Start prostacyclin analogue
E. Pulmonary hypertension specific therapy is inappropriate

chapter
8.4
PULMONARY HYPERTENSION
ANSWERS

1. D. Pulmonary arterial hypertension (PAH) is a diagnosis that requires a mean pulmonary artery pressure (mPAP) > 20 mmHg and pulmonary arterial wedge pressure (PAWP) ≤ 15 and a PVR of > 2 WU at rest using invasive measurements made during right heart catheterization. Echocardiographic findings can support a diagnosis of precapillary PH, but cannot confirm the diagnosis. If chronic thromboembolic lesions are present the diagnosis cannot be PAH. Severe lung disease can also cause precapillary PH (normal wedge pressure) but again excludes PAH. An elevated wedge confirms a left heart cause of PH, thus excluding PAH.

2. A. The echocardiogram in PH may provide evidence of the underlying aetiology and left heart disease related PH is the most prevalent cause. Left atrial dilatation is a red flag for left heart disease. Systemic disease processes, such as connective tissue disease, can underlie pulmonary arterial hypertension. Scleroderma is the most common connective tissue disease causing PAH. Proximal pulmonary artery thrombus can form in situ due to sluggish flow when the pulmonary arteries are dilated, especially in patients with the Eisenmenger syndrome, and is occasionally seen in acute pulmonary emboli.

3. C. The diagnostic work up should be started as soon as PH is suspected including bed side tests as ECG, chest X-ray, echocardiography, and lung function testing before cardiac catheterization or referral to PH specialist centre. PAH specific therapies (e.g. sildenafil) should be only started after PAH is confirmed by a specialist centre. Anticoagulation should not be routinely used in the absence of a clinical indication. Diuresis is helpful in the management of symptomatic heart failure. Currently there is no evidence for ACEI in RV failure.

4. C. This description fits with a diagnosis of chronic thromboembolic PH (CTEPH). Patients with thromboembolic disease who remain symptomatic despite 3 months of anticoagulation should be offered echocardiography. If there is evidence of PH, they should be referred for full evaluation and consideration of pulmonary endarterectomy, which is normally 'curative'. Advanced therapies can be considered by a specialist centre for selected patients but surgery remains the first line. Balloon atrial septostomy, which permits the right heart to vent into the left atrium, is used infrequently in selected patients with refractory syncope and heart failure, though not usually in CTEPH because of the risk of paradoxical emboli.

5. D. Computed tomography can provide important information besides the presence or absence of pulmonary emboli. Enlargement of the PA ≥ 30 mm and PA-to-aorta ratio > 0.9 is usually present in PH; it is, however, a non-specific finding commonly found in lung disease.

An enlarged right ventricle right atrium and pulmonary arteries are all typical findings in PH, though normality of these does not exclude PH and their presence is not diagnostic. Abnormal lung parenchyma suggests that PH if present it is due to lung disease. The interventricular septum is best assessed by an echocardiogram or CMR. It is sometimes observed on CTPA studies and deviation to the left suggests elevated RV pressure rather than providing information about atrial pressure. A pericardial effusion is a high-risk feature when present in the setting of pulmonary hypertension.

6. B. Parenteral epoprostenol is a synthetic prostacyclin that has very short life (3–5 minutes) and should not be interrupted. Atrial arrhythmias are not uncommon in patients with PAH, particularly atrial flutter. The loss of atrial transport is poorly tolerated and patients can become severely compromised even at normal ventricular rates. Urgent restoration of sinus rhythm is often required.

Epoprostenol has proven efficacy and mortality benefit and is often used in combination with other therapies. Specialist PH input is required if any changes to the rate of administration are to be made. Parenteral epoprostenol can be switched to a peripheral line if there are any issues with the indwelling catheter.

7. A. Transpulmonary gradient (TPG) is mean PAP − mean PWP and is normally <12 mmHg. Pulmonary vascular resistance is TPG divided by CO. A PWP > 15 mmHg indicates increased left atrial pressure. A vasodilator challenge is performed to identify the small subset of patients with PAH who will benefit from long-term calcium channel blockade. A portion of those with an initially positive response (mPAP ≥10 mmHg to ≤40 mmHg with an increased or unchanged CO), will become refractory to vasodilator provocation (and therefore calcium channel blockade) in the future. Inhaled nitric oxide or IV epoprostenol are commonly used to perform the test.

8. E. Serial multiparameter assessments have an important role in the management of pulmonary hypertension. No single parameter provides sufficient prognostic information in isolation. All of these parameters listed are considered high risk markers.

9. E. Sildenafil, initially marketed for erectile dysfunction, has proven efficacy in PAH patients but can be harmful in patients with PH secondary to left heart disease. Priapism has only been reported when used in sickle cell disease. Since only a minority of patients with pulmonary arterial hypertension respond to a vasodilator challenge (not all of whom will maintain this response) relatively few patients are on calcium channel blockade. Lung transplant is considered for eligible patients. Prostanoids are also available as oral, subcutaneous, inhaled and intravenous preparations.

10. C. Pulmonary hypertension is an important complication in congenital heart disease. Eisenmenger syndrome, defined by reversal of a left-to-right shunt due to the development of pulmonary hypertension. Venesection for patients with Eisenmenger syndrome is now avoided as iron deficiency is poorly tolerated by these patients. A sinus venosus defect (and aberrant pulmonary venous drainage) should be considered in patients with a dilated right heart and PH but no other explanation and can often be missed on TTE. Careful pregnancy counselling should be given to PH patients and family planning is vital. The 6-minute walk test has recognized limitations, particularly in children. A number of factors are therefore looked at for risk assessment.

11. B. Patients with scleroderma have a lifetime risk of developing PAH of approximately 10%. The DETECT algorithm is an evidence based screening tool but has been only validated in asymptomatic patients—this patient is symptomatic. Referral to a specialist centre here is a reasonable next step. Echocardiography is usually abnormal in PH patients, but it may underestimate pulmonary pressures. Starting specific PAH therapies should be done by a specialist centre.

12. A. These recordings indicate precapillary pulmonary hypertension (in this instance most likely due to CTEPH). Ruling out lung, thromboembolic disease, and other miscellaneous causes is required to attribute precapillary PH to PAH. A history of PE may or may not be present in around 25% of patients with CTEPH and so the demonstration of thromboembolic pathology (on CT or conventional pulmonary angiography) is a requirement to establish the diagnosis. Pulmonary veno-occlusive disease is often suspected from CT scan findings (features of centrilobular ground-glass opacities, septal lines, and lymphadenopathy) and is associated with precapillary haemodynamic findings, but cannot be diagnosed on catheter findings alone and is much less common than PAH or CTEPH.

13. A. The data is highly suggestive of heart failure with preserved ejection fraction which is a very common cause of pulmonary hypertension. The peak-to-peak gradient would indicate a degree of aortic stenosis but not severe.

14. E. CTEPH can be only diagnosed following 3 months of anticoagulation for an acute PE. There is therefore little value in early repeat CT scanning or catheterization, and no evidence base for treatment other than continued anticoagulation.

15. A. This can be a typical presentation of idiopathic pulmonary arterial hypertension. Treatment of choice is usually a combination therapy of PDE5I as tadalafil or sildenafil and ERAs as ambrisentan or macitentan in patients without advanced cardiopulmonary compromise (WHO functional class IV, syncope). High-dose calcium channel blockers are only reserved for patients who respond positively to vasodilator testing. The excellent response to medical therapies has rendered transplantation unnecessary in most patients.

16. B. Patients on ambulatory therapy have severe pulmonary arterial hypertension and a possible explanation of the rapid deterioration is pump failure or a blocked line. These patients are usually very good at trouble-shooting pump issues and will have a direct contact numbers for their specialist centre. If failure to administer epoprostenol is suspected then it should given parentrally via a peripheral line immediately at the same dose. Then the specialist centre should be contacted for advice and other causes of deterioration should be considered.

17. E. This is a case of group 3 pulmonary hypertension secondary to chronic lung disease. In patients with lung disease associated PH, it is recommended to optimize treatment of the underlying lung disease.

chapter 8.5

ADULT CONGENITAL HEART DISEASE

QUESTIONS

1. A patient with a Fontan circulation is seen in the Emergency Department. He reports feeling breathless and slightly dizzy. Observations are as follows: heart rate 150 bpm (regular), afebrile, blood pressure 90/60 mmHg, oxygen saturation 94% on air. He takes warfarin, with a consistently therapeutic INR. ECG shows an atrial tachycardia.

What is the best course of action?

A. DC cardioversion
B. Beta blocker
C. IV fluid challenge
D. IV amiodarone
E. Admit and observe

2. A 23-year-old male presents to hospital with 6 weeks of progressive fatigue, breathlessness, and weight loss. He has a history of pulmonary stenosis, balloon pulmonary valvuloplasty as a child, and then implantation of a percutaneous pulmonary valve 1 year ago for severe pulmonary regurgitation.

What is the most likely diagnosis?

A. Infective endocarditis of the prosthetic pulmonary valve
B. Lymphoma
C. Severe pulmonary regurgitation
D. Pulmonary valve obstruction
E. Pericardial effusion

3. A 26-year-old female presents with shortness of breath. CT pulmonary angiography demonstrates a dilated right heart. She goes on to have an echocardiogram which demonstrates an atrial septal defect (ASD) with left-to-right shunt. Further investigation with right heart catheterization shows that the pulmonary vascular resistance (PVR) is 2 WU.

Which of the following is correct?

A. She should be admitted for anticoagulation
B. She should be referred immediately for surgical closure
C. She needs to have a cardiac MRI before any further decisions can be made
D. She is very likely to have another congenital cardiac defect
E. She should be offered device closure if a trans-oesophageal echocardiogram (TOE) demonstrates sufficient rims of tissue around the defect

4. A 30-year-old male with congenitally corrected transposition of the great arteries presents to a district general hospital (DGH) with appendicitis. He is under yearly adult congenital heart disease (ACHD) follow-up at a tertiary centre, and is known to have a moderately impaired systemic right ventricle. The anaesthetic team at the DGH call to discuss his surgical risk, as the surgeons wish to take him for an appendicectomy within the next 48 hours.

Which of these represents the best advice?

A. Continue with surgery as normal and write to ACHD consultant to inform of admission
B. Transfer the patient immediately to the tertiary centre for all ongoing surgical management
C. Advise that the patient must not have surgery as it is too high risk, and that he should be managed conservatively
D. Discuss with the patient's ACHD consultant and a cardiac anaesthetist, then liaise with the treating surgical and anaesthetic teams to balance the risks and benefits of operating locally versus transfer
E. Advise the treating team to delay the operation and that the patient will be discussed at the next ACHD MDT

5. A 35-year-old patient with transposition of the great arteries and an atrial switch operation is seen at her routine ACHD follow-up and reports increasing breathlessness for 6 months with intermittent palpitations. She has had no surgical or interventional procedures after her initial correction, and has been stable for many years. Clinical examination and echocardiogram in clinic are unchanged from previous and 12-lead ECG shows normal sinus rhythm.

What is the most likely cause of her symptoms?

A. Supraventricular tachyarrhythmia
B. Baffle stenosis
C. Baffle leak
D. Heart failure with preserved ejection fraction
E. Interstitial lung disease

6. A 45-year-old male patient with a diagnosis of unrepaired ventricular septal defect (VSD) and Eisenmenger's syndrome comes to clinic for review.

Which of the following findings might typically be present on routine blood tests?

A. Haemoglobin 207 g/dL (normal range 13.5–17.5 g/dL)
B. Platelets 500 × 10^9/L (normal range 150–450 × 10^9/L)
C. Magnesium 0.4 mmol/L (normal range 0.65–1.05 mmol/L)
D. Creatinine 200 micromoles/L (normal range 61.9–114.9 micromoles/L)
E. White cell count 16 x 10^9/L (normal range 4.5–11 × 10^9/L)

7. A female patient with short stature is seen in ACHD clinic for monitoring following childhood repair of coarctation of the aorta.

What is the most likely genetic syndrome linking her appearance and her cardiovascular abnormality?

A. Down syndrome
B. Edwards syndrome
C. Noonan syndrome
D. Turner syndrome
E. DiGeorge syndrome

8. A 25-year-old patient with a history of tetralogy of Fallot repair in childhood presents with shortness of breath on exertion. Transthoracic echo shows moderate to severe pulmonary regurgitation.

What is the best next investigation to clarify the degree of pulmonary regurgitation and determine whether there is a need for intervention/surgery?

A. Cardiac CT
B. Cardiac MRI
C. Diagnostic right heart catheterization
D. Transoesophageal echo
E. Cardiopulmonary exercise test

9. A 19-year-old with Ebstein's anomaly of the tricuspid valve presents to the Emergency Department with dizziness. ECG shows a supraventricular tachycardia. Vagal manoeuvres and adenosine fail to terminate the arrhythmia and she requires one synchronized DC shock. Transthoracic echo shows mild-moderate tricuspid regurgitation and normal RV function.

What is the best definitive management strategy for her arrhythmia?

A. Electrophysiology (EP) study and catheter ablation
B. Amiodarone
C. Beta blocker
D. Pill-in-pocket flecainide
E. Surgical maze procedure

10. A 30-year-old man with Down's syndrome and a history of repaired complete atrioventricular septal defect (AVSD) in childhood comes to clinic for review. His carer reports that he has been 'slowing down' recently with a decrease in energy and slight increase in shortness of breath on exertion.

Which of the following, related to his original defect and repair, might explain his symptoms?

A. Aortic regurgitation
B. Pericardial effusion
C. Pulmonary fibrosis
D. Gastro-oesophageal reflux
E. 2:1 AV block

11. Which of the following congenital abnormalities can be described by sequential segmental analysis as atrioventricular (AV) and ventriculoarterial (VA) discordance?

A. Transposition of the great arteries
B. Congenitally corrected transposition of the great arteries (CCTGA)
C. Tetralogy of Fallot
D. Right atrial isomerism
E. Hypoplastic left heart

12. What follow-up interval would be suggested by ESC guidelines for a 30-year-old patient with a small perimembranous VSD, normal LV size and function, and no symptoms?

A. Every 6 months
B. Every year
C. Every 2 years
D. Every 3–5 years
E. No follow up needed, discharge

13. Regarding DiGeorge syndrome, which of the following is the most frequently occurring congenital cardiac lesion?

A. Conotruncal abnormalities
B. Partial anomalous pulmonary venous drainage
C. Atrioventricular septal defect (AVSD)
D. Bicuspid aortic valve
E. Congenital complete heart block

14. A 25-year-old woman presents with shortness of breath and chest pain on exercise. Echo shows a bicuspid aortic valve with aortic valve Vmax 4.5 m/s. Her case is discussed at MDT and the options of tissue aortic valve, mechanical aortic valve and Ross procedure are considered.

Which of the following investigations would be most helpful (in addition to the transthoracic echo) in assessing her suitability for a Ross procedure?

A. Transoesophageal echo (TOE)
B. Cardiopulmonary exercise test
C. 6-minute walk test
D. Cardiac CT
E. Diagnostic left and right heart catheterization

15. A 40-year-old man presents to the rapid access chest pain clinic with atypical sounding chest pain. He has no conventional cardiovascular risk factors. An echocardiogram shows a dilated right heart with no obvious cause. Cardiac MRI is performed and demonstrates partial anomalous pulmonary venous drainage (right upper pulmonary vein to superior vena cava). Another associated cause of right heart dilation is seen on the MRI. What is this most likely to have been?

A. Pulmonary embolism
B. Sinus venosus atrial septal defect (ASD)
C. Apically displaced tricuspid valve
D. LV systolic impairment
E. Interstitial lung disease

chapter

8.5

ADULT CONGENITAL HEART DISEASE

ANSWERS

1. A. As per ESC guidelines*, DC cardioversion is a Class IC recommendation in this patient: 'sustained atrial arrhythmia with rapid AV conduction is a medical emergency and should be promptly treated with electrical cardioversion.'

*Baumgartner H, De Backer J, Babu-Narayan SV, Budts W, Chessa M, Diller GP, Lung B, Kluin J, Lang IM, Meijboom F, Moons P, Mulder BJM, Oechslin E, Roos-Hesselink JW, Schwerzmann M, Sondergaard L, Zeppenfeld K; ESC Scientific Document Group. 2020 ESC Guidelines for the management of adult congenital heart disease. Eur Heart J. 2021 Feb 11;42(6):563–645. doi: 10.1093/eurheartj/ehaa554. PMID: 32860028.

2. A. Transcatheter pulmonary valve implants (TPVI, e.g. Melody valve) are particularly prone to infective endocarditis. The history in this patient combined with a recent TPVI makes this the most likely diagnosis.

3. E. ESC guidelines state that ASD closure is recommended regardless of symptoms if there is evidence of RV overload (which this patient has), in the absence of pulmonary arterial hypertension (PVR <3 WU). Device closure is the method of choice if technically appropriate.

4. D. ESC guidelines recommend that patients with Fontan circulation, Eisenmenger physiology, or chronic cyanosis undergo non-cardiac surgery in an expert centre. Outside of this, decisions around the appropriate site for non-cardiac surgery will depend on patient factors as well as the experience and skill mix of the team in the treating hospital.

5. A. Although all of the other answers are possible explanations, supraventricular tachyarrhythmia is a common feature following atrial switch operation, and a high level of suspicion should be maintained in such a patient presenting with intermittent palpitations, despite the resting ECG in clinic showing sinus rhythm.

6. A. Patients with chronic cyanosis often have high haemoglobin levels as a compensatory mechanism. Platelet count is frequently low, not high. White cell count is not usually affected. Whilst renal function may become impaired in the context of impaired ventricular function, it is not directly related to cyanosis. Hypomagnesaemia is also not directly linked to cyanosis.

7. D. Typical phenotypic characteristics of Turner syndrome (45XO) include short stature, webbed neck, and broad chest with wide spaced nipples. A significant proportion will have congenital heart disease, of which bicuspid aortic valve, coarctation of the aorta, and aortic dilatation are common. ESC guidelines recommend that every woman with Turner's syndrome is seen at least once by a cardiologist throughout her life.

8. B. Cardiac MRI is the test of choice for quantification of pulmonary valve regurgitant volume and fraction, and also for quantification of right ventricular volumes. ESC guidelines regarding timing of pulmonary valve repair in tetralogy of Fallot patients are based on MRI criteria for pulmonary regurgitation and RV volumes.

9. A. ESC guidelines recommend EP testing following by catheter ablation for patients with symptomatic arrhythmia. If surgical repair of the tricuspid valve is indicated (severe tricuspid regurgitation plus symptoms or objective decrease in exercise capacity) then surgical treatment of arrhythmia can be considered, although in this case the arrhythmia is likely to be mediated by an accessory pathway and surgical treatment of this is challenging. If surgery were to be indicated for tricuspid regurgitation in this particular patient, EP study and ablation prior to tricuspid valve replacement would probably be the best option.

10. E. Due to the abnormal position of the AV node in patients with complete AVSD, in combination with surgery in close proximity to the AV node, patients with repaired (and unrepaired) AVSD are at moderate risk of developing AV block. Systemic AV valve regurgitation is the other major long term complication to be alert to.

11. B. In CCTGA, the morphological right atrium is connected to the left ventricle (sub-pulmonic) which is connected to the pulmonary artery. The pulmonary veins drain into the left atrium, which is connected to the right ventricle (systemic), which is connected to the aorta.

12. D. After surgical repair with no residual issues, guidelines recommend echocardiography every 5 years. After device closure guidelines recommend regularly for 2 years, then every 2–5 years.

13. A. These are the most commonly occurring defects in patients with 22q11 and include truncus arteriosus, tetralogy of Fallot, transposition of the great arteries, and interrupted aortic arch.

14. D. The Ross procedure involves using the patient's native pulmonary valve to replace their aortic valve. A tissue pulmonary valve is then placed in the pulmonary position. In order for this to be technically possible, the pulmonary and aortic valves need to be of similar size. The annulus of each valve can be accurately measured on CT. Exercise testing is useful in asymptomatic patients with severe aortic stenosis. TOE is unlikely to add much above and beyond the transthoracic echo. Cardiac catheterization is not usually required if the echo data is sufficiently conclusive regarding the severity of aortic stenosis and data on coronary arteries can be obtained non-invasively by CT.

15. B. Partial anomalous pulmonary venous drainage may be seen in isolation, but it can also be associated with other congenital lesions, most frequently a sinus venosus ASD. Patients may be asymptomatic or present with symptoms of shortness of breath, palpitations, and reduced exercise capacity during adulthood. The chest pain in this patient is likely to be unrelated rather than caused by the defect.

chapter 8.6

CARDIOVASCULAR DISEASE IN PREGNANCY

QUESTIONS

1. **A woman attends for pre-pregnancy counselling. She has moderate residual coarctation after surgical repair in infancy. Her blood pressure is 140/90mmHg. She is taking bisoprolol 5mg od.**

   What is the biggest risk if she becomes pregnant at this stage?

   A. Heart failure
   B. Pre-eclampsia
   C. Fetal loss
   D. No complications
   E. Prematurity

2. **A woman presents with severe asymptomatic aortic stenosis with a peak velocity of 4.1 m/s across the valve and a valve area of 1.0 cm^2. She is asymptomatic and currently 16 weeks pregnant.**

   Which of the following is part of appropriate management?

   A. Termination of pregnancy
   B. Aortic valve surgery before the third trimester
   C. Admission to hospital with delivery before 30 weeks
   D. Multidisciplinary approach and careful frequent follow up with echocardiography and clinical review in a tertiary centre
   E. Caesarean section rather than vaginal delivery

3. **A woman with previous peripartum cardiomyopathy 2 years ago, currently on an ACE inhibitor, beta-blocker, and spironolactone, with a LV ejection fraction of 55%, wants to embark on another pregnancy.**

   Which of the following is correct?

   A. The woman can safely undergo pregnancy once her ACE inhibitor and medication has been replaced with hydralazine and a nitrate
   B. The risk of complications is reduced as her LV function has returned to normal
   C. Further pregnancy is contraindicated
   D. Dilated cardiomyopathy is a more likely diagnosis and pregnancy is safe
   E. She should proceed with pregnancy and not change any medication

4. You review a 27-year-old woman with tetralogy of Fallot in the follow-up clinic and note that her pulmonary regurgitation has deteriorated such that it is now graded as severe. Which of the following is NOT a known predictor of an increased risk of cardiac events for this patient?

A. Ventricular dyssynchrony
B. Previous arrhythmia
C. Impaired and progressive RV dysfunction
D. Impaired LV function
E. Severe PR

5. You are providing pre-pregnancy counselling to a 26-year-old woman with a mechanical mitral valve in-situ.

What is the safest approach for managing her anticoagulation during pregnancy?

A. Warfarin throughout pregnancy
B. Low molecular weight heparin (LMWH) throughout pregnancy
C. A direct oral anticoagulant throughout pregnancy
D. Low-molecular weight heparin from weeks 6 to 12, followed by warfarin from weeks 12–36, then back onto LMWH until post-partum
E. Warfarin until week 12 and then switch to LMWH until post-partum

6. A 37-year-old woman who is 34 weeks pregnant is admitted with an anterior STEMI.

How would you proceed?

A. Aspirin, clopidogrel, heparin, and primary PCI
B. Aspirin, clopidogrel, heparin, and conservative management
C. Aspirin, prasugrel, heparin, and primary PCI
D. Thrombolysis
E. Aspirin, prasugrel, heparin, and conservative management

7. You are asked for advice on the management of a young woman with Marfan syndrome and an aorta measuring 40mm at the sinuses of Valsalva who has become pregnant.

What is the best management option?

A. Termination of pregnancy
B. Aortic root surgery
C. Careful monitoring of the aorta during pregnancy and a vaginal delivery under epidural cover with a passive second stage and instrumentation
D. Angiotensin receptor blocker to reduce the risk of further dilation/dissection
E. Careful monitoring of the aorta during pregnancy and a caesarean section at 38 weeks

8. Which of the following is the best advice to give a young woman with Marfan syndrome contemplating pregnancy who has a dilated aorta with sinuses of Valsalva measuring 46 mm and no aortic regurgitation?

A. Pregnancy is safe as long as there is no family history of dissection
B. Pregnancy is safe as long as regular monitoring occurs
C. Beta-blocker medication will reduce the risk of further dilation/dissection
D. Valve sparing root surgery is indicated
E. Pregnancy is contraindicated, but she should not have surgery until the aorta measures 50 mm

9. A 25-year-old pregnant women presents to the Emergency Department with SVT. Blood pressure is 70/50 mmHg and she is breathless.

What is the first-line of treatment?

A. IV amiodarone
B. IV labetalol
C. IV adenosine
D. DC cardioversion
E. IV verapamil

10. What are normal cardiovascular findings during pregnancy?

A. Stroke volume increases 35–50%
B. Increase in heart rate up to 10–20 bpm
C. Increased LV/RV volumes
D. Decrease in GLS during third trimester
E. All of the above

11. You are running a pre-pregnancy counselling clinic for patients with adult congenital heart disease.

In which of the following situations should pregnancy be discouraged?

A. Cyanotic congenital heart disease
B. Systemic ventricular dysfunction with an ejection fraction <30%
C. Pulmonary hypertension
D. Symptomatic severe aortic stenosis
E. All of the above

12. Which of these options are correct in regards to pregnancy and congenital heart disease?

A. There may be low uteroplacental flow perfusion
B. Fontan patients have less successful pregnancies due to a high rate of miscarriages
C. Thromboembolic events are more common in cyanotic and complex congenital heart disease
D. There is an increased risk of arrhythmias
E. All of the above

13. You are reviewing the birthing plan for patients in your congenital heart disease pregnancy clinic.

In which of the following is vaginal delivery not the best option?

A. Marfan with aorta measuring 40 mm
B. Mechanical valve on oral anticoagulation
C. Moderate mitral regurgitation
D. Moderate aortic regurgitation
E. Dilated cardiomyopathy with EF 50%

14. Which drug is not safe during pregnancy?

A. Aspirin
B. Irbesartan
C. Clexane
D. Bisoprolol
E. Nifedipine

15. A 26-year-old woman with Ebstein's anomaly and asymptomatic severe tricuspid regurgitation has asked for advice regarding her options for becoming pregnant.

Which of these statements is true?

A. Pregnancy is not recommended
B. The risk of a cardiac event during pregnancy is low in the presence of previous atrial arrhythmias
C. Pregnancy is well tolerated in the absence of cyanosis, right heart failure, and arrhythmias
D. Left ventricular non-compaction should be sought
E. All of the above

chapter

8.6

CARDIOVASCULAR DISEASE IN PREGNANCY

ANSWERS

1. B. The majority of patients with coarctation of the aorta have had an intervention prior to pregnancy. In these women, pregnancy is fairly well tolerated, although there is an increased risk of hypertension and pre-eclampsia. If there is a residual gradient there is a theoretical risk of a small-for-dates baby. Coarctation results in high upper body hypertension with a lower perfusion of the distal aorta resulting in uteroplacental insufficiency. There is limited data on pregnancy in unrepaired coarctation, but it is advised that these women are repaired first. There is an association with bicuspid aortic valve (BAV) and aortopathy. If the woman has Turner Syndrome (some are mosaic and can become pregnant), there is an increased risk of aortic dissection of the aorta, and even if the heart is structurally normal. Therefore, strict blood pressure control is warranted to avoid maternal complications as well as placenta hypoperfusion in those with residual coarctation.

2. D. Appropriate pre-cardiac assessment is extremely important for women with cardiac conditions before embarking on pregnancy so that they are aware of the risks to themselves and the fetus, and are prepared for the type of medical follow-up and delivery that will be required. It also allows for detailed assessment of the condition and optimization of haemodynamics as well as assessing whether or not medication will need to be changed or stopped and the risk of continuing medication in pregnancy. In the case of aortic stenosis individual assessment will allow for elective procedures to be performed before pregnancy, especially in symptomatic women with severe AS. Asymptomatic aortic stenosis, however, even if severe, is well tolerated in pregnancy, though high risk by definition. Obstructive heart lesions are aggravated by the increase in stroke volume occurring with pregnancy, and are therefore of particular concern. Ideally, an exercise test should be done before pregnancy in order to unmask any symptoms or blood pressure drop, which would indicate surgery. Severe and symptomatic lesions should be corrected prior to pregnancy as they carry a substantial risk of heart failure and higher rates of cardiac hospitalizations. The ESC advises that 'Pregnancy should not be discouraged in asymptomatic patients, even with severe aortic stenosis, when left ventricular size and function and the exercise test is normal. There should also be no recent progression of aortic stenosis.' There is an increased risk of prematurity, IUGR, and low birth weight.

Cardiac surgery carries a significant risk of fetal mortality and should only be performed if urgent and the fetus is not mature enough to be delivered. Caesarean delivery carries with it larger and more sudden haemodynamic shifts and so vaginal delivery is preferred with passive instrumental delivery under epidural.

3. B. PPCM is defined as new-onset cardiomyopathy with systolic dysfunction (LV ejection fraction <45%) without a reversible cause presenting near the end of pregnancy or in the postpartum period in a woman without known heart disease and is a significant cause of maternal morbidity and mortality. Pre-pregnancy counselling is imperative. The risk of recurrence with cardiac decompensation and maternal death must be discussed.

If LV dysfunction or dilation persists more than 6 months after diagnosis, pregnancy is not advised as the risk of deterioration is higher. Pre-pregnancy counselling requires unsafe anti heart failure medication to be stopped (in this case spironolactone and the ACE inhibitor) and further assessment with echocardiography and exercise testing off medication.

4. A. Patients with repaired tetralogy of Fallot usually tolerate pregnancy well (WHO risk class II). Nonetheless, predictors of clinical events in TOF are an important clinical target pre-pregnancy. Cardiac complications have been reported in 8% of repaired patients; arrhythmias and HF are the most common complications. Abnormal ventricular performance pre-pregnancy can increase the risk of heart failure and arrhythmias during pregnancy and post-partum period. Moderate to severe pulmonary regurgitation is also a risk factor. Previous pregnancy may be associated with a persisting increase in RV size and long-term cardiac events. Dyssynchrony has not been associated with an increase in cardiac events in pregnanct Fallot patients.

5. A. A pregnant patient with a mechanical valve is a high risk patient. Pregnancy is a hypercoagulability state. The risk is higher in mitral valves compared to aortic valves, as well as in other clinical situations, such as previous history of thromboembolism, atrial fibrillation, and ventricular dysfunction. The risk of developing a thromboembolic event or bleeding is high, even if anticoagulation levels are well controlled. The ESC ROPAC registry quoted a maternal mortality rate of 1.4%, valve thrombosis 4.7% (versus 0% in bioprosthetic valves), and haemorrhagic events 23% (vs 5.1% in bioprosthetic valves). However, this was selected registry data. In a UKOSS study of real world data, the mortality rate was 9%.

Warfarin crosses the placenta and can cause fetal embryopathy (highest risk in weeks 6–12) and bleeding, which results in an increased risk of miscarriage, intra-uterine death, and stillbirth. LMWH does not cross the placenta but has been associated with an increased risk of valve thrombosis and maternal mortality. The 'sandwich' approach of using LMWH for weeks 6–12, then warfarin for weeks 12–36, then LMWH until postpartum avoids the risk of embryopathy, but it carries the risk of valve thrombosis when changing regimens and when on LMWH and needs to be monitored carefully. A woman cannot have a vaginal delivery on warfarin as the anticoagulated fetus would suffer trauma in the birth canal.

Women choosing to take LMWH require weekly anti-Xa trough and peak levels and frequent echocardiography. Pre-pregnancy and ideally pre-surgical counselling is essential in these women. In 2023 the British Society of Hypertension published a guideline recommending a higher dose of LMWH than had previously been used. It remains to be seen whether or not this reduces the risk of valve thrombosis and what effect this has on bleeding.

6. A. Myocardial infarction accounts for >20% of all maternal cardiac deaths. Though atherosclerotic coronary artery disease is increasingly common in older mothers, spontaneous coronary artery dissection (P-SCAD) is a major cause of MI in pregnancy.

Clinical presentation is as with non-pregnant population and should be treated in the same way with aspirin, heparin, and PPCI. Low-dose aspirin is safe and there is limited evidence to support the safe use of clopidogrel. However, there is very little data on newer anti-platelet agents and therefore these should be avoided. Heparinization is safe.

P-SCAD occurs most commonly in late pregnancy and early post-partum, and most often involves the left-sided coronaries. Multi-vessel involvement and cardiogenic shock are not uncommon. Thrombolysis should be avoided because of the possibility of P-SCAD as the cause. Care should be taken with catheter manipulation because of the risk of iatrogenic dissection, which is significantly increased in pregnancy.

7. C. The overall risk of a woman with Marfan syndrome having an aortic dissection associated with pregnancy is 3–4%. Aortic size is a major determinant of risk, but other risk factors must be taken into account at the time of risk stratification, such as family and/or personal history of dissection, uncontrolled hypertension, rapid growth progression (defined as more than 3 mm in a year) and genotype (haploinsufficiency of the protein results in a more aggressive phenotype than the dominant negative genotype). All Marfan pregnancies are high risk by definition: type B dissection can occur in the presence of a normal ascending aorta. Despite scarce data, pregnancy should be avoided in Marfan patients with an aortic root diameter >45 mm as there is an increased risk of dissection. When the aorta is 40–45 mm, other factors should be considered as described above.

Strict blood pressure control is advised, and antihypertensive treatment that is safe for the fetus should be initiated if necessary. Beta-blocker therapy throughout pregnancy should be considered in women with Marfan syndrome and other heritable thoracic aortic diseases, though there is no data in pregnancy to show their efficacy (class IIa level C). Angiotensin receptor blockers are contraindicated in pregnancy.

8. D. Dilatation of the ascending aorta may be seen in presence of a connective tissue disease, such as Marfan syndrome, bicuspid aortic valve, vascular Ehlers–Danlos syndrome, Loeys–Dietz syndrome and non syndromic hereditary thoracic aortopathies (HTA).

Prophylactic surgery should be considered during pregnancy if the aorta diameter is >45 mm and increasing rapidly (Class IIA level C). Pregnancy is not recommended in patients with severe dilatation of the aorta (HTA, Marfan syndrome with aorta >45 mm, bicuspid aortic valve with aorta >50 mm, or Turner syndrome with aortic size index (ASI) >25 mm/m^2). (Class III level C).

Prophylactic aortic surgery (valve sparing or personalized external aortic root support (PEARS)) can be carried out with relatively low mortality and is indicated in this case.

9. D. Treatment of any arrhythmia has to be driven based on the haemodynamic situation. If haemodynamically stable, vagal manoeuvres followed by IV adenosine are the best first-line treatment. IV beta-blockers can also be used. Amiodarone should be avoided due to the effect on the fetal thyroid.

Synchronized DC cardioversion is indicated if there is haemodynamically significant supraventricular tachycardia, atrial fibrillation, or ventricular tachyarrhythmia, as with non-pregnant patients. Concurrent monitoring of the fetus is not required but fetal heart Doppler should be performed post cardioversion.

10. E. Pregnancy leads to major physiological changes in the cardiovascular system, to accommodate adequate blood flow to the uteroplacental unit and meet the metabolic and physiological demands of the mother and the growing fetus.

The endocrine changes in pregnancy (i.e. a huge increase in progesterone but also a rise in estrogen and relaxin) lead to a 30–50% increase in blood volume and up to 80% decrease in systemic vascular resistance. Subsequent cardiovascular changes occur as a response to this haemodynamic adaptation, such as augmentation of left ventricular end-diastolic diameter (LVEDD), left ventricular mass, thickness of the posterior LV wall, a transitory decrease in LV systolic function based on a systolic stress index, and reduced longitudinal strain at the end of the second trimester.

11. E. Cyanotic congenital heart disease: Maternal risk during pregnancy depends on whether or not pulmonary hypertension is present or not. In the presence of pulmonary hypertension, maternal mortality increases dramatically. Maternal outcomes depend mainly on ventricular function and oxygen saturation. Maternal complications (HF, thrombosis, arrhythmias, and endocarditis) occur in >15% of cyanotic pregnant patients.

Fetal outcomes depend on maternal oxygen levels. If oxygen saturation is >90%, then there is usually a better outcome (10% fetal loss). If oxygen saturation is <85%, fetal growth restriction, prematurity, and fetal death are common, and pregnancy should be discouraged (live birth rate of only 12%).

Ventricular function (either subpulmonary or systemic) is of the utmost importance in successfully carrying a pregnancy. Pregnancy is poorly tolerated in some women with pre-existing ventricular dysfunction, with the potential for further deterioration.

Predictors of maternal mortality are NYHA class III/IV and EF <40%. Highly adverse risk factors include EF <20%, MR, RV failure, AF, and/or hypotension. The European Society of Cardiology 2018 guidelines advise avoiding pregnancy when the ejection fraction is less than 30%.

Pulmonary hypertension: pregnancy is contraindicated in women with PHT due to the high mortality rate (can be as low as 20% with meticulous care in a specialist centre). The greatest period of risk is the puerperium and early post-partum. The RV cannot cope with the volume load of pregnancy and this is exacerbated when the profound volume shifts occur at the at the time of delivery. Targeted pulmonary vasodilators and aggressive diuresis in intensive care postpartum can reduce the risk of mortality.

Symptomatic severe aortic stenosis: surgery, not pregnancy is indicated in this clinical scenario. There is a high rate of heart failure (26.3% vs 6.3% in asymptomatic women) as well as a high rate of hospitalization.

12. E. Though congenital heart disease patients are a highly heterogenous group, the above findings have been found to be correct. The chances of successful pregnancy to term in a Fontan circulation patient are less than 50%; maternal complications are not common but miscarriage and severe IUGR are the norm. Management should be in a specialist centre.

13. B. Elective caesarean section carries no maternal benefit and results in earlier delivery and lower birth weight. Vaginal delivery is associated with less blood loss and lower risk of infection, venous thrombosis, and embolism, and should be advised for most women. Caesarean section should be suggested for obstetric indications and for patients presenting in labour on oral anticoagulants, with aggressive aortic pathology or acute intractable heart failure. Some advocate caesarean section for pulmonary hypertension but vaginal delivery is preferred by some experts. The reason for caesarean delivery in Marfan's with a severely dilated aortic root is so that the patient can be in theatre if there is an acute emergency. It is usually done in the cardiac or general theatres, not in the obstetric centre. When a woman is on oral anticoagulation for a mechanical heart valve this is changed to low-molecular weight heparin for the last few weeks of pregnancy. If she comes in in labour on oral anticoagulation the baby must be delivered by Caesarean section as it is anticoagulated.

14. B. The physiological changes of pregnancy affect drug absorption, action, and metabolism. In the second and third trimester, drugs mainly affect either fetal growth and functional development, and they have direct toxicity to the tissues. Fetal affects are dependent on the amount of drugs that crosses the placenta tissue, which is directly related to the molecular size of the drug. On average, the fetus is exposed to no more than 10% of maternal levels.

When using drugs during pregnancy the benefits and risks need to be weighed up carefully. Use of the previous FDA Classification system is now discouraged in favour of careful weighing up of the evidence available for an individual drug. Aspirin is safe and often used used to reduce the risk of pre-eclampsia. Clexane does not cross the placenta. Nifedipine is often used for hypertension in pregnancy and bisoprolol is relatively safe. Higher doses can cause IUGR. Angiotensin receptor blocker inhibitors and ACE inhibitors are contraindicated as they result in oligohydramnios and fetal contractures.

15. C. In women with uncomplicated Ebstein's anomaly, pregnancy is often tolerated well (WHO risk class II). Women with cyanosis, right heart failure, or persistent arrhythmias should be counselled against pregnancy until further investigation and appropriate treatment. Cyanosis could be due to ASD or patent foramen ovale, and it could be treated percutaneously if there is no severe tricuspid regurgitation (TR) or surgically if so. Right ventricular failure can be either due to progression of the myopathy or due to the TR. Atrial arrhythmias commonly recur in pregnancy and warrant further investigation in Ebstein's due to the association with accessory pathways (20%). Left heart lesions are common in Epstein (occur in about 39% of cases). These include mitral valve abnormalities and in particular hyper trabeculation of the left ventricle associated with reduced function.

chapter

9

THE CARDIOLOGICAL CONSULTATION

chapter

9.1

THE PATIENT UNDERGOING NON-CARDIAC SURGERY

QUESTIONS

1. **You are asked to review a 76-year-old gentleman in clinic prior to laparoscopic cholecystectomy. He has a past medical history of dilated cardiomyopathy with an ejection fraction of 39% (last echo was 6 months ago). His medications include ramipril 5 mg od, bisoprolol 2.5 mg od, eplenerone 25 mg od, and dapagliflozin 10 mg od. The surgical team are concerned about the degree of LV impairment. His heart rate is 67 bpm, BP 128/68 mmHg, saturations 98% on air. He appears euvolaemic and asymptomatic.**

   What would you advise?

   A. Delay surgery until you have an up to date echocardiogram
   B. Optimize heart failure medications with the introduction of sacubitril/valsartan
   C. Optimize heart failure medications with the addition of ivabradine
   D. Arrange for a CRT-P
   E. Advise patient is on adequate prognostic therapy and should be able to proceed from a cardiac perspective

2. **You are called by the anaesthetic team regarding a 78-year-old male who is due to undergo elective AAA repair tomorrow. He had a routine ECG which shows bifascicular block. The anaesthetist is concerned about increased risk of cardiac arrhythmia. The patient is otherwise asymptomatic.**

   What would you advise?

   A. Delay surgery and advise getting a Holter monitor and echo
   B. Arrange for a TPW
   C. List for pacemaker given the evidence of significant conduction abnormality
   D. Advise proceeding with surgery but with chronotropic drugs and transcutaneous pacing skills/equipment available
   E. Organize a CT coronary angiogram

3. A 72-year-old man is due to undergo carotid endarterectomy. He has ischaemic heart disease, chronic kidney disease, type 2 diabetes, and had a TIA 3 years ago. The vascular team would like your opinion regarding any cardiac tests prior to surgery.

What would you suggest?

A. Do nothing
B. Organize a CT coronary angiogram plus/minus invasive coronary angiogram
C. Organize a nuclear myocardial perfusion scan
D. Organize an ECG, blood tests including troponin/BNP, and assess functional capacity
E. Organize a stress echocardiogram

4. You are called by the urology registrar regarding a 76-year-old gentleman who is due to undergo a transurethral resection of the prostate (TURP) and who has a history of IHD with a previous angiogram 4 years ago revealing a 50% distal LAD lesion. The registrar would like the patient to be optimized from a cardiovascular point of view prior to surgery. The patient himself has been angina-free for a number of years. His current medications include aspirin 75 mg od atorvastatin 20 mg od.

What would you advise?

A. Nothing to be done. Can proceed to surgery
B. Delay surgery and arrange a functional scan to look for ischaemia
C. Start anti-anginal medication in the form of bisoprolol prior to surgery
D. Arrange for an angiogram prior to surgery

5. You are called by the surgical registrar regarding a 74-year-old male who is about to undergo emergency surgery for a perforated duodenal ulcer. He recently underwent PCI to his distal circumflex artery 7 weeks ago for stable angina. He is currently on aspirin 75 mg and clopidogrel 75 mg od. The surgical team would like to advice regarding discontinuing dual anti-platelet therapy (DAPT).

What would you advise?

A. Must continue DAPT; may need to consider delaying surgery
B. Continue with aspirin therapy if bleeding risk allows
C. Switch to IV heparin
D. Stop all anti-platelet agents
E. Switch to a DOAC

6. **You are asked to review a 69-year-old gentleman who has presented this morning with an acute abdomen and is about to undergo urgent laparotomy. He has known symptomatic severe aortic stenosis. His last echocardiogram showed a peak gradient across the aortic valve of 84 mmHg, mean 56 mmHg, and aortic valve area of 0.8 cm^2.**

   What would you advise?

   A. Proceed with surgery as it is an emergency
   B. Consider deferring surgery and refer for valve replacement
   C. Discuss with the interventional team regarding the possibility for an urgent balloon aortic valvuloplasty or TAVI prior to surgery
   D. Do nothing patient is very high risk and has a high chance of death. Consider palliation
   E. Re-do an echo to see if the gradients have improved

7. **A 64-year-old male on the surgical ward is about to undergo thyroidectomy for a non-malignant nodule. He suddenly develops a central chest discomfort whilst lying in bed. ECG showed some inferior T-wave inversion. Serial troponins are mildly elevated. His heart rate is 88 bpm and his BP is 134/86 mmHg. He mentions he has had the odd episode of chest discomfort over the last 6 months.**

   What would be your management?

   A. Start antianginal therapy in the form of bisoprolol and isosorbide mononitrate. If pain-free can proceed to surgery
   B. Treat as ACS and arrange an IP angiogram
   C. Arrange an inpatient CTCA and depending on this treat as ACS
   D. Delay surgery, start antianginal therapy, and arrange an outpatient CTCA
   E. Think about a drug eluting balloon

8. **You are asked to review an 84-year-old gentleman prior to prostatectomy for an enlarged prostate. Incidentally his ECG shows Mobitz II AV block. He is, however, asymptomatic from a cardiac perspective. His surgery has been scheduled for tomorrow. The anaesthetist is concerned.**

   What would you advise?

   A. Arrange a transvenous temporary pacemaker
   B. Proceed with surgery but have transcutaneous pacing available should he need it
   C. Delay surgery until a permanent pacemaker has been implanted
   D. Proceed with surgery as he is asymptomatic and reassure that cardiology cover will be provided should he need it
   E. Organize a 24-hour tape to assess the burden of block

9. You are called regarding a 76-year-old lady who is due to undergo a left knee replacement. She underwent PCI to her proximal LAD 10 months ago following an NSTEMI. She had no bystander disease. She has been pain-free since and takes aspirin and clopidogrel. The surgeon would like to know whether the anti-platelet therapy can be adjusted prior to surgery.

What would you advise?

A. Can stop anti-platelets and proceed to surgery as it has been over 6 months. But to restart aspirin as soon as it is safe from a bleeding perspective
B. Delay surgery until 12 months post procedure as it is a non-urgent procedure
C. Stop clopidogrel and proceed with surgery
D. Delay surgery until after 12 months post procedure, then arrange a functional scan prior to surgery

10. A 79-year-old patient is admitted following an NSTEMI. She undergoes PCI to her proximal LAD. The next day she develops what she describes as black tarry stools. She is haemodynamically stable and her haemoglobin level has dropped 1 unit. The ward doctor is concerned she is bleeding and wants to stop her dual anti-platelet therapy (DAPT).

What would you advise?

A. Stop dual DAPT and arrange an urgent endoscopy
B. Continue DAPT and arrange urgent endoscopy
C. Stop DAPT and commence and IV heparin infusion
D. Stop aspirin only and arrange endoscopy
E. Stop clopidogrel only and arrange endoscopy

11. You are asked to review a 74-year-old gentleman in clinic prior to surgery. He has a past medical history of type 2 diabetes on insulin, chronic kidney disease, and he is an ex-smoker. He is otherwise asymptomatic from a cardiovascular perspective. He has had and ECG and biomarkers checked and has a poor functional capacity (<4 METS) when tested in clinic.

Which of the following factors would make you want to investigate further to assess his pre-operative risk?

A. If his surgery were a total knee replacement
B. Previous history of diabetes mellitus
C. If his surgery were a fem-pop bypass
D. A PR interval of 200 ms on ECG
E. His age

12. Which of the following procedures would carry the highest risk of cardiac complications?

A. Mastectomy
B. TURP
C. Cystectomy
D. Renal transplant
E. Laparotomy for perforated bowel

13. You are asked to review a 72-year-old gentleman who has developed cardiac sounding chest pain. He has dynamic T-wave changes in the inferior leads. Troponins are elevated. He was due to undergo a left hip replacement. This was due to be an expedited procedure due to significant pain on mobilizing.

What you your management plan be?

A. Treat with a balloon angioplasty prior to surgery
B. Consider PCI with a bare metal stent
C. Consider PCI with a new generation drug eluting stent (DES)
D. Treat medically for one year; suggest surgery after this
E. Thrombolysis

14. A 45-year-old gentleman is due to undergo ankle surgery. He has significant cardiac risk factors including diabetes mellitus, hypertension, and a positive family history of IHD. He also smokes 15 cigarettes per day. He denies any chest pain.

What would be your approach prior to surgery?

A. Organize a calcium score prior to surgery
B. Organize an exercise tolerance test
C. Organize a MIBI scan
D. Start bisoprolol prior to surgery
E. Do nothing

15. A 67-year-old gentleman is about due to undergo an elective open iliac bypass procedure. He has a CKD with a baseline eGFR of 45, diabetes mellitus type 2, and IHD. He is an ex-smoker. He has no symptoms of angina or shortness of breath but is unable to climb two flights of stairs. You are asked to review his cardiovascular risk prior to surgery. He has had a normal ECG in clinic.

Prior to surgery what would your approach be?

A. He is asymptomatic—do nothing
B. Start bisoprolol and a statin
C. Arrange an invasive angiogram prior to surgery
D. Arrange a CT coronary angiogram
E. Arrange a dobutamine stress echocardiogram

16. A 70-year-old patient is due to undergo urgent bowel resection secondary to malignancy. He underwent PCI with a DES to his mid circumflex 6 months ago for stable angina. He is on DAPT. The surgeons want to stop antiplatelet therapy due to bleeding risk.

What would you advise?

A. Stop both aspirin and clopidogrel
B. Stop clopidogrel and start heparin
C. Stop clopidogrel and continue aspirin
D. Delay surgery
E. Organize a functional scan prior to altering DAPT

17. You are asked to review a 56-year-old lady who is due to undergo a cholecystectomy in the next day or so. She underwent PCI to her LAD 2 years ago and has been asymptomatic since. She is on aspirin 75 mg, atorvastatin 80 mg, amlodipine 5 mg od, and isosorbide mononitrate 10 mg bd. Her heart rate is 80 bpm and in sinus rhythm. The surgical team would like her cardiovascular medications to be optimized prior to surgery.

What would you advise?

A. Start bisoprolol 2.5 mg od
B. Start Ivabradine 5 mg bd
C. Recommend a CTCA
D. Recommend an exercise tolerance test
E. Do nothing

18. A 76-year-old lady is seen in pre-op clinic. Her functional capacity is two flights of stairs with some breathlessness.

What would her MET equivalent be?

A. 1 MET
B. 2 METS
C. 4 METS
D. 6 METS
E. 7 METS

chapter

9.1

THE PATIENT UNDERGOING NON-CARDIAC SURGERY

ANSWERS

1. E. Patient appears to be on optimal medical therapy. There would be no indication for further pharmacological therapy unless symptoms worsen. Device therapy is currently not indicated.

2. D. A permanent system may be considered but generally patients with bifascicular block can proceed with non-cardiac surgery with appropriate provisions.

3. D. The patient has significant cardiac risk factors and known CVD and will be undergoing what is considered to be intermediate-risk surgery so should have an ECG, biomarkers, and functional capacity checked plus/minus echocardiography.

4. A. A TURP would be classed as a low-risk procedure therefore further assessment is not warranted.

5. B. This patient needs to undergo emergency surgery: delay is not an option. His PCI was performed for stable angina, so a shorter duration of DAPT could be acceptable given the urgency of the clinical picture. The shortest duration for a new generation DES is typically 1 month of DAPT.

6. C. This patient needs an emergency procedure but is also at high risk of cardiac decompensation. Percutaneous aortic valve intervention should be explored.

7. B. The patient has had an acute coronary syndrome and should be treated as you would if there wasn't a need for surgery.

8. C. The patient has an indication for a pacemaker. The surgical procedure isn't an emergency life-threatening one. Temporary pacing should be reserved for situations where the non-cardiac surgery is time-sensitive and the bradyarrhythmia is haemodynamically compromising despite chronotropic drugs or is leading to ventricular tachyarrhythmias.

9. B. This lady has undergone a PCI to her proximal LAD following an NSTEMI. The recommended duration would be 1 year of DAPT. This can be shortened to 6 months for high-risk bleeding, but for a non-urgent procedure the safer option would be to delay.

10. B. It is too soon to consider stopping DAPT. This would significantly increase the risk of stent thrombosis. She is not haemodynamically unstable and hasn't dropped her haemoglobin level significantly. Risk vs benefit would be more in favour of keeping DAPT.

11. C. If this gentleman were to undergo a high-risk procedure, such as a fem-pop bypass, non-invasive stress imaging should be considered due to his risk factor profile.

12. E. The following are considered high-risk procedures: aortic and major vascular surgery, symptomatic carotid artery stenting, open lower limb revascularization or amputation, duodeno-pancreatic surgery, liver resection or bile duct surgery, repair of perforated bowel, total cystectomy, oesephagectomy, adrenal resection, pneumonectomy, and pulmonary or liver transplant.

13. C. This patient should be treated as an ACS. PCI if indicated should be undertaken with a new generation DES. Post ACS, elective non-cardiac surgery should be delayed for 12 months. For time sensitive non-cardiac surgery, consider at least 3 months of DAPT.

14. E. This patient is due to undergo a low-risk procedure. Although he has risk factors, routine imaging would not be indicated. He should be advised to stop smoking.

15. E. The patient is due for a high-risk procedure. He has significant cardiac risk factors which would carry a higher peri-operative risk of a cardiac event. Although symptom-free, stress imaging would help risk stratification.

16. C. This patient needs to undergo urgent surgery, delaying may not be an option. It has been 6 months post PCI for stable angina. In newer drug eluting stents, DAPT can be discontinued after 3 months and potentially 1 month if the bleeding risk is high. Aspirin should, however, be continued if possible according to the bleeding risk.

17. E. The patient is due to undergo an intermediate risk procedure. Whilst a beta blocker may be indicated for her CAD, commencing a beta-blocker immediately prior to surgery can increase the likelihood of haemodynamic instability.

18. C. 4 METS is equivalent to climbing two flights of stairs.

chapter

9.2

THE PATIENT WITH NEUROLOGICAL SYMPTOMS

QUESTIONS

1. A 31-year-old female is 24 weeks pregnant. She experiences symptoms of vertigo, nausea and diplopia shortly after strenuous exertion. Examination reveals her to be ataxic; she has bilaterally swollen calves. Her MRI brain scan reveals infarcts in the right cerebellum and pons as well as the left thalamus.

Which of the following factors raises the most suspicion of patent foramen ovale (PFO) as the cause of her stroke?

A. She is pregnant
B. Her stroke affected the posterior circulation
C. Her symptoms occurred after exertion
D. Infarcts affected both right and left cerebral hemispheres
E. She has bilateral calf swelling

2. An 82-year-old male presents with three recent episodes of pre-syncope. He is diabetic and also has a history of hypertension and benign prostatic hypertrophy. His medications include atenolol, losartan, and tamsulosin. His symptoms have all occurred first thing in the morning and are short-lived. His ECG shows first-degree heart block, heart rate 64 bpm. He suffers from occasional palpitations.

Which of the following is the most likely cause of his pre-syncope?

A. Vasovagal presyncope
B. Drug-induced orthostatic hypotension
C. Chrontropic incompetence with sinus bradycardia
D. Ventricular arrhythmias
E. Autonomic failure

3. **An 81-year-old male is admitted with a left middle cerebral artery stroke (infarct). He is in sinus rhythm but is hypertensive. He is a lifelong smoker and refuses to give up. His carotid Doppler shows at least 90% stenosis of his left internal carotid artery and so a CT angiogram is arranged which confirms that the artery is completely occluded.**

   Which is the most appropriate management strategy?

   A. Monotherapy with clopidogrel 75 mg
   B. Dual antiplatelet therapy with aspirin 75 mg and clopidogrel 75 mg
   C. Urgent carotid endarterectomy
   D. Routine carotid endarterectomy
   E. Carotid stenting

4. **The following symptoms are more common with posterior circulation strokes than anterior circulation strokes EXCEPT:**

   A. Vomiting
   B. Diplopia
   C. Inattention (neglect)
   D. Ataxia
   E. Vertigo

5. **A 45-year-old male presents with right arm weakness and numbness along with right sided facial drooping. He is a smoker and has a history of hypertension. His symptoms last for 3 hours in total with complete resolution thereafter. His MRI brain scan is normal. His ECG shows atrial flutter with 3:1 block.**

   Which of the following is the appropriate strategy for ongoing thromboprophylaxis?

   A. Anticoagulation with warfarin immediately
   B. Anticoagulation with warfarin at 72 hours
   C. Aspirin 75 mg and clopidogrel 75 mg
   D. Anticoagulation with DOAC agent immediately
   E. Anticoagulation with DOAC agent at 72 hours

6. **An 81-year-old male presents to the Emergency Department after waking up with left arm and leg weakness and numbness and a mild left facial droop. His speech and vision are unaffected. He is a type 2 diabetic with poor glycaemic control but is otherwise well. CT scan confirms a right middle cerebral artery infarct.**

   How would his stroke be classified according to the Bamford Criteria?

   A. Total anterior circulation infarct (TACI)
   B. Partial anterior circulation infarct (PACI)
   C. Lacunar stroke (LACI)
   D. Posterior circulation stroke (POCI)
   E. Watershed Infarct

7. An 88-year-old woman from a nursing home is admitted to the Emergency Department with sudden onset right arm and leg weakness, right facial droop, dysphagia, and dysarthria. She is usually bed bound and is hoisted for transfers, but enjoys communicating with staff, although she is disorientated to her surroundings. She has a background of vascular dementia, ischaemic heart disease, hypertension, and diabetes. A CT head shows early changes consistent with a left middle cerebral artery infarction.

Which of the following is NOT an appropriate component of her management?

A. Aspirin 300 mg od for 2 weeks followed by clopidogrel 75 mg od
B. 24-hour heart recording to investigate for atrial fibrillation
C. Physiotherapy and occupational therapy
D. Carotid imaging to assess for carotid stenosis and need for endarterectomy
E. Optimal glycaemic control

8. A 54-year-old man, previously fit and well, is admitted with sudden onset left-sided weakness, left facial droop, and dysarthria. He has associated headache and vomiting with decreased GCS documented at 13/15. A CT head reveals a large right basal ganglia haemorrhage with surrounding oedema and mass effect. He is discussed with the neurosurgical team who advise medical management but to re-discuss should he deteriorate. His blood pressure is 242/115 mmHg. His swallow has not yet been assessed.

How do you manage his hypertension?

A. Do nothing in the acute period and monitor his hypertension
B. Insert a nasogastric tube to enable administration of amlodipine
C. 10 mg amlodipine orally
D. Give a bolus of IV labetalol and set up an infusion if no response
E. Use GTN via transdermal patch

9. Which of the following statements regarding cardioembolic stroke is INCORRECT?

A. PFO is found in up to 40% of patients with cryptogenic stroke
B. AF is associated with doubled risk of ischaemic stroke compared to being in sinus rhythm
C. LV thrombus complicating MI merits anticoagulation for at least 3 months
D. Stroke complicates infective endocarditis in approximately 10% of cases
E. Cardioembolic strokes tend to affect cortical rather than subcortical brain tissue

10. With regards to patients with cardiac involvement of neuromuscular dystrophies (NMDs), which of the following statements is false?

A. Genetic testing is crucial to the diagnostic workup
B. LV systolic dysfunction can often be present without symptoms
C. Asymptomatic patients with LV dilation or dysfunction or arrhythmia (e.g. supraventricular tachycardia, ventricular ectopy) should be re-evaluated at least 3 yearly
D. Cardiac transplantation may be considered in carefully selected patients with NMD and end-stage HF
E. Conduction system involvement is not a feature of Duchenne (DMD) and Becker muscular dystrophies (BMD)

11. An inpatient on the cardiology ward is being treated for native-valve spontaneous bacterial endocarditis of the mitral valve. On the morning ward round five days into his admission, he appears confused and has word finding difficulties which were not present the previous day. Neurological examination also confirms a left homonymous hemianopia. An urgent CT head scan shows multiple bilateral hypodense areas consistent with infarction.

Which of the following is the most appropriate next step in management?

A. Intravenous thrombolysis
B. Refer for mechanical thrombectomy
C. Aspirin 300 mg
D. Dual antiplatelet therapy
E. Extending the duration of IV antibiotic therapy

12. A 64-year-old man is admitted with dyspnoea and is found to be in atrial fibrillation with a fast ventricular rate. He first noticed intermittent palpitations 5 days earlier. He has no significant past medical history and takes no regular medications. He is treated with bisoprolol for rate control but remains in atrial fibrillation. The following morning the nurses note a dense right hemiparesis associated with word finding difficulties and calls for an urgent medical review. His National Institutes of Health Stroke Scale (NIHSS) score is calculated to be 18 and a CT head scan is normal.

Which of the following is the most appropriate next step in management?

A. Calculation of CHA_2DS_2-VASc score
B. Establishing eligibility for mechanical thrombectomy
C. Rhythm control (electrical or pharmacological)
D. Commencement of anticoagulation
E. Starting IV thrombolysis

chapter 9.2

THE PATIENT WITH NEUROLOGICAL SYMPTOMS

ANSWERS

1. C. PFOs are found in up to 40% of patients with cryptogenic stroke and may be a conduit for ischaemic stroke via paradoxical embolism. Paradoxical embolism occurs when emboli originating in the venous circulation bypass the normal filtering system of the pulmonary capillaries, enter the arterial circulation, and occlude arteries in various organs. Factors which make paradoxical embolism more likely include history of venous thromboembolism (i.e. DVT/PE), Valsalva manoeuvre preceding onset of stroke symptoms (e.g. due to coughing, sneezing, vigorous exercise), and waking up with a stroke.

2. B. The most likely cause of the patient's presyncopal symptoms is orthostatic hypotension (OH) due to polypharmacy—he is on three drugs which are associated with OH in elderly patients. The definition of OH is a sustained reduction of systolic blood pressure of at least 20 mmHg or diastolic blood pressure of 10 mmHg within 3 minutes of standing. Characteristic symptoms include light-headedness, visual blurring, dizziness, generalized weakness, fatigue, cognitive slowing, leg buckling, and gradual or sudden loss of consciousness. Treatment includes encouraging adequate fluid intake, avoidance of large meals or excessive alcohol, dose modification of the offending drugs, compression stockings, and rarely drugs to increase blood pressure such as fludrocortisone.

3. A. In this case the carotid artery is already occluded so the risk of causing further harm by proceeding to carotid endarterectomy outweighs the potential benefits. If the artery is already fully occluded then no further thromboemboli can pass along it and cause a distal obstruction and subsequent stroke. There is no evidence to suggest that dual antiplatelet therapy provides any benefit above monotherapy in this situation, and focus should be on his other modifiable risk factors (hypertension and smoking).

4. C. Inattention (neglect) is a sign associated with strokes affecting the anterior circulation, most commonly involving the middle cerebral artery and subsequent damage to the right (non-dominant) parietal lobe. Vomiting, diplopia, ataxia, and vertigo are all signs consistent with posterior circulation ischaemia, affecting the brain stem and/or cerebellum.

5. D. This patient has clinically experienced a transient ischaemic attack (TIA)—there is no evidence of a completed stroke as evidenced by a normal MRI scan. The patient should be anticoagulated immediately to reduce risk of subsequent stroke. Anticoagulation with a DOAC has been shown to have superior efficacy over with warfarin in reducing stroke or systemic embolization as well as a lower risk of intracranial haemorrhage. There is no suggestion of valvular heart disease which would warrant anticoagulation with warfarin and therefore a DOAC should be the anticoagulation method of choice.

6. C. The Bamford stroke classification divides people with stroke into four categories depending on their signs and symptoms. The criteria can be helpful in understanding the underlying cause of the stroke as well as the expected prognosis.

Total anterior circulation infarct (TACI)—All of: motor and/or sensory deficit, higher cortical dysfunction, hemianopia

Prognosis: 55% mortality at 6 months, 40% modified Rankin Scale (mRS; measures degree of disability/dependence after a stroke) 3–5 at 6 months

Likely cause: Large vessel atherothrombosis, cardiac thromboembolism

Partial anterior circulation infarct (PACI)—Two of: motor and/or sensory deficit, higher cortical dysfunction, hemianopia

Prognosis: 18% mortality at 6 months, 25% mRS 3–5 at 6 months

Likely cause: cardiac thromboembolism

Lacunar infarct (LACI)—Motor and/or sensory deficit only

Prognosis: 8% mortality at 6 months, 25% mRS 3–5 at 6 months

Likely cause: small vessel disease (hypertension, poor glycaemic control, smoking)

Posterior circulation infarct (POCI)—isolated hemianopia, brain stem signs, cerebellar signs

Prognosis: 22% mortality at 6 months, 20% mRS 3–5 at 6 months

Likely case: cardiac thromboembolism, small vessel disease (hypertension, poor glycaemic control, smoking)

7. D. Carotid endarterectomy is an intervention reserved for those patients with good functional baseline, and with good recovery following their stroke. If a patient would not be a surgical candidate then arranging imaging of the carotids is not necessary. Treatment should focus on other means of prevention (e.g. DOAC for atrial fibrillation) and therapy to try to achieve as much improvement in function as possible.

8. D. This patient has an acute haemorrhagic stroke with severe hypertension and his blood pressure should therefore be strictly controlled to prevent further expansion of the haematoma. Strict blood pressure control for haemorrhagic stroke is indicated if within 6 hours of onset aiming for a target BP of <140/90 mmHg. Blood pressure should ideally be maintained at this level for 7 days; common agents used for treatment are intravenous labetalol or nitrate infusions. After the first 24 hours and once an oral route is available, either via safe swallow or nasogastric tube, oral medications such as amlodipine can be used.

9. B. Cardiac embolism often lodges in distal arteries supplying the cerebral cortex as opposed to small-vessel occlusion which affects subcortical tissue; cortical signs such as aphasia or visual field deficits are therefore more likely to be present. AF increases stroke risk by five times compared to those without AF. The finding of LV thrombus merits prompt anticoagulation for a period of at least 3 months; some with poor LV function will require longer (possibly indefinite) anticoagulation. PFO prevalence is up to 40% in patients with cryptogenic stroke, suggesting that it may be a conduit for stroke caused by paradoxical embolism rather than just an incidental finding. Clinically apparent acute brain embolization is estimated to occur in 10% of patients with left-sided infective endocarditis.

10. C. It is important to have a precise genetic diagnosis because this provides vital information about clinical expectations and genetic counselling, and also due to the heterogeneity in cardiovascular manifestations among NMDs. Limitations to movement caused by skeletal muscle disease means early signs of cardiac failure may not appear clinically apparent. Because of the underlying pathogenesis (myocyte disruption attributable to abnormal dystrophin protein), conduction system involvement is not a feature of DMD and BMD as it is with many other NMDs. Asymptomatic DMD/BMD patients with LV dilation or dysfunction or arrhythmia (e.g.

supraventricular tachycardia, ventricular ectopy) should be re-evaluated at least annually—this should be more frequent if symptomatic. Cardiac transplantation may be considered in carefully selected patients with NMD and end-stage HF despite appropriate therapies.

11. C. The rate of neurological complications from bacterial endocarditis is as high as 40%. These include embolic infarction, haemorrhagic transformation of an infarct, mycotic aneurysm formation, brain abscesses, meningitis, and seizures. The management of stroke associated with bacterial endocarditis is difficult due to the extremely high risk of haemorrhagic transformation of infarcts if therapies such as IV thrombolysis or thrombectomy are performed. This patient has evidence of embolic strokes affecting multiple territories and therefore would not be suitable for mechanical thrombectomy. Due to the unclear time of onset IV thrombolysis is contraindicated.

12. B. The patient in question is likely to have had an embolic stroke due to atrial fibrillation. Due to his high NIHSS score, it is likely that he has a large vessel intracranial occlusion causing his symptoms. The patient is outside the time window for IV thrombolysis (4.5 hours) but may be eligible for mechanical thrombectomy. It would be important to arrange a CT angiogram to look for evidence of large vessel occlusion and discuss with the local neuroscience centre regarding suitability for thrombectomy. Anticoagulation in acute stroke is contraindicated, and timing of its commencement depends on the size of the underlying infarct. For larger infarcts anticoagulation is commonly delayed for up to 2 weeks; however, with smaller infarcts this can be done earlier, sometimes as early as a few days after the onset of symptoms. Rhythm control may be considered to be appropriate at a later stage but is not an acute priority, and the duration of the symptoms in this case further complicates the issue.

chapter

9.3

THE PATIENT WITH CHRONIC KIDNEY DISEASE

QUESTIONS

1. A diabetic 75-year-old gentleman with an eGFR of 30 ml/min was noted to have persistent proteinuria of around 1.5 g per day. His blood pressure was 140/80 mmHg. His current medication list includes amlodipine 10 mg daily, metformin 500 mg tds, ramipril 5 mg daily and atorvastatin 20 mg nocte. His serum potassium levels and latest Hba1c results were stable.

Which one of the following would be the next step to optimise his management?

A. Add Valsartan 80 mg daily
B. No change in treatment required
C. Continue Ramipril 5mg daily and add Fineronone 10 mg daily.
D. Increase Ramipril to 10mg daily and consider SGLT2 inhibitor if proteinuria persists
E. Increase Ramipril to 10 mg daily and increase Atorvastatin to 40 mg nocte.

2. A 60-year-old diabetic gentleman with hypertension and an eGFR of 27 ml/min is being reviewed in the renal clinic. He takes a calcium channel blocker and an angiotensin converting enzyme inhibitor for blood pressure control.

With regard to primary prevention for cardiovascular disease, this gentleman

A. Should receive moderate-intensity (atorvastatin 20 mg nocte) statin for primary prevention if at CKD stage IV
B. Should commence statin treatment for primary prevention if established on haemodialysis
C. Should receive high-intensity statin (atorvastatin 40 mg nocte) for primary prevention if at CKD stage IV
D. Should commence aspirin treatment for primary prevention if established if at CKD stage IV
E. Should commence statin and aspirin for primary prevention if established on haemodialysis

3. A 63-year-old woman with treated hypertension and an eGFR of 30 ml/min is being reviewed in the renal clinic. Due to a lack of safety data and risk for toxicity with higher doses of statins in CKD the KDIGO Work Group recommends that prescription of statins in people with CKD should be based on doses that have shown benefit in randomized trials done specifically in CKD population.

What dose would be recommended for this woman?

A. Atorvastatin 40 mg daily
B. Simvastatin/ezetimibe 20 mg/10 mg
C. Atorvastatin 40 mg daily or simvastatin/ezetimibe 20 mg/10 mg
D. Simvastatin/ezetimibe 80 mg/10 mg
E. Atorvastatin 20 mg daily or simvastatin/ezetimibe 20 mg/10 mg

4. A general practitioner contacts tertiary nephrology services for advice about a patient with CKD. He is interested in the role of renin angiotensin blockade in CKD progression and in cardiovascular protection in end-stage kidney disease (ESKD).

You advise him that renin angiotensin system inhibitors should be used in which of the following circumstances?

A. In all adult patients on dialysis
B. In all hypertensive adults with non-dialysis CKD
C. In adults over 65 years of age with non-dialysis CKD
D. In adults with diabetes, proteinuria and non-dialysis CKD
E. In either diabetic or non-diabetic adults with proteinuria and non-dialysis CKD

5. A 60-year-old diabetic male patient with a previous history of ischaemic heart disease and recent haemorrhage from a peptic ulcer is admitted from the dialysis unit. He presented for his regular dialysis treatment 4 kg above his target weight with chest discomfort. Blood tests taken on dialysis showed elevated troponin T (2 × normal value, unchanged from previous value 3 months ago), Hb 75 g/L and platelet 85 × 10^9/L. His ECG shows non-specific T-wave changes.

Which treatment is appropriate?

A. Initiate acute coronary syndrome (ACS) protocol with aspirin and clopidogrel
B. Organise serial troponins and ECGs and reassess need for ACS treatment
C. Monitor Hb but do not transfuse because of risk of fluid overload
D. If he has ongoing chest pain and RRT is required ensure intermittent haemodialysis is used to minimize time on dialysis
E. Initiate acute coronary syndrome (ACS) protocol with aspirin and ticagrelor

6. A 55-year-old gentleman who recently started haemodialysis presents to A&E with acute shortness of breath and orthopnoea. His chest X-ray showed pulmonary oedema, cardiac troponin T tests were elevated but there no significant rise between serial tests while NT-proBNP was >3000 pg/mL. He undergoes an echocardiogram shortly after admission.

What abnormality do you expect to find?

A. Left ventricular hypertrophy
B. Systolic dysfunction
C. Diastolic dysfunction
D. Left ventricular hypertrophy and systolic dysfunction
E. Left ventricular hypertrophy and diastolic dysfunction

7. A 62-year-old lady became suddenly unresponsive 1.5 hours into her 4-hour haemodialysis session. She lost cardiac output and resuscitation attempts were unfortunately unsuccessful.

Which of the following statements is correct?

A. Sudden cardiac death is typically associated with left ventricular dysfunction in dialysis patients
B. Implanted cardioverter-defibrillator devices are effective in reducing mortality in dialysis patients dialyzing via permanent lines.
C. The majority of patients with sudden cardiac death do not have reduced ejection fraction.
D. There is a strong relationship between severity of coronary artery disease and sudden cardiac death among CKD patients.
E. Dialysing against a low-potassium dialysate may prevent sudden cardiac death.

8. A 65-year-old lady was noted to develop paroxysmal atrial fibrillation (AF) while on haemodialysis.

With regard to non-valvular AF in patients with CKD and ESKD, which of the following is true:

A. Anticoagulation with warfarin is recommended in dialysis patients with a CHA_2DS_2-VASc score of >1
B. Routine anticoagulation in dialysis patients with atrial fibrillation is not recommended
C. Novel oral anti-coagulants (NOACs) are used in preference to warfarin in dialysis patients with a CHA_2DS_2-VASc score of >1
D. Routine anticoagulation does not lower risk of thromboembolic events in patients with CKD stage 3 or higher.
E. As her CHA_2DS-$VASC_2$ score is 1, she does not need routine anticoagulation.

9. A 50-year-old gentleman presents to A&E due to crushing central chest pain. He suffers from type 2 diabetes, hypertension, and CKD stage 3b with an eGFR of 30 ml/min/1.73m^2. His ECG shows new ST depression inferolaterally and his troponin T rose from 55ng/L to 1274ng/L.

Considering ACS treatment in the context of CKD which statement is not correct?

A. Low molecular weight heparins require dose adjustment if eGFR <30 ml/min
B. Glycoprotein IIb/IIIa inhibitors (eptifibatide) do not require dose reduction
C. Aspirin and clopidogrel may carry a greater bleeding risk on CKD
D. Beta-blockers may need dose reduction
E. Care is needed to manage contrast-induced nephropathy risk during angiography

10. A 60-year-old male diabetic patient with CKD stage 4 (eGFR 28 ml/min) is planned for coronary angiography.

Which of the following interventions is not useful to reduce the risk of contrast nephropathy?

A. Optimize fluid balance and ensure adequate hydration peri-procedure
B. Monitor renal function tests
C. Minimize contrast dose if possible
D. Organize dialysis line insertion and treatment post procedure to remove contrast agent.
E. Use of non-ionic, iso- or low-osmolal contrast agents

chapter 9.3

THE PATIENT WITH CHRONIC KIDNEY DISEASE

ANSWERS

1. D. The standard of care in proteinuric CKD is RAS blockade. This has been shown to be of clear benefit especially in patients with diabetic nephropathy. All patients recruited into CREDENCE were on stable maximally tolerated RAS blockade, as were 97% of DAPA-CKD participants. Therefore the recommendation is to prescribe RAS blockade and ensure clinically appropriate dosing alongside any SGLT-2 inhibitor use. It is recommended to use single agent RAS blockade, as combination therapy (i.e. dual blockade with ACEi plus ARB) has been found to increase the risk of serious hyperkalaemia or acute kidney injury, and has not been shown to importantly slow CKD progression (30).

2. A. A statin is recommended for all patients with T1D or T2D and CKD, moderate intensity for primary prevention of ASCVD or high intensity for patients with known ASCVD and some patients with multiple ASCVD risk factors. The dosage of the statin also needs to be adjusted to the degree of renal impairment. Aspirin is not recommended for primary prevention in diabetic and/or CKD patients without ASCVD.

3. E. Statins have been shown to reduce adverse cardiovascular events both when used as primary prevention in CKD patients without established atherosclerotic cardiovascular disease and as secondary prevention in patients who have already suffered adverse cardiovascular events. The best data supporting the use of statins for primary prevention of cardiovascular events in patients with non-dialysis CKD come from the SHARP trial as described above. The role of statins in dialysis patients is less clear, however, in a subgroup analysis of the 4-D trial, haemodialysis patients with LDL-cholesterol concentrations >145 mg/dL assigned to atorvastatin 20 mg daily had a reduction in composite primary outcome consisting of cardiovascular, death, nonfatal MI, and stroke. Atorvastatin is typically used in CKD patients because renal dosing is not required as it undergoes hepatic clearance.

4. E. Multiple randomized controlled trials have shown that renin angiotensin blockade has a beneficial, nephroprotective effect in both proteinuric non-diabetic and diabetic CKD with improved proteinuria and slower progression of renal disease. They do not have clear advantages over calcium channel blockers or diuretics in diabetic or non-diabetic CKD without proteinuria. Renin angiotensin blockade also plays a major cardioprotective role in patients with heart failure (especially HFrEF) and CKD, just like in non-CKD heart failure, but close monitoring and a multi-disciplinary approach are advised. It has not been established whether renin angiotensin blockade confers cardiovascular benefits to patients on haemodialysis and may be associated with adverse events, such as suppression of erythropoiesis, hyperkalaemia, and anaphylactoid reactions with certain haemodialysis membranes. Renin angiotensin blockade has, however, been associated with reduced loss of native renal function in patients receiving peritoneal dialysis.

5. B. Acute coronary syndrome is common in patients on haemodialysis and is typically caused by myocardial ischaemia secondary to epicardial coronary atherosclerotic plaque rupture (type 1 myocardial ischaemia). However in up to 27% of patients, myocardial ischaemia could be due to an imbalance between myocardial oxygen supply and demand (type 2 myocardial ischaemia). It is likely that this gentleman is suffering from such an event due to the following risk factors: volume overload leading to both high wall tension in the left ventricle leading to increased oxygen demand and the risk of intradialytic hypotension and reduced myocardial perfusion due large ultrafiltration volumes, and anaemia leading to inadequate oxygen supply to the myocardium. Left ventricular hypertrophy is highly prevalent in haemodialysis patients and this also contributes to an imbalance between oxygen supply and demand by increasing cardiac work and reducing capillary density. In fact, most patients with CKD and ESKD have elevated baseline troponin levels, probably secondary to underlying structural heart disease and chronic myocardial injury. A serial change in troponin concentrations over three to six hours after presentation should be used to define an acute myocardial infarction, rather than a single value obtained at presentation. Continuous haemofiltration offers more haemodynamic stability than intermitted haemodialysis and hence it is preferable in patients with an acute myocardial infarction. Given that this gentleman is probably suffering from type 2 myocardial ischaemia and in light of the recent GI bleed and low platelet count, anti-platelet therapy as per ACS protocol is not recommended.

6. E. Patients with CKD and end-stage kidney disease (ESKD) have a high prevalence of left ventricular hypertrophy (LVH) and it is found in up to 80% of haemodialysis patients. Potential causes for LVH in these patients include hypertension, anaemia, vascular calcification, vascular non-compliance, and volume overload. LVH leads to left ventricular (LV) stiffness, increased LV filling pressures, and abnormal diastolic filling, leading to diastolic dysfunction. Indeed, while 85–90% of ESKD patients have preserved left ventricular systolic function on echocardiograms, up to 40% of incident ESKD patients present with circulatory congestion due to heart failure with preserved ejection fraction within the first year.

7. C. Left ventricular hypertrophy increases the risk of cardiac arrhythmias and sudden cardiac death which accounts for 25% of dialysis patients' deaths, and has an annual incidence rate of 5.5%. Although in the general population ischaemic cardiomyopathy with reduced ejection fraction often underlies sudden cardiac death (SCD), up to 75% of haemodialysis patients who suffered a SCD had ejection fractions >35%. Left ventricular mass index has been shown to be the best predictor of SCD over time. Chronic hypertension, anaemia, microvessel disease, and repetitive myocardial injury caused by hypoperfusion during dialysis may account for this disease pattern. It is advisable to avoid large shifts in fluids and electrolytes during haemodialysis as these can trigger arrythmias. Low potassium dialysates have been associated with an increased SCD risk.

8. B. Despite the increased prevalence of atrial fibrillation in haemodialysis patients, observational studies have shown that anticoagulation with either warfarin or NOAC in this population of patients may increase the risk of bleeding and may not reduce the risk of thromboembolic cerebrovascular events. In view of this, the decision to start anti-coagulation in a haemodialysis patient will require risk stratification using the CHA_2DS_2-VASc score, and a discussion of risks and benefits between the clinician and the patient. Hence, routine anticoagulation in dialysis patients with non-valvular AF is not recommended. For patients with stages 1 to 3 CKD and CHA_2DS_2-VASc score >1, a NOAC is recommended over warfarin as NOACs have been shown to be associated with similar or lower rates both of ischaemic stroke and major bleeding compared to adjusted dose warfarin. Although patients with CKD stage 4 have been poorly represented in clinical trials, if the embolic risk outweighs bleeding risk it is also reasonable to anticoagulate these patients with a NOAC.

9. B. Chronic kidney disease is an independent risk factor for ACS and it is associated with worse outcomes, including mortality and bleeding. Patients with CKD have, however, been largely underrepresented in randomized controlled trials investigating pharmacotherapy in ACS hence there is a lack of robust evidence-based guidance for the management of ACS in these patients. Standard recommendations state that patients with CKD benefit from evidence-based medications routinely used in all patients presenting with ACS, taking into consideration the degree of creatinine clearance as calculated by the Cockcroft–Gault equation and making the appropriate dose-adjustments of cardiovascular medications. Glycoprotein IIb/IIIa inhibitors do need dose reduction as do low molecular weight heparins and beta-blockers. Contrast-induced nephropathy needs to be considered but should not limit use of coronary angiography.

10. D. The risk of contrast-induced acute kidney injury (CI-AKI) is higher with procedures involving the arterial administration compared with venous administration of contrast, either due to phenotypic differences in patient populations or to nephrotoxicity of the intra-arterial contrast load. The incidence of CI-AKI is also higher among patients with CKD, especially in those with diabetes, and increases with the severity of kidney dysfunction hence precautions need to be taken to prevent CI-AKI. These include avoidance of volume depletion, pre-hydration with isotonic saline if appropriate, using the lowest effective dose possible of contrast, ideally non-ionic, iso- or low-osmolal agents, and close monitoring of renal function post-procedure. N-acetylcysteine has not been observed to improve outcomes in high-risk patients undergoing elective angiography hence its role remains uncertain. There is no evidence to support immediate dialysis after intravascular contrast administration.

chapter

9.4

THE PATIENT WITH PULMONARY DISEASE

QUESTIONS

1. **A 67-year-old male with pharmacological optimized systolic heart failure (left ventricular ejection fraction 40%) has been complaining of excessive daytime sleepiness (Epworth sleepiness score 14) and poor sleep quality. A sleep study has revealed 32 central apnoea/hypopnea episodes per hour and Cheyne–Stokes respiration.**

   Which of the following is the first line therapeutic treatment option?

   A. Theophylline
   B. Continuous positive airway pressure (CPAP)
   C. Bilevel positive airway pressure (BiPAP) with a backup rate
   D. Adaptive servo-ventilation (ASV)
   E. Supplemental nocturnal oxygen

2. **A patient attends heart failure clinic for annual review. She is 67 years old with a long-standing diagnosis of heart failure with reduced ejection fraction (left ventricular function 30%). She is an ex-smoker with a 45 pack per year history and a diagnosis of COPD. After reading an article on the internet, she is concerned that her heart failure medication is making her breathing worse. In comorbid chronic systolic heart failure and obstructive airway disease (COPD or asthma) which of the following is true:**

   A. Beta-blockers should be avoided in COPD as they can cause bronchoconstriction
   B. Beta-blockers increase mortality in COPD
   C. Beta-blockers improve survival rates in COPD
   D. Beta-blockers can be used freely in severe asthma
   E. Selective beta-2 receptor blockers are preferred in COPD

3. A 55-year-old severely obese, smoker, who is a lorry driver complains about nocturnal choking. The patient does not complain about daytime sleepiness and his Epworth sleepiness score is 8 (normal <11). The cardiovascular examination reveals elevated blood pressure. Subsequently, a cardiac echo is performed which is in normal range and a spirometry which suggests restrictive ventilatory defect.

Which of the following is the most appropriate next diagnostic procedure?

A. Chest X-ray
B. Overnight oximetry
C. Referral to a specialist for consideration of appropriate testing
D. Polysomnography
E. Follow up in 3 months

4. A 60-year-old male smoker (50 packs per year) complains about breathlessness on exertion. The cardiovascular evaluation is within normal limits. Laboratory investigation which included full blood count, N-terminal pro-BNP, blood glucose, urea, creatinine, electrolytes, calcium, phosphate, and thyroid stimulating hormone, were normal. Which one of the following is the most appropriate next investigation?

A. Overnight oximetry
B. Polysomnography
C. Spirometry pre and post bronchodilation
D. High resolution computed tomography
E. Cardiopulmonary exercise test

5. A 70-year-old female, diagnosed with COPD, has an FEV_1, % pred = 49%, mMRC score = 3, and had one exacerbation in the previous year when she was treated as an outpatient with oral corticosteroid and antibiotic.

Which of the following GOLD and Group categories does this patient fit in?

A. Gold 1, Group B
B. Gold 3, Group B
C. Gold 3, Group C
D. Gold 4, Group D
E. Gold 3, Group D

6. A 45-year-old male, BMI 35 kg/m^2, on medication for hypertension with a history of loud intrusive snoring, poor sleep quality, and excessive daytime sleepiness was assessed for possible sleep apnoea and underwent polysomnography. The sleep study revealed 22 obstructive sleep apnoea (OSA)/hypopnoea episodes per hour.

What is the severity of the patient's OSA?

A. None, he does not have OSA
B. Mild
C. Moderate
D. Severe
E. Very Severe

7. A 52-year-old obese male with moderate obstructive sleep apnoea syndrome attends sleep clinic for review and discussion for possible treatment. Which one should be the most appropriate initial treatment?

A. Conservative (diet and exercise advice alone)
B. Oral appliance
C. Upper airway surgery
D. Continuous positive airway pressure (CPAP)
E. Bi-level positive airway pressure (BiPAP)

8. A 62-year-old woman with COPD is being considered for anti-inflammatory therapy.

Which of the following is NOT true regarding anti-inflammatory therapy in COPD?

A. Long therapy monotherapy with inhaled corticosteroid (ICS) should not be used
B. Long-term treatment with ICS should be considered in association with long-acting bronchodilator (LABA) for patients with a history of exacerbations despite appropriate treatment with long-acting bronchodilators
C. Long-term therapy with oral corticosteroids should be considered
D. Statin therapy is not recommended for prevention of exacerbation
E. Antioxidant mucolytics should be used only in selected patients

9. A 42-year-old male, who has been an occasional smoker in the past, but without any significant exposure to biomass fumes, complains about dyspnoea on exertion. Clinical examination reveals remarkably reduced breathing sounds bilaterally. Spirometry shows severe obstructive ventilator defect (post bronchodilation, FEV_1/FVC: 53% and FEV_1, %pred: 44%). Chest radiograph shows emphysema predominant in the lower zones.

Which one is the most probable diagnosis?

A. Asthma
B. Cystic fibrosis
C. Chronic bronchitis
D. Alpha 1-antitrypsin deficiency
E. Obesity related respiratory function impairment

10. You are asked to review a 55-year-old male with an established diagnosis of COPD. He has confirmatory spirometry with an FEV_1 of 75% and is established on an inhaled bronchodilator therapy with a long-acting anti-muscarinic. He is able to walk for 5–10 minutes on the flat but is breathless on a moderate incline (MRC score 3). He has had two exacerbations requiring community therapy and one requiring admission to hospital but not critical care in the past 12 months. He stopped smoking 6 months ago with a 50 pack per year history.

Which one of the following is the best predictor of future acute exacerbations of COPD?

A. FEV_1
B. History of previous treated events
C. mMRC score
D. Smoking status
E. Current inhaler management

11. You see a 64-year-old male with a history of heart failure with reduced ejection fracture. He was recently reviewed due to poor sleep quality and daytime fatigue. He complains of sleep onset insomnia with frequent awakenings overnight and episodes of paroxysmal nocturnal dyspnoea. He is clinically euvolaemic with well-controlled blood pressure and a recent echocardiogram showing stable left ventricular function. An overnight respiratory sleep study has demonstrated mild central sleep apnoea.

Which one of the below are first line treatment of central sleep apnoea in heart failure in this patient?

A. ASV
B. CPAP
C. Sleep hygiene
D. Nocturnal oxygen
E. Optimal medical management (ACEi, B-blockers, digoxin and diuretics)

12. Whilst covering the cardiology on call you are bleeped by the cardio-thoracic ward to review a patient. The patient is a 58-year-old female admitted for lung volume reduction surgery for her severe heterogeneous emphysema. Her pre-operative FEV_1 was 35% predicted. Post-operatively she has required oxygen therapy and periods of non-invasive ventilation for hypercapnic respiratory failure. She has been persistently tachycardic with an irregular heart rate of 120–140 bpm. The surgical foundation year 1 doctor has called as they are concerned she may have atrial fibrillation but is unsure as they can still see some p waves on the ECG. She is haemodynamically stable without chest pain but is complaining of dyspnoea.

Which of the following is not true regarding the characteristics of cardiac dysrhythmias in COPD?

A. COPD increases the risk of cardiac dysrhythmias during thoracic surgery
B. Risk factors includes hypoxemia, acidosis, and reduced FEV_1
C. Multifocal atrial tachycardia is common in COPD patients
D. COPD acute exacerbation increases the risk for cardiac dysrhythmias
E. Presence of multifocal atrial tachycardia in COPD does not affect mortality rate

13. In outpatient clinic you review a 48-year-old male with hypertension. He has a BMI of 38kg/m^2 and co-morbid type 2 diabetes and OSA. His diabetes is controlled with a HbA1c of 52 mmol/mol (6.9%) and he uses his CPAP therapy for over 4 hours per night with good symptomatic relief. He would like to better understand his individual cardiovascular risk in the coming years.

Which of the following vascular risk factors and vascular disease markers is related to OSA?

A. Hypertension
B. Decreased high density lipoproteins
C. Increased C-reactive protein
D. Increased homocysteine
E. All of the above

14. A 62-year-old man is being treated for obstructive sleep apnoea and requires continuous positive airway pressure (CPAP).

Which of the following statement is true regarding the effect of CPAP on cardiovascular physiology?

A. Generates negative intrathoracic pressure
B. Reduces left ventricular stroke volume
C. Increases left ventricular preload
D. Increases left ventricular transmural pressure
E. Improves left ventricular diastolic relaxation

15. A 32-year-old man presents to the Emergency Department short of breath and is found to have a large goitre compressing his upper airway.

Which of the following statements is true regarding the effect of an obstructed upper airway on the heart?

A. Generates positive intrathoracic pressure
B. Generates negative intrathoracic pressure
C. Decreases left ventricular transmural pressure
D. Decreases right ventricular preload
E. Decreases left ventricular afterload

chapter

9.4

THE PATIENT WITH PULMONARY DISEASE

ANSWERS

1. B. CPAP is the preferred first-line therapy for symptomatic patients with hyperventilation-related central sleep apnoea, including those with heart failure. In the aforementioned patient group, second-line therapy for those not tolerating or responding to CPAP with nocturnal hypoxemia is the use of supplemental nocturnal oxygen. ASV should not be used in patients with central sleep apnoea due to heart failure with reduced ejection fraction (≤45%) as it has been associated with an increase in mortality in this population. The use of BiPAP with a back-up respiratory rate in patients with central sleep apnoea (CSA) due to heart failure with reduced ejection fraction (≤45%) should be approached with caution due to the similar effect on breathing pattern of ASV and BiPAP with a back-up rate. Theophylline is a respiratory stimulant that can decrease the apnoea/hypopnea episodes per hour in patients with CSA associated with Cheyne–Stokes breathing due to heart failure, but there are no long-term data available.

2. C. Beta-blockers improve survival rates in patients with chronic systolic heart failure and after myocardial infarction, including in those patients with coexisting COPD. Cardio-selective beta-blockers which predominantly block beta-1 receptors are the beta-blockers of choice in this clinical scenario. However, even the use of beta-1-selective drugs should be closely monitor in patients with severe asthma.

3. C. Objective diagnostic testing is necessary to diagnose obstructive sleep apnoea, because the clinical features are non-specific and the diagnostic accuracy of clinical impression alone is poor. In-laboratory polysomnography is the gold standard first-line diagnostic study when obstructive sleep apnoea is suspected. Overnight oximetry followed by home polygraphy may be an alternative first approach. Please note that this patient works in a critical profession and a diagnosis of OSA may have significant implications for their ability to safely and legally perform their role.

4. C. COPD should be considered in any patient who has dyspnoea, chronic cough, or sputum production. Dyspnoea on exertion is the commonest initially reported symptom in COPD. Spirometry is required to make the diagnosis, in a compatible clinical context showing the presence of a post-bronchodilator FEV1/FVC<0.7.

5. B. (see figure 9.4.A1)

Exacerbation History	Groups	
0 to 1 exacerbation per year and no hospitalization for exacerbation	A	B
≥2 exacerbations per year or ≥1 hospitalization for exacerbation	C	D
	CAT score <10 or mMRC grade 0 to 1	CAT score ≥10 or mMRC grade ≥2
	Symptoms	

FEV_1 (%predicted)	
GOLD 1	≥80
GOLD 2	50–79
GOLD 3	49–30
GOLD 4	<30

Figure 9.4.A1 GOLD and Group categories

6. C. OSA severity is measured by the apnea-hypopnea index (AHI):

Mild: patients with an AHI between 5 and 15 respiratory events per hour of sleep.

Moderate: patients with an AHI between 15 and 30 respiratory events per hour of sleep.

Severe: patients with an AHI greater than 30 respiratory events per hour of sleep.

7. D. CPAP is the simplest and most extensive studied of the positive pressure airway administration treatments. Moreover, there is no proven advantage to using BiPAP instead of CPAP for the routine management of OSA. An oral appliance is a reasonable alternative in patients with mild or moderate OSA who decline or do not manage to tolerate positive pressure airway treatment. Finally, there is no consensus regarding the role of surgery in patients with OSA of varying degrees of severity, nor is it known which patients are most likely to benefit from surgery. Lifestyle advice should be given to all patients with OSA including sleep hygiene, weight management, caffeine reduction, and smoking cessation where appropriate. However, in symptomatic patients with moderate to severe OSA this should not be used as the sole management strategy.

8. C. Short course (5–7 days) of systemic glucocorticoids is used to treat acute exacerbations of COPD. However, long-term systemic glucocorticoid therapy can have significant side effects and has been related with increased morbidity and mortality and should only be used under specialist supervision.

9. D. Clinical features that should lead clinicians to test for alpha1-antitrypsin deficiency are:

- Emphysema in a young adult (e.g. age ≤45 years)
- Emphysema in a non-smoker or occasionally smoker
- Emphysema not characterized by predominant upper zone changes on radiological examination
- Familial emphysema and/or liver disease
- Unexplained chronic liver disease

10. B. Exacerbations become more frequent and more severe as the severity of underlying COPD increases. The most important determinant of frequent exacerbations is a history of exacerbations.

Patients who are more subject to frequent exacerbations have a distinct susceptibility phenotype. This is relatively stable over time and can be identified on the history of previous treated events.

11. E. Medical therapy directed at congestive heart failure, followed by CPAP (commenced gradually under supervision) and/or supplemental oxygen should be considered. Recent data suggests an increase risk in patients with a poor left ventricular ejection fraction, symptomatic heart failure, and central sleep apnoea treated with adaptive-servo ventilation and therefore this therapy should not be used outside expert guidance. Optimal pharmacological therapy of heart failure can decrease the likelihood of periodic breathing and CSA. Heart failure treatment improves cardiac function due to reverse remodelling. Consecutively, stroke volume increases and pulmonary capillary pressure and oedema reduces, and stimulation to the J receptors decreases. As stroke volume increases and cardiopulmonary blood volume decreases, effective arterial circulation time should decrease. The effect of these changes is a trend towards limiting tachypnoea and so reverting hypocapnia to eucapnia. Cardiac resynchronization by biventricular pacing and heart transplantation may also alleviate CSR/CSA.

12. E. COPD clearly increases the risk of cardiac dysrhythmias and a high rate of rhythm disturbances exists in patients with COPD even while stable. The causes of cardiac dysrhythmias in COPD is multifactorial and includes a number of risk factors such as hypoxemia, acidosis, and reduced FEV1. The risk is more profound during acute exacerbation or thoracic surgery. Multifocal atrial tachycardia (MAT) is often found in COPD and has been frequently described during times of exacerbation. Note that the mortality rate of patients with COPD and MAT is high.

13. E. An increased risk for cardiovascular events related to coronary heart disease, independent of other shared risk factors has been noted in OSA. Furthermore, OSA is a risk factor for worse outcomes in patients with established coronary heart disease.

14. E. CPAP increases intrathoracic pressure and can augment stroke volume and cardiac output. CPAP also decreases left ventricular preload and afterload by decreasing left ventricular transmural pressures during diastole and systole. Additionally, attenuates the sympathetic nervous activity and increases cardiac vagal modulation of the heart with improved blood pressure regulation. The effects of inter-related factors such as elimination of both nocturnal hypoxaemia and nocturnal sympathetic surges, improvement in LV diastolic relaxation properties, and decreased LV afterload may restore the balance between endothelial vasoactive mediators with the application of CPAP.

15. B. Obstructed upper airway may produce negative intrathoracic pressure that increases left ventricular transmural pressure and left ventricular afterload. The negative pressure also draws more blood into the thorax and thus increases right ventricular preload. Moreover, intermittent hypoxia related to OSA may also impair cardiac function during systole and diastole.

chapter 9.5

THE PATIENT WITH RHEUMATIC DISORDERS

QUESTIONS

1. A 60-year-old woman with rheumatoid arthritis (RA) being treated with tocilizumab is found to have increased lipid levels. She asks whether this might be associated with her RA and what relevance this has to her choice of medication.

Which of the following advice about lipids, cardiovascular risk, and RA treatments would incorrect?

A. Patients with RA with active disease tend to have lower serum total cholesterol and low-density lipoprotein-cholesterol (LDL-C) levels compared with the general population, while their CVD risk is increased

B. Corticosteroid use is associated with a dose-dependent and duration-dependent increased risk of CVD in RA, and recommendations advise their use should be kept to a minimum

C. Tocilizumab, an IL-6 inhibitor, increases serum lipids, including TC/HDL-C and triglycerides, and is associated with an increase in CVD.

D. In RA, tumour necrosis factor inhibitor (TNFi) use has been associated with a 30–50% reduction in CVD compared to non-users.

E. NSAID use in RA should be prescribed with caution, especially for patients with known CVD or CV risk factors.

2. A 52-year-old female with RA, who has never smoked and has no history of diabetes mellitus, presents to clinic enquiring about her latest lipid checks; total cholesterol 4.5 mmol/L, HDL-C 1.6mmol/L. She does no exercise, but eats at least five portions of fruit and vegetables a day. Her blood pressure is 159/87. Her RA disease activity score (DAS 28) is 2.5.

What would you do and advise?

A. Advise her to undertake more aerobic exercise but leave her treatments unchanged.

B. Calculate her 10-year CV risk score and multiply risk by 1.5, advise patient regarding lifestyle changes to improve CV risk profile, and commence pharmacotherapy for primary prevention if appropriate

C. Advise patient regarding lifestyle changes to improve CV risk profile. Calculate her 10-year CV risk score using the QRisk 3.0 calculator and commence pharmacotherapy for primary prevention if appropriate.

D. Commence a statin and advise patient regarding lifestyle changes to improve CV risk profile, and refer to rheumatologist for better RA control

E. Reassure patient of low CV risk and reassess in 5 years

3. A 45-year-old man with ankylosing spondylitis (AS) presents with increasing dyspnoea on exertion. He was diagnosed with AS 15 years ago and is managed on adalimumab (tumour necrosis factor inhibitor) and PRN naproxen (NSAID). He is an ex-smoker, and his recent total cholesterol was 4.5 mmol/L and HDL-C was 1.4 mmol/L. His blood pressure was 156/70 mmHg. Auscultation of his heart sounds reveals an early diastolic murmur, and his lungs were clear. A chest radiograph is normal. An ECG reveals occasional ventricular ectopics.

What is the most likely cause of his symptoms?

A. Ischaemic heart disease
B. Apical lung fibrosis
C. Aortic insufficiency
D. Conduction defect
E. Myocarditis

4. A 52-year-old female who has had a diagnosis of primary Sjogren's syndrome (pSS) for 10 years presents with persistent chest pain worse lying flat. She has a history of Raynaud's phenomenon for over 15 years along with xerostomia and xerophthalmia. She is a non-smoker with no history or diabetes mellitus, or dyslipidaemia. An examination is unremarkable except for an erythematous scaly skin lesion with evidence of follicular plugging on her right arm, with no chest wall tenderness and normal heart sounds. An ECG and chest radiograph are normal. Initial blood tests reveal a mild lymphopenia (0.9 $\times 10^9$/L), CRP 15mg/L, and she is strongly positive for anti-Ro(SS-A) and anti-Sm antibodies.

What is the most likely diagnosis?

A. Pericarditis secondary to pSS
B. Ischaemic heart disease
C. Costochondritis
D. Gastro-oesophageal reflux
E. Pericarditis secondary to systemic lupus erythematosus

5. A 45-year-old male non-smoker with a 5-year history of polymyositis (CpK 3200 at presentation) is referred by the respiratory team following investigation of exertional breathlessness on inclines and a dry cough. A high-resolution CT thorax has revealed evidence of basal non-specific interstitial pneumonia affecting approximately 15% of the lungs. Routine blood sample has revealed a CpK of 225 and a troponin T level of 40. The patient denies any history of recent anterior chest pain or palpitations. His only medications are prednisolone 5 mg daily and mycophenolate mofetil 1 g twice daily. The blood pressure is 135/80. The ECG and echocardiogram are normal. The most likely explanation for the raised troponin T level is:

A. Ischaemic heart disease related to accelerated atherosclerosis secondary to his polymyositis
B. Myocarditis
C. Expression of troponin T from regenerating skeletal muscle fibres
D. Cor pulmonale
E. Mycophenolate mofetil-induced cardiac myopathy

6. A 36-year-old lady presents with ST-elevation myocardial infarction (MI). She is an ex-smoker (5 pack per year history). There is no significant family history of ischaemic heart disease. She is married with two healthy children, one of whom was born at 33 weeks gestation following an episode of pre-eclampsia. There is no past medical history of venous or atrial thrombosis. Past medical history includes mild, well-controlled asthma for inhaled salbutamol on an as needed basis. Her migraines have been more problematic of late and she has been using her sumatriptan daily.

Which of the following tests might help elucidate a cause for her presentation?

A. Plasma homocysteine levels
B. Anticardiolipin antibodies and lupus anticoagulant
C. 13N-ammonia PET scanning to exclude sumatriptan-induced myocardial perfusion defects
D. Genetic studies for factor V Leiden heterozygosity
E. Protein C and protein S levels

7. A 25-year-old man presents with a 6-month history of skin thickening over his arms, legs, face, and trunk, with Raynaud's phenomenon and digital ulceration. He reports breathlessness on exertion, fatigue, and palpitations. He has never smoked and has no history of hypertension. His blood pressure is 144/75. A high resolution CT chest reveals widespread ground-glass change with some basal fibrotic change, consistent with pulmonary function tests (transfer factor 59%). An ECG is normal. An echocardiogram reveals a pulmonary artery systolic pressure of 24 mmgHg and mild diastolic dysfunction only. He is diagnosed with rapidly progressive diffuse cutaneous systemic sclerosis (dcSSc) and commenced on IV pulsed cyclophosphamide with methylprednisolone.

What would be the next most appropriate course of action?

A. Check troponin, CK and NTproBNP, perform stress-perfusion CMR and 24-hour ECG monitoring, considering an external (or implantable) loop recorder if normal
B. Check troponin, CK and NTproBNP, and perform 24-hour ECG monitoring, considering an external (or implantable) loop recorder if normal
C. Monitor closely, and repeat pulmonary function tests and HRCT chest after completion of IV cyclophosphamide course
D. Check troponin, CK and NTproBNP, and perform stress-perfusion CMR
E. Check troponin, CK, and NTproBNP, and perform an endomyocardial biopsy

8. A 64-year-old man with systemic sclerosis is found to have developed a cardiomyopathy.

Which of the following statements about SSc cardiomyopathy is incorrect?

A. Features associated with SSc-cardiomyopathy include male sex, anti-topoisomerase antibody positivity, rapid skin thickness progression, age of onset >65 year, and digital ulceration
B. IV cyclophosphamide has shown to be more effective in the treatment of SSc-cardiomyopathy over steroids and other oral disease modifying anti-rheumatic therapy (DMARDs)
C. β-Blockers are contraindicated in severe dcSSc
D. CMR studies frequently show late gadolinium enhancement sparing the subendocardium
E. Severe organ involvement in dcSSc most often occurs in the first three years of disease

9. A 29-year-old male is admitted with acute central chest pain. He reports a 2-month history of generalized malaise, unintentional weight loss, and low grade fever. He works as a kitchen fitter and has noticed increased aching in his left arm whilst at work, particularly when fitting units. He smokes approximately 20 cigarettes per day. His ECG has revealed ST elevation of the anterior leads and his troponin T level is 91. Blood tests at his surgery the previous week revealed a CRP of 87.

What is the most likely diagnosis?

A. Acute viral myocarditis
B. Kawasaki's arteritis
C. Subacute bacterial endocarditis
D. Buerger's disease
E. Takayasu's arteritis

10. A 22-year-old previously fit and well male presents to the emergency department complaining of worsening dyspnoea over the last 24 hours. He reports having felt unwell for the preceding 2 weeks with pharyngitis and fever. He has developed pain in his wrists and ankles, particularly when getting up in the morning. Clinical examination reveals evidence of mitral regurgitation and pulmonary oedema. The CRP is 138 with a neutrophil count of 13.1. His PR interval is prolonged but the ECG is otherwise normal.

Which test is most likely to help yield a diagnosis?

A. Genetic studies for Marfan's syndrome
B. HLA B27
C. Anti-streptolysin-O titre
D. Blood cultures for *Streptococcus viridans*
E. Troponin I to identify evidence of viral myocarditis

11. A 31-year-old female presents with intermittent palpitations. The echocardiogram has revealed evidence of mitral regurgitation and left atrial enlargement. She has recently been assessed by the rheumatologists for long-standing joint pain affecting her elbows, knees, and fingers that first became apparent as a teenager after she dislocated her patella. These symptoms have worsened in recent months since the birth of her daughter and have affected her ability to nurse her baby. The pregnancy proceeded without complication until the third trimester when she developed significant pain in her symphysis pubis.

What is the most likely diagnosis?

A. Ehlers–Danlos syndrome
B. Acute rheumatic fever
C. Subacute bacterial endocarditis
D. Marfan's syndrome
E. Systemic lupus erythematosus

12. A 32-year-old female non-smoker presents with acute anterior chest pain. Her ECG has revealed widespread anterior lead ST segment elevation. Her blood pressure is 152/95. She is currently 32/40 gestation in her third pregnancy. She has had two previous first trimester miscarriages. Her CRP is elevated at 48. The Hb is reduced at 96g/L with a lymphopenia (0.9). Her urine dip has revealed 2+ protein and 1+ blood. Systems review reveals a recent history of fever, inflammatory arthralgia, mouth ulceration and fatigue.

What is the most likely diagnosis?

A. Pre-eclampsia
B. Rheumatoid arthritis
C. Acute viral myocarditis
D. Acute myocardial infarction
E. Systemic lupus erythematosus

13. A 35-year-old woman is diagnosed with systemic lupus erythematosus (SLE). The woman is interested to know what factors might lead to cardiac problems associated with her SLE.

Which of the following factors is NOT associated with the potential development of cardiac manifestations in SLE?

A. Atherogenic lipid profile
B. Antimalarial therapy with hydroxychloroquine
C. Methotrexate therapy
D. Cumulative glucocorticoid exposure
E. Persistently elevated inflammatory response

14. A 56-year-old lady with a history of myelodysplasia presents with acute mitral valve regurgitation. On examination, she is noted to have marked erythema of her right ear. She has also noticed some recent hoarseness and joint pain. She has been feeling generally more under the weather of late and her CRP is noted to be elevated at 27. Her FBC is abnormal with a Hb 87, lymphopenia 0.6, and a platelet count of 110. Her white cell count differential is otherwise normal.

What is the most likely unifying diagnosis?

A. Subacute bacterial endocarditis
B. SLE complicated by Libman–Sacks Endocarditis
C. Ehlers–Danlos Syndrome
D. Relapsing polychondritis
E. Acute rheumatic fever

15. A 48-year-old man with a history of gout and psoriasis is newly diagnosed with ankylosing spondylitis.

What advice would be incorrect to give to the patient?

A. Patients with spondyloarthopathies are at increased risk of atherosclerotic heart disease
B. Patients with psoriasis demonstrate a greater prevalence of metabolic syndrome
C. HLA-B27 positivity has been associated with conduction defects in ankylosing spondylitis
D. Ankylosing spondylitis associated conduction defects can improve with NSAIDs
E. In patients with gout and hyperuricaemia, urate-lowering medication is advocated in the treatment of hypertension

chapter

9.5

THE PATIENT WITH RHEUMATIC DISORDERS

ANSWERS

1. C. Tocilizumab, an IL-6 receptor inhibitor, can cause increases in lipid levels. However, there is no evidence currently to suggest that the risk of future risk of CVD is increased, but perhaps the risk is actually reduced. Serum lipids levels tend to negatively correlate with systemic inflammation, therefore, in patients with active RA lipid levels may be low, although their CV risk remains higher than those without RA. In RA the TC/HDL-C ratio, rather than individual lipid components, is superior in the prediction of CVD risk. Corticosteroid use is associated with a dose-dependent and duration-dependent increased risk of CVD, even with addressing confounding by indication, and therefore EULAR recommendations advise minimizing corticosteroid use with frequent review to address the possibility of tapering the dose. Disease-modifying anti-rheumatic therapy (DMARDs, synthetic or biological) has been shown to reduce the risk of CVD, thought secondary to the reduction in disease activity and systemic inflammation. Methotrexate has been reported to reduce the risk by 20–30%, whereas TNFi use studies report a reduction by 30–50%. In 2015, a meta-analysis reported an increase in all CV events (relative risk 1.18) and strokes, but no increase of MI with the use of NSAIDs in RA; however, this included the use of rofecoxib (now withdrawn). Therefore, EULAR recommendations suggest using NSAIDs with caution, especially in those thought to be at higher risk of CVD.

2. C. Patient with RA are at increased risk of CVD and the 2016 EULAR (European League against Rheumatism) advised multiplying CV risk scores by 1.5 to reflect this. Earlier EULAR guidance had advised only doing this for those with certain RA-specific features (seropositivity, lengthy disease duration, and extra-articular features) but their new guidance in 2016 recognizes there is little evidence to support such an approach, with increased risk of CVD observed in early RA. The newer QRisk 3.0 calculator incorporates RA as a domain and this result can now be used to determine whether primary preventative treatment is required (without multiplying their risk scores by 1.5). It is not currently recommended that all patients with RA are given lipid-lowering therapy irrespective of their CV risk score, and a DAS28 of 2.5 indicates disease remission and adequate control of RA. Current recommendation is to reassess CV risk at least once every 5 years if CV risk is deemed low after full assessment.

3. C. The long disease duration of AS, wide pulse pressure, and auscultation findings suggest aortic insufficiency as the cause of his symptoms. Patients with AS are at greater risk of cardiovascular disease, but his 10-year CV score is fairly low at 6.5% making the presence of ischaemic heart disease less likely. Apical lung fibrosis occurs rarely in AS, and the normal chest examination and chest radiograph help exclude this. Histological studies demonstrate the fibrotic process involved in the pathogenesis of aortic regurgitation in AS can extend into the interventricular conduction system making conduction defects a common occurrence in AS. Therefore, 24-hour ECG monitoring should be considered in this patient, but the normal ECG helps exclude significant disease. Myocarditis is rare in AS, and less likely given the above examination findings. Cardiac magnetic resonance imaging can help exclude this.

4. E. The clinical features of discoid lupus, lymphopenia, and pericarditis, and positive immunology fulfil the American College of Rheumatology (ACR) criteria for systemic lupus erythematosus (SLE). Although pericardial effusions are commonly described in pSS, symptomatic pericarditis is less so. Therefore, other causes for pericarditis should be considered, and in this case SLE is more likely. There is no clear evidence to support an increase in ischaemic heart disease (IHD) in pSS, together with clinical history and the absence of traditional CV risk factors makes IHD unlikely. Chest pain associated with costochondritis would be reproducible by palpation of the costochondral joints on examination. Although dysphagia can be seen in pSS due to xerostomia, gastro-oesophageal reflux is not a common feature of the disease.

5. C. Regenerating skeletal muscle fibres can express and release troponin T in polymyositis. Troponin I is a more reliable biomarker of myocardial injury. Accelerated atherosclerosis polymyositis is not as well established as other autoimmune rheumatic diseases (e.g. rheumatoid arthritis and SLE) although the risk of myocardial infarction appear higher than the general population. The additional clinical features in this case are not suggestive of coronary artery disease. His ILD provides a reasonable explanation for his breathlessness and dry cough but is not sufficiently severe to cause cor pulmonale. Myocarditis can occur in polymyositis but his troponin is only modestly elevated and the normal echocardiogram is reassuring. There is no known association between mycophenolate mofetil and cardiomyopathy.

6. B. Acute MI in young patients without traditional cardiovascular risk factors should prompt further assessment to exclude a pro-coaguable state. There are a number of features of antiphospholipid syndrome (APS) including her history of pre-term delivery following pre-eclampsia (occurs in 10–15% of patients with APS) and history of poorly controlled migraine (20% of patients with APS). Homocysteinuria can result in accelerated atherosclerosis and thrombotic events but typically presents at a younger age with musculoskeletal or CNS complications. Sumatriptan can promote coronary vasospasm in people with angina but would not usually result in acute MI. Factor V Leiden studies and protein C and S deficiency should be undertaken in all young patients presenting with acute MI but the clinical features and past medical history make APS the more likely diagnosis in this instance.

7. A. In the context of rapidly progressive dcSSc disease, particularly in someone who complains of cardiac symptoms (shortness of breath and palpitations) or with abnormalities on echocardiogram, the possibility of SSc-cardiomyopathy should be considered. Serum markers such as troponin, CK, and NTproBNP may be raised; however, the gold standard to assess for systemic sclerosis (SSc)-cardiomyopathy is CMR providing information not only on cardiac function, but also myocardial inflammation, fibrosis and perfusion. Arrhythmias are frequently described in SSc, particularly in those with poor prognostic features for SSc, such as the diffuse subtype, and are associated with sudden death. Routine electrophysiology tests such as ECG and 24-hour ECG monitoring may be normal, and longer studies should be considered, including the possible use of an implantable loop recorder. There is limited evidence to support the need for endomyocardial biopsy, but if still required after non-invasive testing and multi-disciplinary assessment this may be considered. It is standard practise to repeat pulmonary function tests and HRCT after completion of pulsed cyclophosphamide to assess response; however, in this scenario, the presence of SSc-cardiomyopathy should be excluded in the meantime.

8. B. There is no robust evidence for the treatment of SSc-cardiomyopathy with immunosuppression. It is accepted that the general poor prognostic markers for SSc are also associated with SSc-cardiomyopathy. Beta-blockers may exacerbate Raynaud's phenomenon but are not contraindicated.

Focal fibrosis on CMR (as measured by late gadolinium enhancement) is frequently seen to spare the subendocardium suggesting alternative pathology to atherosclerosis. In dcSSc, it is recognized that severe organ involvement occurs in early stages of disease.

9. E. Takayasu's arteritis (TAK) is the most likely diagnosis given the patient demographics and clinical history. TAK is a large vessel autoimmune vasculitis that typically presents in the third decade. Acute myocardial ischaemia can follow aortic aneurysmal dilation occluding the coronary ostia, focal coronary arteritis, or coronary aneurysm formation. The recent symptoms in his left arm are consistent with limb claudication and may represent subclavian stenosis. Kawasaki's arteritis is a medium-sized vessel vasculitis that can affect the coronary arteries but typically presents in childhood and should not result in limb ischaemia. Buerger's disease would be unusual at this age and should not be associated with constitutional symptoms of ill health. Subacute bacterial endocarditis and acute viral myocarditis can present with constitutional symptoms of ill health but do not usually present with an acute ischaemic event.

10. C. Acute rheumatic fever (ARF) typically presents with arthritis, carditis, and cutaneous changes (such as nodules or erythema nodosum). It usually follows Group A streptococcal pharyngitis and the anti-streptolysin-O titre is typically elevated during the acute phase of the illness. ECG changes include a prolonged PR interval (which forms part of disease classification criteria). Valvulitis is common in ARF and usually affects the mitral valve. Cardiac failure can occur secondary to acute valve disease or primary myocardial involvement. Viral myocarditis would not be expected to result in valve disease. Subacute bacterial endocarditis should be excluded but would not be the most likely diagnosis given the clinical picture and demographics. Regurgitant valve disease can be a late feature of ankylosing spondylitis (often HLA B27 positive) and collagen vascular disorders (such as Marfan's) but the clinical picture is not suggestive of these diagnoses.

11. A. Ehlers–Danlos syndrome (EDS) is a collagen vascular disease associated caused by abnormalities in collagen structure and function within the connective tissues. Exertional arthralgia secondary to joint hypermobility can occur. Skin laxity can occur in some forms. Valve disease often affects the mitral valve, sometimes requiring valve replacement. No features are presented to raise concerns regarding infective endocarditis, acute rheumatic fever, SLE, or Marfan's (although all can be associated with mitral valve disease).

12. E. The most likely diagnosis is systemic lupus erythematosus (SLE) complicated by acute pericarditis. Pregnancy can be associated with the new presentation or disease flares of pre-existing SLE. The prodromal symptoms are suggestive of SLE. The history of recurrent first trimester miscarriage might indicate the presence of secondary anti-phospholipid syndrome. Pericarditis can occur in rheumatoid arthritis, although this usually improves during pregnancy. Acute viral myocarditis would not explain the urinary sediment. Pre-eclampsia can present with elevated BP and urinary sediment but would not normally be associated with clinical and ECG evidence of cardiac disease.

13. C. Methotrexate is not associated with cardiac manifestations of SLE. The atherogenic lipid profile, persistently elevated inflammatory response and cumulative glucocorticoid exposure have all been implicated in the development of accelerated atherosclerosis in SLE. Anti-malarial therapies such as hydroxychloroquine (HCQ) are often used in the management of SLE. HCQ has beneficial effects on the pro-atherogenic lipid profile but can occasionally result in the development of HCQ-induced cardiomyopathy.

14. D. Each of the options can be associated with regurgitant mitral valves. Her age would make acute rheumatic fever unlikely. Both her age and inflammatory response would make Ehlers–Danlos unlikely. Whilst SBE and SLE complicated by Libman–Sacks endocarditis would need to be excluded, the history of erythema of the ear and myelodysplasia makes relapsing polychondritis the most likely unifying diagnosis.

15. E. Although hyperuricaemia has been associated with hypertension and cardiovascular disease (CVD), there is no clear evidence to support the routine use of urate-lowering medication in the treatment of hypertension or CVD.

chapter
10

GENETICS AND CLINICAL PHARMACOLOGY

chapter

10.1

GENETICS

QUESTIONS

1. **You are reviewing an 18-year-old male in outpatients who has recently been diagnosed with hypertrophic cardiomyopathy (HCM) and fitted with a defibrillator. He is asking about family screening as his older sister is a professional athlete.**

   Which of the following is the most appropriate genetic test?

   A. Whole genome sequencing
   B. Whole exome sequencing
   C. Gene panel testing
   D. Sanger sequencing
   E. Array CGH (comparative genomic hybridisation)

2. **A 19-year-old male has Duchenne muscular dystrophy (DMD). His two younger brothers are both affected. His parents are both fit and well, as are his grandparents and the extended family.**

   What is the most likely mode of inheritance?

   A. Autosomal dominant
   B. Autosomal recessive
   C. De novo
   D. X-linked dominant
   E. X-linked recessive

3. **A 33-year-old male has recently had genetic testing which shows he has a pathogenic variant causative of arrhythmogenic right ventricular cardiomyopathy (ARVC). His sister was diagnosed 6 months earlier with ARVC after collapsing whilst playing sport at university, precipitating familial testing of her five siblings. He is very anxious about developing the condition as severely as his sister. You explain that despite having the same variant, family members often display a different clinical course. Specifically, in ARVC, relatives detected on family screening are often more mildly affected.**

   This is an example of which of the following?

   A. Heteroplasmy
   B. Variable expression
   C. Mosaicism
   D. Genetic heterogeneity
   E. Reduced penetrance

4. **A 33-year-old female presents with sudden loss of consciousness to the Emergency Department. Her ECG shows first degree atrioventricular (AV) block and she is seen to have short runs of ventricular tachycardia (VT) in the emergency department so is transferred to the coronary care unit. Her full blood count, electrolytes, and troponin are normal. Overnight telemetry shows further VT. An echocardiogram the next day shows a mildly dilated left ventricle (LV) and mild global LV systolic impairment. A CT coronary angiogram reveals normal coronaries and cardiac MRI shows no features of myocarditis or ischaemia. On further questioning, it appears that her father and paternal uncle both died in their 30s of suspected heart attacks.**

   Given the likely diagnosis of familial dilated cardiomyopathy (DCM) in this patient, which of the following genes is the most likely cause?

   A. *LMNA*
   B. *TTN*
   C. *MYH7*
   D. *TNNT2*
   E. *DSP*

5. **Which of the following are NOT diagnostic of Fabry disease (FD)?**

   A. A pathogenic variant in the *GLA* gene
   B. Interventricular septal diameter >1.6 cm
   C. Low alpha galactosidase levels in male patients
   D. Increased plasma lysosomal Gb3
   E. A family member with a definite FD diagnosis

6) Which of the following regarding HCM is FALSE?

A. A genetic cause is found in around 60%
B. Variants that code for the sarcomere tend to have earlier disease onset and a higher risk of sudden cardiac death
C. 15% of families have two sarcomeric variants, resulting in a more severe phenotype
D. Can be associated with Pompe disease and Noonan syndrome
E. *PRKAG2* variants are additionally associated with Wolf–Parkinson–White syndrome

7. Which of the following genetic disorders do NOT cause a restrictive cardiomyopathy?

A. Haemochromatosis
B. Pseudoxanthoma elasticum
C. Hereditary TTR amyloid
D. Gaucher disease
E. William's syndrome

8) A 19-year-old female originally from Greece presents with palpitations and an episode of pre-syncope. On examination she has woolly hair and thickened skin on the palms of her hands and soles of her feet. The ECG shows T-wave inversion in leads V1-V4. Echocardiography shows a dilated right ventricle (RV) with impaired RV function.

Which of the following is FALSE regarding this condition?

A. It is autosomal dominant
B. It is caused by a variant in plakoglobin
C. Sudden death occurs due to VT originating in the right ventricle
D. Inferior T-wave inversion suggests LV involvement
E. Penetrance is in the region of 90%

9. A 45-year-old female is resuscitated after a cardiac arrest at home. On admission to hospital her ECG shows a QTc of 520ms and there are runs of torsades de pointes on the cardiac monitor. She does not take any regular medication.

What is the likelihood that her daughter is also affected?

A. 1 in 2
B. 1 in 4
C. 1 in 8
D. 1 in 10
E. Zero

10. Which of the following statements regarding long QT syndrome (LQTS) is FALSE?

A. Arrhythmic events in long QT 1 are often triggered by exercise
B. Arrhythmic events in long QT 2 are often triggered by sounds, such as alarm clocks
C. Variants in genes coding for sodium channels account for the majority of LQTS cases
D. Patients with Anderson–Tawil syndrome may have a prominent U wave
E. A negative genetic test for LQTS does not exclude the diagnosis

11. A 37-year-old male was suffering from an upper respiratory tract infection and was noticed to have agonal breathing whilst asleep, consistent with cardiac arrest. He had successful bystander CPR and was transferred to hospital. On arrival, the ECG showed sinus rhythm with coved ST elevation in V2 and V3 followed by T-wave inversion. The remainder of the ECG was normal. He was pyrexial at 38.9°C with a CRP of 96 mg/L.

Which of the following is NOT a risk factor for SCD in this condition?

A. Atrial fibrillation
B. Sinus node disease
C. Spontaneous type 1 ECG pattern of coved ST elevation followed by T-wave inversion
D. Family history of SCD
E. LV systolic dysfunction

12. Which of the following arrhythmias are least commonly encountered in patients with Brugada Syndrome?

A. Atrial fibrillation
B. SVT
C. AV block
D. VT
E. Sinus node disease

13. A 16-year-old boy complains of palpitations whilst running in a cross-country race. He collapses and an ambulance is called. An ECG performed pre-hospital showed bi-directional VT. His resting ECG is normal. His echocardiogram and cardiac MRI are also normal.

A variant in which of the following genes is most likely to be the cause?

A. *RYR2*
B. *CASQ2*
C. *CALM1*
D. *TRDN*
E. *KCNQ1*

14. Which of the following conditions are NOT caused by variants in the fibrillin (*FBN1*) gene?

A. Marfan syndrome
B. MASS syndrome (**M**itral valve prolapse, **A**ortic root dilatation, **S**kin striae, **S**keletal features)
C. Familial mitral valve prolapse
D. Loeys–Dietz Syndrome
E. Familial ectopia lentis

15. Which of the following is NOT true of Loeys–Dietz syndrome?

A. There is a risk of uterine rupture in pregnancy
B. There may be widespread aneurysmal disease which may be best detected using magnetic resonance angiography
C. The risk of aortic dissection is lower than in Marfan syndrome
D. Patients may share similar facial and musculoskeletal appearances to Marfan syndrome
E. Loeys–Dietz syndrome patients may have associated atrial septal defects (ASD)

16. You are asked to a review a 20-year-old female in the Emergency Department who has presented with interscapular and abdominal pain. On examination, you note a small lower jaw, a narrow nose, quite prominent eyes, and her skin is slightly translucent such that her veins are highly visible on her chest wall. The CT scan confirms aortic dissection.

In which gene is the causative variant likely to be?

A. *FBN1*
B. *COL3A1*
C. *SMAD2*
D. *TGFBR1*
E. *TGFBR2*

17. A 26-year-old female presents with exertional breathlessness and chest pain to the Emergency Department. There are signs of right heart strain on the ECG and so a CT pulmonary angiogram is requested which shows no pulmonary emboli but there is a suggestion of an enlarged right ventricle and pulmonary trunk. Echocardiography confirms pulmonary hypertension and the remainder of her investigations show no secondary cause.

Which of the following is TRUE of this condition?

A. When inherited, it is a highly penetrant condition
B. Men are more often affected than women
C. Individuals with a *BMPR2* variant are more likely to benefit from calcium channel blockers
D. The inherited form can be easily clinically distinguished from acquired causes
E. 75% are due to *BMPR2* variants

18. A 39-year-old male presents with an acute coronary syndrome. His total cholesterol is 10.9 mmol/L and it is noted that his father also had a heart attack around age 40. You notice papules on the dorsal aspect of his hands and yellow raised papules around his eyes.

Which of the following is TRUE regarding this condition?

A. Most patients do not have a family history
B. *PCSK9* variants are the most common cause
C. Homozygous patients have a milder phenotype
D. Cholesterol testing should only commence in adulthood for genetically confirmed family members
E. It is the most common inherited cause of premature cardiovascular disease

19. Which of the following is NOT associated with cardiac tumours?

A. Tuberous sclerosis
B. Von Hippel Lindau syndrome
C. Gorlin syndrome
D. Carney complex
E. LAMB syndrome

20. Which of the following is NOT true of Di George syndrome?

A. Caused by a 22q11.2 microdeletion
B. Deletion of *TBX1* is largely responsible for the cardiac manifestations
C. Gene panel testing is the most appropriate test
D. Hypocalcaemia is a feature
E. Patients can have a cleft palate

chapter 10.1 GENETICS

ANSWERS

1. C. A group of genes known to cause HCM are tested for using a gene panel. Sanger sequencing is a reliable way of testing for a single known variant in a specific gene, such as if we were to subsequently test his sister for a variant detected in him. Genome and exome sequencing are used in the search for variants after negative panel testing, or in research.

2. E. DMD is inherited in an X-linked recessive fashion. One in three cases are due to a de novo variant, the rest being inherited from a carrier mother. In this case, the children will have received the dystrophin variant from the mother's X chromosome, with their Y chromosome coming from the father. The mother has two X chromosomes and hence is usually unaffected in an X-linked recessive condition. Sometimes, female carriers of dystrophin variants can develop a mild form of cardiomyopathy and should therefore have regular clinical screening with echocardiography.

3. B. Variable expression refers to the different clinical course that occurs within individuals in a family carrying the same variant. Reduced penetrance is where some relatives who carry a pathogenic variant may be only mildly affected or sometimes display no clinical features. Mosaicism is where the variant arises after several cell divisions in the fertilized egg so not all cells in the body are affected. Genetic heterogeneity is where the same phenotype can be caused by different variants in different genes or by different genetic mechanisms. For example, dilated cardiomyopathy may be caused by many a variant in *TTN* or *RBM20* (amongst others) but the clinical features may look extremely similar. Heteroplasmy is where mitochondrial genomes amongst different cells within the same individual have different DNA, hence the severity of mitochondrial disease can be variable.

4. A. *LMNA* is the most likely causative gene in this case. It classically presents with AV block (first, second and third) at a young age and left ventricular impairment. Ventricular arrhythmias can occur when LV impairment is only mild. LV impairment and conduction disease are both markers of increased risk of ventricular arrhythmias and should inform decision making about an ICD. It is autosomal dominant which is consistent with her family history of three affected relatives over two generations. *TTN*, *MYH7*, and *TNNT2* all cause DCM, but it would be unusual to have this degree of VT with relatively mild LVSD and AV block is not a common feature. Variants in Filamin C, Phospholamban and Desmin all produce DCM with a high risk of ventricular arrhythmias. DSP causes ARVC and some cases of ALVC but AV block is much more suggestive of *LMNA*.

5. B. Fabry disease accounts for around 1% of unexplained LVH but septal hypertrophy on its own is not diagnostic.

6. C. Only 5% of families have two sarcomeric variants, but they do often have a more severe phenotype, with earlier onset and a higher risk of adverse cardiac events, heart failure symptoms, and need for cardiac transplantation.

7. E. Patients with William's syndrome commonly have supra-valvular aortic stenosis due to a deletion on chromosome 7 which contains the elastin (*ELN*) gene.

8. A. Naxos disease is an autosomal recessive form of ARVC, found specifically in Greek islanders, originally described in Naxos as the name suggests. A similar presentation is seen in Indian and Ecuadorian families and is known as Carjaval syndrome, in which LVSD often predominates.

9. A. Long QT syndrome (LQTS) is most commonly autosomal dominant. Seventy percent of families with LQTS have a genetic variant identified. Jervell–Lange–Nielsen syndrome is an autosomal recessive condition characterized by LQTS and congenital sensorineural deafness, caused by heterozygous variants in *KCNQ1*.

10. C. Long QT 1 and 2 are caused by variants in potassium channels (*KCNQ1* and *KCNH2*) and make up 40–45% of LQT syndrome. LQT3 is cause by gain-of-function variants in the *SCN5A* gene (loss-of-function variants in SCN5A cause Brugada syndrome).

11. E. This is a typical presentation of Brugada syndrome (BrS), in this case the malignant ventricular arrhythmia (VA) is likely to have been precipitated by a febrile illness. All of these are risk factors for SCD in BrS except LV systolic dysfunction. SCD in BrS typically occurs at night, during sleep. The average age of VF presentation is 41 +/- 15 years. Malignant VA occurs in 13.5% of patients per year in those with a previous cardiac arrest, 3.2% in patients with previous syncope, and 1% in asymptomatic patients.

12. B. SVT is not classically associated with Brugada syndrome. AF and sinus node disease are common and are associated with an increased risk of SCD. Progressive cardiac conduction disease (Lev–Lenègre syndrome) presenting as AV block leading to syncope or SCD is not uncommon in Brugada families.

13. A. A to D are all associated with CPVT, which is the most likely diagnosis. The variant is most likely to be found in the *RYR2* gene as *RYR2* variants cause CPVT in 60% of cases. Variants in the *CASQ2* gene (which regulates the *RYR2* receptor) are autosomal recessive but cause a more severe phenotype and make up about 5% of positive tests. Variants in *CALM1* and *TRDN* are extremely rare causes of CPVT. *KCNQ1* causes long QT type 1, where polymorphic VT is typically triggered by exercise, swimming, or emotion.

14. D. Loeys–Dietz syndrome (LDS) is caused by a pathogenic variant in any of six LDS genes (*SMAD2*, *SMAD3*, *TGFB2*, *TGFB3*, *TGFBR1*, *TGFBR2*), although there may be phenotypic similarities with Marfan syndrome. It is inherited in an autosomal fashion, although 75% of LDS patients have a de novo variant. The other conditions listed all may be caused by variants in *FBN1*.

15. C. In LDS, aortic dissection tends to occur at a younger age and at smaller aortic dimensions than Marfan syndrome.

16. B. The history and examination findings are suggestive of vascular Ehlers–Danlos syndrome (vEDS), caused by variants in *COL3A*1. vEDS is autosomal dominant and has almost 100% penetrance. *FBN1* is the cause of Marfan syndrome as well as isolated heritable thoracic aortic aneurysm and dissection (TAAD) syndrome. Variants in *SMAD*2, *TGFBR1*, and TGFBR2 may cause Loeys–Dietz syndrome or heritable TAAD.

17. E. Penetrance is low with 40% in females and 10% in men. Although it is autosomal dominant, the low penetrance means that far fewer than 50% of offspring ever develop clinical features. Women are more likely to develop clinical features than men. Those with *BMPR2* variants are less likely to respond to calcium channel blockers. The genetic and acquired causes present in an identical fashion and thus cannot be distinguished from each other clinically, other than by finding a secondary cause.

18. E. De novo variants are uncommon and familial hypercholesterolaemia (FH) is autosomal dominant, so most patients have a family history. In most cases it is due to a variant in the LDL receptor gene (*LDLR*) which tends to have a more severe phenotype than when caused by pathogenic variants in other genes including *APOB* and *PCSK9*. Homozygotes typically need coronary artery bypass surgery before adulthood, and some develop severe aortic stenosis. Cholesterol testing in genetically confirmed family members is recommended over age 10.

19. B. Tuberous sclerosis is caused by variants in the tumour suppressor genes tuberous sclerosis complex 1 (*TSC1*/hamartin) and tuberous sclerosis complex 2 (*TSC2*/tuberin). As a result, hamartomas form in multiple organ systems including rhabdomyomas in the heart in up to half of tuberous sclerosis patients. More than one cardiac rhabdomyoma is diagnostic of tuberous sclerosis. Cardiac fibromas occur in a small minority (5%) of patients with Gorlin syndrome, although much more commonly than in the general population. Carney complex is characterized by atrial myxomas as well as non-cardiac tumours. Lentigines, Atrial myxoma, Mucocutaneous myxomas Blue naevi (LAMB) is a rare myxoma syndrome. Von Hippel Lindau Syndrome is caused by variants in the *VHL* gene (another tumour suppressor) where young adults present with both malignant and non-malignant tumours. Haemangioblastomas are a typical finding and, whilst themselves benign, may occur in the brain or spinal cord. Pancreatic neuroendocrine tumours, renal cell carcinoma, and phaemochromocytoma are also common.

20. C. Gene panel testing would not be the most appropriate test for a microdeletion. Chromosomal microarray would be more appropriate but fluorescent in-situ hybridization (FISH) could also be used. Most 22q11.2 microdeletion patients have cardiac malformations including tetralogy of Fallot, interrupted aortic arch, VSDs, truncus arteriosus, vascular ring, ASDs, hypoplastic left heart, or other left ventricular outflow abnormalities.

chapter 10.2

CLINICAL PHARMACOLOGY

QUESTIONS

1. **You are considering various medication options for a patient. The pharmacokinetic factors describing the passage of the drug and its metabolites through the body can be summarized as:**

A. Administration, doseage, metabolites, excretion
B. Absorption, distribution, metabolism, excretion
C. Absorption, bioavailability, doseage, excretion
D. Ingestion, digestion, action, egestion
E. Absorption, doseage, metabolism, excretion

2. **You are considering anti-arrhythmic drug therapy for a patient with Brugada syndrome.**

Which of the following statements is true?

A. Long-term use of class I anti-arrhythmics is helpful as it both reduces risk of arrhythmia and confirms the diagnosis of Brugada syndrome
B. Any anti-arrhythmic medications are safe and should be used to reduce risk of dangerous arrhythmia
C. Brugada syndrome is a mutation of K^+ channels and therefore Class III anti-arrhythmics should be avoided
D. The commonest forms of Brugada syndrome involve dysfunction of Na^+ channels and therefore class I anti-arrhythmics should be avoided
E. Drug therapy should be avoided altogether in favour of ICD implantation

3. **You are picking an anti-arrhythmic drug to treat a 70-year-old woman who has developed symptomatic palpitations after a myocardial infarction who has moderate left ventricular systolic dyscfunction (ejection fraction estimated at 40–45%). Rhythm analysis has showed these to be occasional ventricular ectopics.**

What anti-arrhythmic medication would you offer?

A. Flecainide
B. Verapamil
C. Bisoprolol
D. Amiodarone
E. Atenolol

4. You are treating a 28-year-old female athlete with paroxysmal atrial fibrillation (AF) with a 'pill in the pocket' strategy using as required flecainide.

With regards to administration advice, which of the following is true?

A. She should double the dose every 2 hours until the arrhythmia subsides
B. She should try vagal manoeuvres before taking the flecainide
C. She should always co-administer a dose of bisoprolol before taking the flecainide
D. She should take an anticoagulant tablet during the episodes of AF
E. A rhythm control strategy will assure better long term outcomes

5. The cardiac devices team email you about an active patient with a dual chamber pacemaker for AV block who is having symptomatic episodes of paroxysmal AF. Regarding digoxin:

A. It's likely to provide significant symptomatic relief as part of a rhythm control strategy
B. Its positive inotropic effect will prevent the patient from developing pacing-mediated cardiomyopathy
C. It's a poor choice as not only will blocking the AV node have little effect, but the shortening of atrial refractory period may make AF episodes more likely
D. Digoxin use is safe in the presence of electrolyte abnormalities such as hypokalaemia
E. The 'DIG' trials showed long-term use of digoxin reduces mortality

6. A 77-year-old's patient has a remote download from their ICD demonstrating prolonged episodes of atrial fibrillation. They have a CHA_2DS_2VASc score of 3 but no active bleeding. A valid reason not to anticoagulate would be:

A. The patient is already taking dual antiplatelet therapy for a recent PCI
B. A significantly raised HASBLED score
C. There are important bleeding risk factors which cannot be modified
D. The patient has a history of dementia and falls
E. A homeopathic alternative is available

7. In patients requiring triple therapy following PCI who have co-existent atrial fibrillation, in general:

A. The default strategy is a tapering of therapy with cessation of aspirin after 1 week, clopidogrel after 12 months, and lifelong anticoagulant monotherapy
B. The ESC guidelines suggest ticagrelor is a safe alternative to clopidogrel in the context of triple therapy
C. If there is ongoing angina then aspirin should be used on an as required basis
D. Warfarin is preferred to non-vitamin K oral anticoagulant (NOAC) therapy
E. The bleeding risk should not alter the duration of combined antiplatelet and anticoagulant treatment

8. A patient with a previous intracranial haemorrhage is admitted with a STEMI. There is no evidence of current bleeding. On the way to the catheter lab, you decide to load the patient with:

A. Aspirin and ticagrelor
B. Aspirin
C. Aspirin and prasugrel
D. Nothing for now
E. Aspirin and clopidogrel

9. You are on-call overnight in a district general hospital looking after a patient with NSTEMI. They are awaiting angiography in the morning and have a markedly raised troponin.

Regarding the use of glycoprotein IIb/IIIa inhibitors, which of the following is true?

A. They can be used in patients with a high bleeding risk as the half-life is short
B. They can be used as a temporising measure to avoid the need for emergent PCI
C. They should be used routinely in NSTEMI/STEMI if thrombotic risk is high
D. They can be used in high-risk PCI alongside dual antiplatelet therapy
E. If bleeding risk is high, the oral form should be used

10. You are asked to provide an opinion as to whether the medical team should thrombolyse a patient with a new diagnosis of pulmonary embolism.

Which of the following statements is true?

A. Evidence of right ventricular strain on echocardiography indicates the patient will have a better outcome with thrombolysis
B. In a normotensive patient with hypoxia and tachycardia, the benefits of thrombolysis outweigh the bleeding risk
C. Thrombolysis should be co-administered with low-molecular weight heparin (LMWH) or a direct oral anti-coagulant (DOAC)
D. Current evidence only supports overall benefit from thrombolysis in patients with refractory hypotension
E. Features of right ventricular strain cannot be diagnosed on cross-sectional CT scanning

11. You are initiating pharmacological therapy for a patient with a new diagnosis of heart failure with reduced ejection fraction (HFrEF). Which of the following medications has NOT been shown to improve prognosis?

A. Angiotensin receptor neprilysin inhibitors (ARNIs)
B. ACE inhibitors
C. Mineralocorticoid receptor antagonists
D. Digoxin
E. Beta-blockers

12. You receive a telephone referral from a General Practitioner regarding a 82-year-old female patient with heart failure. The enquiry is whether to start sacubitril-valsartan therapy.

Regarding sacubitril-valsartan, which of the following statements is NOT correct?

A. Sacubitril-valsartan has been shown to improve morbidity and mortality in HFrEF patients
B. If the patients has been taking an ACE-inhibitor, a washout period should be observed between treatments
C. It can be used, at a lower dose, in patients with an eGFR <30 ml/min
D. There is established evidence of significant benefit in those with heart failure with preserved ejection fraction (HFpEF)
E. Sacubitril-valsartan should be used in patients with HFrEF who remain symptomatic of heart failure despite a period of optimal medical therapy

13. You review a 43-year-old Ghanaian man with hypertension in the general cardiology clinic.

Which of the following statements is NOT correct?

A. Secondary causes of hypertension should be excluded
B. UK NICE guidelines suggest dihydropyridine calcium channel blockers should be considered as first-line therapy
C. ACE-inhibitors should be started as first-line therapy if he is <55 years old
D. Early use of combination drug therapy is recommended by ESC guidelines
E. Early aggressive management of hypertension in young patients is associated with improved long-term outcomes

14. An 83-year-old gentleman with heart failure was admitted to hospital 5 days ago with an acute decompensation. After 3 days of successful diuresis, he is switched to oral furosemide 40 mg bd. His weight begins to rise and his renal function deteriorates.

Which of the following statements is true?

A. The impaired renal function is likely secondary to dehydration and furosemide should be stopped
B. Oral and intravenous furosemide are equally likely to provide effective diuresis in the presence of gut oedema
C. Studies suggest that ongoing congestion, but not worsening renal function, is associated with worse outcomes in acute heart failure
D. Lower doses of furosemide are associated with improved outcomes overall
E. The diagnosis is likely incorrect and he should undergo a CT pulmonary angiogram imaging

15. A 28-year-old woman with an acute myocarditis is in cardiogenic shock secondary to heart failure, with a significant acute kidney injury.

Which cardiac inotrope is most appropriate first-line therapy?

A. Adrenaline
B. Dobutamine
C. Noradrenaline
D. Milrinone
E. Digoxin

16. A 51-year-old woman is taking atorvastatin 80 mg od following a recent STEMI and PCI. She reports uncomfortable muscle aches and is keen to stop taking the medication.

What course of action do you suggest?

A. Stopping the statin and substituting for ezetimibe
B. Stopping the statin and trying aggressive dietary measures to lower cholesterol
C. Reducing the dose by half and assessing response
D. Measure creatine kinase (CK) and act based on results
E. No action

17. A 47-year-old male patient in the general cardiology clinic has a random total cholesterol of 11 mmol/L.

Which of the following is true regarding PCSK9 inhibitor therapy?

A. It is not indicated in primary hypercholesterolaemia for patients who have not responded to first-line therapies (i.e. high-intensity statins and combination medications)
B. It is not administered subcutaneously
C. It is not indicated in established cardiovascular disease without adequate lipid control despite use of first-line therapies
D. It is not considered safe in pregnancy to reduce risk of cardiovascular events
E. Side effects do not include arthralgia, injection-site reactions, and back pain

18. You are seeing a 63-year-old male patient with stable angina in the chest pain clinic. They have arrived with a list of questions.

Which of the following statements regarding anti-anginal therapy is correct?

A. Anti-anginal therapy provides prognostic rather than symptomatic benefit
B. Developing a tolerance to the effects of nitrates over time is not a recognized issue
C. Potential side effects of nicorandil therapy does not include skin or gastrointestinal ulceration and can be used in those with diverticular disease
D. Ivabradine is not an effective treatment for those with atrial fibrillation and angina
E. Ranolazine has no potential to cause QT prolongation

19. Ivabradine is indicated in which of the following patient groups?

A. A young man admitted with acute decomensated heart failure
B. A gentleman with long-standing stable heart failure with reduced ejection fraction
C. An elderly lady with angina and atrial fibrillation
D. An elderly gentleman on anti-dementia medication intermittently affected by sinus node disease and hypotension
E. A young man with liver failure

20. You have been asked by the medical team to review a 32-year-old female patient with congenital long QT syndrome who has been admitted with a Colles' fracture after a fall. She is having occasional ventricular ectopics on cardiac telemetry. The medical team are querying whether to start anti-arrhythmic therapy.

Which of the following anti-arrhythmics is most appropriate to reduce her ectopic burden?

A. Intravenous amiodarone
B. Oral amiodarone loading followed by regular oral amiodarone
C. Sotalol
D. Flecainide
E. Bisoprolol

chapter 10.2

CLINICAL PHARMACOLOGY

ANSWERS

1. B. ADME refers to absorption (how the drug enters the body), distribution (how the drug moves between compartments), metabolism (how the drug is changed to a different molecule), and excretion (how the drug is removed from the body).

2. D. The commonest genetics variants of Brugada syndrome involve dysfunction of Na^+ channels responsible for the rapid upstroke of the cardiac action potential. Class I anti-arrhythmics can further exacerbate this dysfunction. Indeed, ajmaline and flecainide can be used as part of provocation testing to demonstrate a type 1 Brugada ECG pattern. With regards to ICD implantation for patients with Brugada Syndrome, the 2015 ESC guidelines for Ventricular Arrhythmias and the Prevention of Sudden Cardiac Death recommend:

- ICD is implanted in patients with a diagnosis of Brugada syndrome who (a) are survivors of an aborted cardiac arrest and/or (b) have documented spontaneous sustained VT (*IA*)
- ICD should be considered in patients with a spontaneous diagnostic type I ECG pattern and history of syncope (*IIA*)
- ICD may be considered in patients with a diagnosis of Brugada syndrome who develop VF during EP study with two or three extrastimuli at two sites (*IIB*)

3. C. It's likely that bisoprolol would provide the most favourable safety profile here. Flecainide is contraindicated in patients with coronary artery disease or heart failure (in light of the CAST trial). Verapamil is negatively inotropic and can worsen heart failure. Amiodarone is associated with significant adverse effects and so would need a strong indication of benefit from treatment; atenolol is less cardio-specific than bisoprolol.

4. C. It's important that an AV-node blocking drug such as bisoprolol is co-administered with flecainide. This reduces the likelihood of 1:1 atrioventricular (AV) conduction in the event of a macro-reentrant atrial tachycardia such as atrial flutter, and the resulting dangerous ventricular tachycardia. Vagal manoeuvres will not provide adequate sustained AV-nodal slowing. Use of anti-coagulants should be guided by thromboembolic risk scores, such as CHA_2DS_2VASc or electrical cardioversion. Rhythm control, while potentially improving symptoms, has not been shown in any trial to improve outcomes, such as morbidity or mortality, over a rate-control approach. Early studies, such as AFFIRM and RACE-II, actually suggested significant adverse effects associated with rhythm control medication (such as flecainide, sotalol, and amiodarone) and that aiming for an average heart rate in AF of 110,bpm is the 'sweet spot' of minimizing tachycardia-mediated cardiomyopathy versus adverse drug events.

5. C. Digoxin is a negative dromotrope, slowing conduction at the AV node, and thus likely to have little effect in this case. Due to effects on the atrial effective refractory periods (ERP), it may actually promote formation of AF and increase the likelihood of episodes occurring. All other answers are incorrect.

6. C. Although useful to quantify bleeding risk, the HASBLED risk score shares many common points with CHA_2DS_2-VASc. ESC guidelines for the management of atrial fibrillation suggests a shift towards using this to address and correct reversible risk factors to allow safe anticoagulant therapy. A history of falls is not an independent predictor of bleeding on oral anticoagulation (a modelling study estimated that a patient would need to fall 295 times per year for the benefits of ischaemic stroke reduction with oral anticoagulation to be outweighed by the potential for serious bleeding), according to the 2020 AF guidelines.

7. A. The default strategy in this patient group is 1 week of triple therapy with dual anti-platelet therapy and a NOAC, reduced to single antiplatelet therapy and NOAC to 12 months, then NOAC only long-term. This may be further personalized to the individual patient: the duration of triple therapy may be extended to 1 month in the presence of high ischaemic risk and low bleeding risk, whilst the duration of single antiplatelet with NOAC may be reduced to 6 months in high-bleeding-risk, low-ischaemic-risk patients. In general, clopidogrel is preferred to aspirin as the single antiplatelet therapy used in combination with NOAC. The ESC also advises the use of clopidogrel as opposed to ticagrelor or prasugrel, in the context of triple therapy, due to a lower relative bleeding risk, and NOAC therapy is now preferred to warfarin.

8. E. Ticagrelor is contraindicated in patients with a history of intracranial bleeding. While this patient has an indication for dual antiplatelet therapy, prasugrel is contraindicated as the coronary anatomy is not known; if this patient were to need coronary artery bypass grafting, prasugrel is associated with a higher cardiac surgical bleeding risk. Prasugrel is also contraindicated in those with a history of stroke.

9. D. Use of glycoprotein IIb/IIIa inhibitors is associated with excess bleeding risk and ESC NSTEMI guidelines 2020 only recommend its use for bail-out if there is evidence of no-reflow or a thrombotic complication, in association with dual antiplatelet therapy. Importantly, treatment with GP IIb/IIIa antagonists in patients in whom coronary anatomy is not known is not recommended. The oral form was discontinued due to excess mortality.

10. D. Current evidence (largely based on the PEITHO study into fibrinolysis for intermediate-risk PE) supports an overall benefit of fibrinolysis only in those with PE causing refractory hypotension. In those with intermediate-risk PE or other compromising features but absence of shock, any potential haemodynamic benefits are weighed against very significant bleeding risks. CT scanning can often show indicators of right ventricular strain, such as flattening or bowing of the interventricular septum. Fibrinolysis should be used with caution if at all in the presence of DOAC therapy as this may be associated with excess bleeding—LMWH is advised.

11. D. The other options have all been shown to improve mortality in systolic heart failure. Digoxin may provide symptomatic relief, as may loop diuretic therapy, but neither have been shown to provide prognostic benefit.

12. D. While the PARADIGM trial showed significant benefit of sacubitril-valsartan therapy in those with HFrEF, unfortunately the PARAGON therapy failed to show similar benefit for those with HFpEF. Benefit was marginal and limited only to small subgroups (the most prominent of which was, indeed, those with evidence of a degree of systolic dysfunction). A 36-hour washout period is recommended between ACE-inhibitor therapy and commencement of sacubitril-valsartan, which is not required if switching from an angiotensin receptor blocker. Sacubitril-valsartan is acceptable at lower doses in patients with chronic kidney disease, alongside close observation of renal function.

13. C. All other statements are correct. In individuals who are black African or of African-Caribbean family origin, hypertension is less likely to be renin-mediated. Therefore in these individuals, ACE-inhibitors are unlikely to be effective. Early use of combination therapy is guideline recommended, creating a synergistic effect and increased treatment efficacy.

14. C. This common clinical scenario reflects the point at which the administered dose of diuretic is not having the required diuretic effect. This may be due to an insufficiently high dose, or the oral route proving ineffective in the presence of an oedematous gut. The resultant venous congestion can cause renal and hepatic derangement.

15. B. Dobutamine acts mainly as a β1 agonist, increasing heart rate and cardiac contractile force. Adrenaline and noradrenaline cause significant peripheral vasoconstriction which may be unhelpful in this situation. Milrinone may have been a reasonable choice, but in this case the significant renal impairment increases the risk of drug toxicity. Another potential option would be a calcium sensitizer such as levosimendan which increases myocardial contractility without a significant increase in myocardial oxygen demand. Digoxin has no role in the described clinic scenario.

16. D. Statin therapy has multiple benefits, many of which are independent of lipid lowering. Studies show a large proportion of reported muscle symptoms may result from a 'nocebo' effect. However, the ESC dyslipidaemia guideline suggests measurement of CK. Based on results of this, options involve statin washout and re-challenge, use of a second statin, or in cases of rhabdomyolysis, use of a maximally tolerated dose.

17. D. PCSK9 inhibitors are contraindicated in pregnancy due to a lack of data and risk of toxicity. All other answers are valid indications or recognized side effects. Although early concerns included an increased risk of infection, meta-analyses failed to show any increased risk.

18. D. Ivabradine will not be effective in atrial fibrillation as it acts primarily by slowing the rate of pacemaker activity at the sinoatrial node. It should also be avoided in bradycardia or acutely following myocardial infarction. There is limited evidence of prognostic benefit of anti-anginal drugs in the stable angina population. However, there is evidence of prognostic benefit of beta-blockers in the post-MI patient population.

19. B. Ivabradine is indicated in the treatment pathway of heart failure with reduced ejection fraction (when in sinus rhythm and remain symptomatic despite optimal medical therapy, including maximally tolerated beta-blocker therapy and a heart rate ≥ 70 bpm or when beta-blocker therapy is contraindicated), or in the treatment of angina. It is ineffective in the presence of atrial fibrillation, and contraindicated in advanced age, hypotension, bradycardia or conduction disease, or liver failure.

20. E. Bisoprolol, while effective at suppressing ectopy, is least likely to lead to adverse drug-related events in this lady. Amiodarone, sotalol, and flecainide are all associated with drug-induced QT-prolongation and thus likely to be pro-arrhythmogenic. It is important to note that whilst most potent anti-arrhythmic medications alter the cardiac action potential in such a way that while they reduce the risk of certain arrhythmia mechanisms, they also increase the potential for others.

INDEX

For the benefit of digital users, indexed terms that span two pages (e.g., 52–53) may, on occasion, appear on only one of those pages.

Note: Question sections appear in **bold** and answer sections appear in *italics* in the page field.

D

I

S

T